Acute Kidney Injury

Editors

DANA Y. FUHRMAN
JOHN A. KELLUM

CRITICAL CARE CLINICS

www.criticalcare.theclinics.com

Consulting Editor
JOHN A. KELLUM

April 2021 • Volume 37 • Number 2

ELSEVIER

1600 John F. Kennedy Boulevard • Suite 1800 • Philadelphia, Pennsylvania, 19103-2899

http://www.theclinics.com

CRITICAL CARE CLINICS Volume 37, Number 2
April 2021 ISSN 0749-0704, ISBN-13: 978-0-323-76168-0

Editor: Joanna Collett
Developmental Editor: Axell Purificacion

Critical Care Clinics (ISSN: 0749-0704) is published quarterly by Elsevier Inc., 360 Park Avenue South, New York, NY 10010-1710. Months of issue are January, April, July, and October. Business and Editorial Offices: 1600 John F. Kennedy Blvd., Suite 1800, Philadelphia, PA 19103-2899. Customer Service Office: 6277 Sea Harbor Drive, Orlando, FL 32887-4800. Periodicals postage paid at New York, NY and additional mailing offices. Subscription prices are $258.00 per year for US individuals, $890.00 per year for US institutions, $100.00 per year for US students and residents, $287.00 per year for Canadian individuals, $952.00 per year for Canadian institutions, $328.00 per year for international individuals, $952.00 per year for international institutions, $100.00 per year for Canadian students/residents, and $150.00 per year for foreign students/residents. To receive student/resident rate, orders must be accompanied by name of affiliated institution, date of term, and the signature of program/residency coordinator on institution letterhead. Orders will be billed at individual rate until proof of status is received. Foreign air speed delivery is included in all *Clinics* subscription prices. All prices are subject to change without notice. POSTMASTER: Send address changes to *Critical Care Clinics*, Elsevier Periodicals Customer Service, 11830 Westline Industrial Drive, St. Louis, MO 63146. **Customer Service: 1-800-654-2452 (US). From outside of the US, call 1-314-447-8871. Fax: 1-314-447-8029. E-mail: journalscustomerservice-usa@elsevier.com (for print support) or journalsonlinesupport-usa@elsevier.com (for online support).**

Reprints. For copies of 100 or more of articles in this publication, please contact the Commercial Reprints Department, Elsevier Inc., 360 Park Avenue South, New York, NY 10010-1710. Tel.: 212-633-3874; Fax: 212-633-3820; E-mail: reprints@elsevier.com.

Critical Care Clinics is also published in Spanish by Editorial Inter-Medica, Junin 917, 1er A, 1113, Buenos Aires, Argentina.

Critical Care Clinics is covered in *MEDLINE/PubMed (Index Medicus), EMBASE/Excerpta Medica, Current Concepts/ Clinical Medicine, ISI/BIOMED, and Chemical Abstracts.*

Contributors

CONSULTING EDITOR

JOHN A. KELLUM, MD, MCCM
Professor, Critical Care Medicine, Medicine, Bioengineering and Clinical and Translational Science, Director, Center for Critical Care Nephrology, The Clinical Research, Investigation and Systems Modeling of Acute Illness (CRISMA) Center, Vice Chair for Research, Department of Critical Care Medicine, University of Pittsburgh School of Medicine, Pittsburgh, Pennsylvania, USA

EDITORS

DANA Y. FUHRMAN, DO, MS
Assistant Professor, Department of Critical Care Medicine and Pediatrics, UPMC Children's Hospital of Pittsburgh, The Center for Critical Care Nephrology, Pittsburgh, Pennsylvania, USA

JOHN A. KELLUM, MD, MCCM
Professor, Critical Care Medicine, Medicine, Bioengineering and Clinical and Translational Science, Director, Center for Critical Care Nephrology, The Clinical Research, Investigation and Systems Modeling of Acute Illness (CRISMA) Center, Vice Chair for Research, Department of Critical Care Medicine, University of Pittsburgh School of Medicine, Pittsburgh, Pennsylvania, USA

AUTHORS

SEAN M. BAGSHAW, MD, MSc, FRCPC
Professor and Chair, Department of Critical Care Medicine, Faculty of Medicine and Dentistry, University of Alberta, Edmonton, Alberta, Canada

VIKRAM BALAKUMAR, MD
Department of Critical Care Medicine, Mercy Hospitals, Springfield, Missouri, USA; Department of Critical Care Medicine, Center for Critical Care Nephrology, University of Pittsburgh School of Medicine, Pittsburgh, Pennsylvania, USA

LAKHMIR S. CHAWLA, MD
Department of Medicine, Veterans Affairs Medical Center, San Diego, California, USA

GASPAR DEL RIO-PERTUZ, MD
Department of Critical Care Medicine, Center for Critical Care Nephrology, Department of Critical Care Medicine, The Clinical Research, Investigation and Systems Modeling of Acute Illness (CRISMA) Center, University of Pittsburgh School of Medicine, Pittsburgh, Pennsylvania, USA; Department of Internal Medicine, Texas Tech University Health Sciences Center, Lubbock, Texas, USA

FRANCOIS DURAND, MD
Hepatology and Liver Intensive Care, Hospital Beaujon, University of Paris, Clichy, France

KEVIN W. FINKEL, MD, FACP, FASN, FCCM
Professor and Director, Division of Renal Diseases and Hypertension, Chief, Section of Critical Care Nephrology, Department of Internal Medicine, The University of Texas Health Science Center at Houston, McGovern Medical School, Houston, Texas, USA

CLAIRE FRANCOZ, MD, PhD
Hepatology and Liver Intensive Care, Hospital Beaujon, Clichy, France

DANA Y. FUHRMAN, DO, MS
Assistant Professor, Pediatrics, Critical Care Medicine, and Nephrology, Department of Critical Care Medicine, The Center for Critical Care Nephrology, University of Pittsburgh School of Medicine, University of Pittsburgh Medical Center, UPMC Children's Hospital of Pittsburgh, Pittsburgh, Pennsylvania, USA

HERNANDO GOMEZ, MD, MPH
Assistant Professor, Department of Critical Care Medicine, Center for Critical Care Nephrology, Department of Critical Care Medicine, The Clinical Research, Investigation and Systems Modeling of Acute Illness (CRISMA) Center, University of Pittsburgh School of Medicine, Pittsburgh, Pennsylvania, USA

JENNIFER G. JETTON, MD
Clinical Associate Professor of Pediatrics, Division of Pediatric Nephrology, Dialysis, and Transplantation, Stead Family Department of Pediatrics, University of Iowa, Iowa City, Iowa, USA

JAYA KALA, MD, FASN
Assistant Professor of Medicine, Division of Renal Diseases and Hypertension, Department of Internal Medicine, The University of Texas Health Science Center at Houston, McGovern Medical School, Houston, Texas, USA

SANDRA L. KANE-GILL, PharmD, MSc, FCCM, FCCP
Professor, Department of Pharmacy and Therapeutics, School of Pharmacy, Faculty, Center for Critical Care Nephrology, School of Medicine, University of Pittsburgh, Pittsburgh, Pennsylvania, USA

CONSTANTINE J. KARVELLAS, MD, SM, FRCPC
Division of Gastroenterology (Liver Unit), Department of Critical Care Medicine, University of Alberta, Edmonton, Alberta, Canada

KEEGAN J. KAVANAUGH, MD
Pediatric Resident, Stead Family Department of Pediatrics, University of Iowa, Iowa City, Iowa, USA

JOHN A. KELLUM, MD, MCCM
Professor, Critical Care Medicine, Medicine, Bioengineering and Clinical and Translational Science, Director, Center for Critical Care Nephrology, The Clinical Research, Investigation and Systems Modeling of Acute Illness (CRISMA) Center, Vice Chair for Research, Department of Critical Care Medicine, University of Pittsburgh School of Medicine, University of Pittsburgh Medical Center, Pittsburgh, Pennsylvania, USA

ALISON L. KENT, BMBS, FRACP, MD
Adjunct Professor of Pediatrics, Division of Neonatology, Golisano Children's Hospital, University of Rochester School of Medicine, Rochester, New York, USA; Dentistry and Honorary Professor, College of Health and Medicine, Australian National University, Canberra, Australian Capital Territory, Australia

SARO KHEMICHIAN, MD
Division of Gastroenterology/Liver, Keck School of Medicine of USC, University of Southern California, Los Angeles, California, USA

WIN KULVICHIT, MD
Division of Nephrology, Faculty of Medicine, Chulalongkorn University, Excellence Center for Critical Care Nephrology, King Chulalongkorn Memorial Hospital, Pathum Wan, Bangkok, Thailand

CARLOS L. MANRIQUE-CABALLERO, MD
Department of Critical Care Medicine, Center for Critical Care Nephrology, Department of Critical Care Medicine, The Clinical Research, Investigation and Systems Modeling of Acute Illness (CRISMA) Center, University of Pittsburgh School of Medicine, Pittsburgh, Pennsylvania, USA

CHRISTINA MASSOTH, MD
Department of Anesthesiology, Intensive Care, and Pain Medicine, University Hospital Münster, Münster, Germany

MELANIE MEERSCH, MD
Department of Anesthesiology, Intensive Care, and Pain Medicine, University Hospital Münster, Münster, Germany

RAGHAVAN MURUGAN, MD, MS, FRCP, FCCM
Department of Critical Care Medicine, Center for Critical Care Nephrology, University of Pittsburgh School of Medicine, Professor of Critical Care Medicine and Clinical and Translational Science, Department of Critical Care Medicine, The Clinical Research, Investigation, and Systems Modeling of Acute Illness (CRISMA) Center, University of Pittsburgh School of Medicine, University of Pittsburgh, Pittsburgh, Pennsylvania, USA

MITRA K. NADIM, MD, FASN
Division of Nephrology and Hypertension, Keck School of Medicine of USC, University of Southern California, Los Angeles, California, USA

JAVIER A. NEYRA, MD, MSCS
Assistant Professor of Medicine, Director of Critical Care Nephrology, Department of Internal Medicine, Division of Nephrology, Bone and Mineral Metabolism, University of Kentucky Medical Center, Lexington, Kentucky, USA

ZACCARIA RICCI, MD
Department of Cardiology and Cardiac Surgery, Pediatric Cardiac Intensive Care Unit, Bambino Gesù Children's Hospital, IRCCS, Rome, Italy; Department of Health Science, University of Florence, Florence, Italy

STEFANO ROMAGNOLI, MD, PhD
Department of Anesthesiology and Intensive Care, Azienda Ospedaliero-Universitaria Careggi, Department of Health Science, University of Florence, Florence, Italy

CLAUDIO RONCO, MD
International Renal Research Institute of Vicenza (IRRIV), Department of Nephrology, Dialysis and Transplantation, San Bortolo Hospital, Vicenza, Italy

NATTACHAI SRISAWAT, MD, PhD
Division of Nephrology, Faculty of Medicine, Chulalongkorn University, Pathumwan, Excellence Center for Critical Care Nephrology, King Chulalongkorn Memorial Hospital, Pathum Wan, Bangkok, Thailand; Department of Critical Care Medicine, Center for

Critical Care Nephrology, The CRISMA Center, University of Pittsburgh School of Medicine, Pittsburgh, Pennsylvania, USA; Critical Care Nephrology Research Unit, Chulalongkorn University, Academy of Science, Royal Society of Thailand, Tropical Medicine Cluster, Chulalongkorn University, Excellence Center for Critical Care Medicine, King Chulalongkorn Memorial Hospital, Bangkok, Thailand

SIDDHARTH VERMA, MD
Department of Medicine, Renal-Electrolyte Division, University of Pittsburgh Medical Center, Center for Critical Care Nephrology, University of Pittsburgh Medical Center, Pittsburgh, Pennsylvania, USA

RON WALD, MDCM, MPH, FRCPC
Associate Professor, Division of Nephrology, St. Michael's Hospital, University of Toronto, Li Ka Shing Knowledge Institute of St. Michael's Hospital, Toronto, Ontario, Canada

ALEXANDER ZARBOCK, MD
Department of Anesthesiology, Intensive Care, and Pain Medicine, University Hospital Münster, Münster, Germany

Contents

> Acute kidney injury (AKI) is a syndrome of impaired kidney function asso-
> ciated with reduced survival and increased morbidity. International
> consensus criteria were developed based on changes in serum creatinine
> and urine output. Based on these definitions, epidemiologic studies have
> shown strong associations with clinical outcomes including death and
> dialysis. However, numerous limitations exist for creatinine and urine vol-
> ume as markers of AKI and novel biomarkers have been developed to
> detect cellular stress or damage. Persistent AKI and acute kidney disease
> are relatively new concepts that explore the idea of AKI as a continuum
> with chronic kidney disease.

> Acute kidney injury (AKI) occurs frequently after cardiac surgery and is
> associated with high morbidity and mortality. Although the number of
> cardiac surgical procedures is constantly growing worldwide, inci-
> dence of cardiac surgery–associated AKI is still around 40% and has
> a significant impact on global health care costs. Numerous trials at-
> tempted to identify strategies to prevent AKI and attenuate its detri-
> mental consequences. Effective options remained elusive. Current
> evidence supports a multimodal risk-stratification approach with
> biomarker-guided management of high-risk patients, perioperative
> administration of dexmedetomidine, and implementation of a care
> bundle as recommended by the Kidney Disease: Improving Global Out-
> comes group.

> Sepsis-associated acute kidney injury (S-AKI) is a common and life-
> threatening complication in hospitalized and critically ill patients. It is char-
> acterized by rapid deterioration of renal function associated with sepsis.
> The pathophysiology of S-AKI remains incompletely understood, so
> most therapies remain reactive and nonspecific. Possible pathogenic
> mechanisms to explain S-AKI include microcirculatory dysfunction, a dys-
> regulated inflammatory response, and cellular metabolic reprogramming.
> In addition, several biomarkers have been developed in an attempt to
> improve diagnostic sensitivity and specificity of S-AKI. This article dis-
> cusses the current understanding of S-AKI, recent advances in

pathophysiology and biomarker development, and current preventive and therapeutic approaches.

Sandra L. Kane-Gill

Drugs are the third leading cause of acute kidney injury (AKI) in critically ill patients. Nephrotoxin stewardship ensures a structured and consistent approach to safe medication use and prevention of patient harm. Comprehensive nephrotoxin stewardship requires coordinated patient care management strategies for safe medication use, ensuring kidney health, and avoiding unnecessary costs to improve the use of nephrotoxins, renally eliminated drugs, and kidney disease treatments. Implementing nephrotoxin stewardship reduces medication errors and adverse drug events, prevents or reduces severity of drug-associated AKI, prevents progression to or worsening of chronic kidney disease, and alleviates financial burden on the health care system.

Saro Khemichian, Claire Francoz, Francois Durand, Constantine J. Karvellas, and Mitra K. Nadim

Development of acute kidney injury in patients with chronic liver disease is common and portends a poor prognosis. Diagnosis remains challenging, as traditional markers, such as serum creatinine, are not reliable. Recent development of novel biomarkers may assist with this. Pathophysiology of this condition is multifactorial, relating to physiologic changes associated with portal hypertension, kidney factors, and systemic inflammatory response. Mainstay of treatment remains use of vasoconstrictors along with albumin. Recent guidelines streamline the selection of patients that will require simultaneous liver and kidney transplantation. Posttransplant kidney injury is common relating to multiple factors.

Zaccaria Ricci, Stefano Romagnoli, and Claudio Ronco

Cardiorenal syndrome (CRS) describes a specific acute and chronic clinical picture in which the heart or the kidney are primarily dysfunctioning and secondarily affect each other. CRS is divided into five classes: acute and chronic CRS, acute and chronic renocardiac syndromes, and secondary dysfunction of heart and kidneys. This article specifically details the classification and the epidemiology, some risk factors, and the pathophysiology of CRS. Some emerging aspects of CRS are also discussed, such as CRS in patients with end-stage heart failure, with mechanical ventricular assistance, and after heart transplantation. Finally, some aspects of pediatric CRS are detailed.

Keegan J. Kavanaugh, Jennifer G. Jetton, and Alison L. Kent

The study of neonatal acute kidney injury (AKI) has transitioned from small, single-center studies to the development of a large, multicenter cohort.

The scope of research has expanded from assessment of incidence and mortality to analysis of more specific risk factors, novel urinary biomarkers, interplay between AKI and other organ systems, impact of fluid overload, and quality improvement efforts. The intensification has occurred through collaboration between the neonatology and nephrology communities. This review discusses 2 case scenarios to illustrate the clinical presentation of neonatal AKI, important risk factors, and approaches to minimize AKI events and adverse long-term outcomes.

Current advances in cancer chemotherapeutics have remarkably helped in rapid and definitive treatment options. However, these potent chemotherapeutics have been associated with severe renal toxicities that later impact treatment options. Acute kidney injury is common in patients with cancer. In hospitalized patients with cancer, acute kidney injury is associated with increased morbidity, mortality, length of stay, and costs. This article provides an overview of acute kidney injury caused by cancer or its treatment, including prerenal, tubular, glomerular diseases, infiltrative disease, tumor lysis syndrome, anticancer drug nephrotoxicity, hematopoietic stem cell transplantation–related acute kidney injury, and cancer-associated thrombotic microangiopathy.

Biomarkers have become a pillar of precision medicine in acute kidney injury (AKI). Traditional markers for diagnosis of AKI are insensitive and insufficient to provide comprehensive information for prognostication. Several emerging biomarkers have shown promising results in large-scale clinical studies. These novel markers likely will be beneficial for personalized AKI prevention and treatment.

Renal functional reserve (RFR) is described as the difference between a glomerular filtration rate (GFR) measured at baseline and after protein stimulation. The percent change in GFR after a protein load varies based on differences in experimental conditions, with the use of an oral meat protein stimulus and a creatinine clearance method to quantify GFR showing the greatest RFR. A decline in RFR has been found in numerous patient groups. Recent investigations have suggested that a lower RFR may be associated with an increased risk of acute kidney injury and eventual chronic kidney disease.

Kidney replacement therapy (KRT) is a core organ support in critical care settings. In patients suitable for escalation in support, who develop acute kidney injury (AKI) complications and urgent indications, there is consensus that KRT should be promptly initiated. In the absence of such urgent indications, the optimal timing has been less certain. Current clinical practice guidelines do not present strong recommendations for when to start KRT for patients with AKI in the absence of life-threatening and urgent indications. This article discusses how best to provide KRT to critically ill patients with severe AKI.

Vikram Balakumar and Raghavan Murugan

Emerging evidence from observational studies suggests that both slower and faster net ultrafiltration rates during kidney replacement therapy are associated with increased mortality in critically ill patients with acute kidney injury and fluid overload. Faster rates are associated with ischemic organ injury. The net ultrafiltration rate should be prescribed based on patient body weight in milliliters per kilogram per hour, with close monitoring of patient hemodynamics and fluid balance. Randomized trials are required to examine whether moderate net ultrafiltration rates compared with slower and faster rates are associated with reduced risk of hemodynamic instability, organ injury, and improved outcomes.

Javier A. Neyra and Lakhmir S. Chawla

Acute kidney injury (AKI) and chronic kidney disease are common interconnected syndromes that represent a public health problem. Acute kidney disease (AKD) is defined as the post-AKI status of acute or subacute kidney damage/dysfunction manifested by persistence of AKI beyond 7 to 90 days after the initial AKI diagnosis. Limited clinical data exist regarding AKD epidemiology but its incidence is observed in ~25% of AKI survivors. Useful risk-stratification tools to predict risk of AKD and its prognosis are needed. Interventions on fluid management, nephrotoxic exposure, and follow-up care hold promise to ameliorate the burden of AKD and its complications.

CRITICAL CARE CLINICS

SERIES OF RELATED INTEREST

Emergency Medicine Clinics
https://www.emed.theclinics.com/

THE CLINICS ARE AVAILABLE ONLINE!
Access your subscription at:
www.theclinics.com

Preface

Acute Kidney Injury in the Intensive Care Unit: Advances in the Identification, Classification, and Treatment of a Multifactorial Syndrome

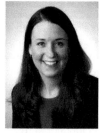 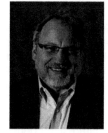

Dana Y. Fuhrman, DO, MS   John A. Kellum MD, MCCM
Editors

Acute kidney injury (AKI) remains an epidemic in the intensive care unit (ICU), occurring in more than 50% of patients and with a mortality of 20% to 25%.[1] With the development of a standard for defining AKI with the Kidney Disease: Improving Global Outcomes (KDIGO) criteria in 2012,[2] arguably no other area of study in critical care medicine has seen as rapid a rise in research efforts when compared with critical care nephrology. In 2020, there is no indication that these efforts are slowing, with still much work to be done.

A unified definition of AKI has allowed us to maintain consistency and provide a standard for defining AKI in research studies and in clinical practice. Study results in neonates, children, and adults have made it clear that we need to include oliguria when defining AKI.[3–5] Given that worsening kidney function can occur over hours, refining our ability to predict changes in serum creatinine and urine output is crucial. The quest for the biomarkers to detect AKI early, determine progression and need for renal replacement therapy (RRT), and prediction of long-term outcomes continues. It has become increasingly clear that no single biomarker can fill these diverse roles, but instead, different biomarkers will be needed for different intended uses.

It is now evident that AKI is a syndrome with multiple causes. Recognizing that AKI "behaves" differently in different patient groups, investigators have focused their efforts on studying potentially vulnerable patients. The recent multicenter AWAKEN study has alerted us to the myriad of issues related to AKI in the neonatal period,

Crit Care Clin 37 (2021) xiii–xv
https://doi.org/10.1016/j.ccc.2021.01.001
0749-0704/21/© 2021 Published by Elsevier Inc.

including the need for RRT devices for our smallest patients.[3] In addition, exciting recent advances in the pathophysiology of sepsis-associated AKI have shown us that AKI in the setting of systemic infection should be regarded as a "sepsis-defining event," occurring in the absence of signs of renal hypoperfusion.[6] Importantly, research efforts dedicated to patients with cardiorenal syndrome, hepatorenal syndrome, and oncologic diseases have expanded greatly.

Recent advancements have improved our understanding of the management of AKI in the ICU. Satisfying our need for meticulous attention to fluid balance, new technologies to monitor fluid overload in the ICU have become available. Efforts to find the optimal timing for the initiation of RRT continue. The results of the recently published STARRT-AKI trial show no survival benefit to an early compared with delayed strategy for RRT initiation in patients without an urgent indication.[7] In addition, once the decision to initiate RRT is made, there is emerging evidence showing the association of ultrafiltration rates that are too fast or too slow with mortality.[8]

Importantly, the AKI research community has developed a commitment to exploring the impact of this syndrome on patients once they leave the ICU. We have learned that a longer duration of AKI is associated with worse outcomes when compared with AKI that rapidly resolves. The KDIGO AKI Work Group first proposed a definition equivalent to chronic kidney disease occurring before 90 days, termed acute kidney disease.[2] More recently, the Acute Disease Quality Initiative expanded this by proposing AKI-based staging for patients with acute kidney disease arising from AKI.[9] Understanding that we should not be reassured by a return of normal renal function by serum creatinine, a renewed interest in concepts like renal functional reserve has emerged.

This issue of *Critical Care Clinics* provides a comprehensive review of current advances in the identification, classification, and treatment approaches to AKI. We wish to thank the outstanding group of experts that contributed their work. For those caring for patients with AKI in the ICU, we hope that this issue will serve as a guide of the current evidence and a source of excitement for future areas of study in the field of AKI research.

Dana Y. Fuhrman, DO, MS
Department of Critical Care Medicine and
Pediatrics
UPMC Children's Hospital of Pittsburgh
The Center for Critical Care Nephrology
4401 Penn Avenue, Children's Hospital Drive
Faculty Pavilion, Suite 2000
Pittsburgh, PA 15224, USA

John A. Kellum, MD, MCCM
Department of Critical Care Medicine
The Center for Critical Care Nephrology
3347 Forbes Avenue, Suite 220
Pittsburgh, PA 15213, USA

E-mail addresses:
Dana.fuhrman@chp.edu (D.Y. Fuhrman)
kellumja@upmc.edu (J.A. Kellum)

REFERENCES

1. Hoste EA, Bagshaw SM, Bellomo R, et al. Epidemiology of acute kidney injury in critically ill patients: the multinational AKI-EPI study. Intensive Care Med 2015; 41(8):1411–23.
2. KDIGO AKIWG. Kidney Disease: Improving Global Outcomes (KDIGO) clinical practice guideline for acute kidney injury. Kidney Int Suppl 2012;2(1):1–141.
3. Jetton JG, Boohaker LJ, Sethi SK, et al. Incidence and outcomes of neonatal acute kidney injury (AWAKEN): a multicentre, multinational, observational cohort study. Lancet Child Adolesc Health 2017;1(3):184–94.
4. Kaddourah A, Basu RK, Goldstein SL, et al, Assessment of Worldwide Acute Kidney Injury RAaEl. Oliguria and acute kidney injury in critically ill children: implications for diagnosis and outcomes. Pediatr Crit Care Med 2019;20(4):332–9.
5. Amathieu R, Al-Khafaji A, Sileanu FE, et al. Significance of oliguria in critically ill patients with chronic liver disease. Hepatology 2017;66(5):1592–600.
6. Post EH, Kellum JA, Bellomo R, Vincent JL. Renal perfusion in sepsis: from macro-to microcirculation. Kidney Int 2017;91(1):45–60.
7. Bagshaw SM, Wald R, Adhikari NKJ, et al. Timing of initiation of renal-replacement therapy in acute kidney injury. N Engl J Med 2020;383(3):240–51.
8. Murugan R, Kerti SJ, Chang CH, et al. Association of net ultrafiltration rate with mortality among critically ill adults with acute kidney injury receiving continuous venovenous hemodiafiltration: a secondary analysis of the Randomized Evaluation of Normal vs Augmented Level (RENAL) of Renal Replacement Therapy Trial. JAMA Netw Open 2019;2(6):e195418.
9. Chawla LS, Bellomo R, Bihorac A, et al. Acute kidney disease and renal recovery: consensus report of the Acute Disease Quality Initiative (ADQI) 16 Workgroup. Nat Rev Nephrol 2017;13(4):241–57.

Defining Acute Kidney Injury

Siddharth Verma, MD[a,b], John A. Kellum, MD, MCCM[b,c],*

KEYWORDS

- Acute kidney injury • Acute kidney disease • Biomarkers • Electronic alerts

KEY POINTS

- Acute kidney injury (AKI) is associated with an increase in both short-term and long-term mortality, as well as increased costs.
- Epidemiology using standard definitions have shown high incidence of AKI.
- Electronic alert systems implemented for AKI based on standardized definitions have shown variable effects on patient outcomes.
- Cystatin C, PEnk, KIM-1, NGAL, and TIMP2*IGFB7 are some biomarkers of kidney injury that have shown promise in predicting AKI before a rise in serum creatinine.
- Persistent AKI and acute kidney disease are relatively new concepts that explore the idea of AKI as a continuum with chronic kidney disease rather than separate entities.

INTRODUCTION

Acute kidney injury (AKI) is a syndrome with multiple etiologies that can be characterized by a deterioration of kidney function that occurs in a matter of hours to days.[1] Conceptually, it can represent a number of conditions that adversely affect the structure and/or function of the kidney. AKI often occurs in patients with multiple comorbidities and is associated with a significant increase in both short-term and long-term mortality.[2] It is one of the most common causes of organ dysfunction in hospitalized patients, occurring in more than 50% of patients admitted to the intensive care unit (ICU)[3] and as many as 22.7%[2] of hospitalized patients. In the ICU setting, AKI has a mortality rate of 20% to 25%,[3] increasing to 50% to 60% when dialysis is required, with approximately 5% to 20% of the surviving patients requiring dialysis at the

[a] Department of Medicine, Renal-Electrolyte Division, University of Pittsburgh Medical Center, 3550 Terrace Street, Pittsburgh, PA 15213, USA; [b] Center for Critical Care Nephrology, University of Pittsburgh Medical Center, 3550 Terrace Street, Pittsburgh, PA 15213, USA; [c] Department of Critical Care Medicine, University of Pittsburgh Medical Center, Center for Critical Care Nephrology, 3347 Forbes Avenue, Suite 220, Pittsburgh, PA 15213, USA
* Corresponding author. Center for Critical Care Nephrology, 3347 Forbes Avenue, Suite 220, Pittsburgh, PA 15213.
E-mail address: kellumja@upmc.edu

Crit Care Clin 37 (2021) 251–266
https://doi.org/10.1016/j.ccc.2020.11.001   criticalcare.theclinics.com
0749-0704/21/© 2020 Elsevier Inc. All rights reserved.

time of discharge.[4] Overall, it is estimated that AKI results in the death of more than 7 million people worldwide every year.[5]

AKI is not just associated with mortality and morbidity, but a causal relationship has been established both in animal models and in humans. For example, Singbartl and colleagues[6] found that mice induced to develop AKI either using folic acid injection or secondary to rhabdomyolysis exhibited neutrophil dysfunction, reduced bacterial clearance, and increased mortality when challenged with Pseudomonas aeruginosa. The 6S study randomized 804 patients with sepsis to receive hydroxyethyl starch in Ringer acetate solution (HES) versus Ringer acetate alone.[7] More patients assigned to HES developed AKI and more required dialysis: 87 patients (22%) versus 65 patients (16%) assigned to Ringer acetate (relative risk 1.35; 95% confidence interval [CI] 1.01–1.80; P = .04). At day 90, 201 (51%) of 398 patients assigned to HES had died, as compared with 172 (43%) of 400 patients assigned to Ringer's acetate (relative risk 1.17; 95% CI 1.01–1.36; P = .03). Thus, in patients with sepsis, HES led to increased mortality, principally through increased AKI.

The causal link between AKI and mortality is not surprising. AKI has been associated with various complications, including the uremic syndrome (altered mental status, bleeding diathesis, and increased microvascular permeability), disturbances in fluid, electrolyte and acid-base balance, which can lead to severe cardiac arrhythmias, muscle weakness, and hemodynamic instabilities as well as fluid overload, which can lead to respiratory insufficiency and interstitial edema. Although infections have been a known cause of AKI, in ICU patients, AKI has been found to be a risk factor for infections as well.[8] Kidney dysfunction may be associated with increased morbidity and mortality even if the change does not meet the criteria for acute kidney injury.[9] It is also associated with an elevated risk of cardiovascular mortality and major cardiovascular events, including heart failure and acute myocardial infarction.[10] Other complications include an increased length of stay (LOS), likelihood of admission to critical care, and risk of death.[11] AKI survivors were more likely to be discharged to an extended care facility.[12] This is further burdened by the development of long-term complications, including dialysis dependence, chronic comorbidities, and re-hospitalizations.[13]

As a clinical syndrome, AKI encompasses different etiologies, including systemic conditions directly or indirectly affecting the kidneys, which may include states of low effective arterial blood volume, inflammation and sepsis, autoimmune conditions, glomerulonephritides, and toxic exposures, among others, as well as external pathology including various causes of obstruction. These conditions frequently coexist in an acute setting. Thus, AKI is similar to acute coronary syndrome or acute lung injury,[14] partly due to the similarity of "focal" organ manifestations of a more "global" disease process. In the past, multiple definitions for AKI have resulted in great confusion and discordance when comparing various studies. Consolidation of the current data on AKI to interpret systematic reviews and meta analyses would not have been possible without a single unifying definition, using simple measurable parameters.

HISTORY: ACUTE RENAL FAILURE TO ACUTE KIDNEY INJURY

Acute renal failure was first described in 1802 by William Heberdenin.[15] The definition was then updated and described as Bright's disease in 1827 by Richard Bright[15] as the effect of toxic agents, pregnancy, burns, trauma, or operations on the kidneys. This was used as a "catchall" phrase that included both acute and chronic forms of kidney disease. Bright defined this as a triad of albuminuria, edema, and kidney disease.[16] Lieutenant-Colonel N Raw[17] reported a condition that he named "trench nephritis" due to its clear association with trench warfare conditions in 1915, during the first world war, based on a series of 5 cases. It was recognized as organ-specific, as an irritated kidney, secondary to toxic substances that poisoned this organ and not by direct bacterial invasion. Treatments were mostly conservative, described as "calming" inflammation and "resting" the kidneys.[18]

Bywaters and Beall[19] published a paper in the *British Medical Journal* (1941) on the crush syndrome, which was remarkable for demonstrating a photomicrograph of "pigmented casts" in the renal tubules. But it was actually Homer W. Smith who was credited for the introduction of the term "acute renal failure" in his textbook in 1951.[14] Throughout the remainder of the twentieth century, a specific biochemical definition of ARF was not proposed. Furthermore, until the early twenty-first century, there were approximately 60 definitions of renal failure with a clear lack of consensus. This state of confusion had given rise to a wide variation in the reported incidence of 1% to 25% of ICU patients and a mortality rate between 15% and 60% in different texts.[14]

The first international consensus definition of AKI was described in 2004 at the Second International Consensus Conference of Acute Dialysis Quality Initiative (ADQI), which reviewed animal models and classified them according to their features, usefulness, relevance, and reproducibility.[20] ADQI also developed staging criteria for AKI using the terms Risk, Injury, and Failure for severity and Loss and End-stage kidney disease (RIFLE) as outcomes.[20] These international consensus criteria were later refined by the AKI Network[21] and in 2012, were adopted by Kidney Disease Improving Global Outcomes (KDIGO).[14] AKI is currently considered a broad clinical syndrome that may result from multiple etiologies, of which acute renal failure can be considered to be a part of this spectrum. As the manifestations of AKI can be similar, even though there is a wide variety of possible etiologies, approach to diagnosis becomes crucial to guide treatment.

DEFINING ACUTE KIDNEY INJURY
Creatinine and Urine Output as Parameters

Although glomerular filtration rate (GFR) is considered to be the best reflection of kidney function, low GFR does not provide a specific etiology or a cause for the kidney dysfunction. This needs to be interpreted by the provider based on clinical context. Kidney dysfunction not only gives us an idea of the "state" of kidney damage, and progression toward worsening or recovery, but also guides medication dosing. Although serum creatinine has been a useful parameter to evaluate AKI, it has numerous limitations. It is formed from creatine in the muscles, freely filtered by the glomerulus, and completely cleared by a normally functioning kidney. Severity of AKI can be determined either by the magnitude of increase in serum creatinine or by a decrease in urine output. Short-term and long-term outcomes have been shown to be worse when patients meet both criteria.[22] Both creatinine and urine output act as markers for kidney function, not injury. Due to proximal tubular secretion of creatinine, there is a roughly 10% to 20% overestimation in calculation of GFR when measured by creatinine clearance.

Multiple factors can affect creatinine levels, including muscle mass, age, sex, race, medications, diet, nutritional status, fluid overload, and states of sepsis. Measurements of urine volume are also limited by the inability to obtain accurate urine collections, which has a limited feasibility outside the ICU setting, and its variability in various acute settings. Brief urine collections have shown a good correlation with 24-hour urine collection and are preferred over creatinine in detecting dynamic changes in GFR. States of hyperglycemia and hyperproteinemia can interfere with laboratory assays and give a false elevation in creatinine, whereas the reverse is possible in states of hemolysis and hyperbilirubinemia. In addition, large renal reserves in healthy individuals can delay the detection of a rise in creatinine until more than 50% of GFR is lost.

History of Acute Kidney Injury Definitions

Variations in the definition of AKI lead to heterogeneity, which complicates comparison and interpretation of the results of different studies.[11] The RIFLE criteria[4] were proposed in 2004 and were based on consensus by the ADQI. The RIFLE criteria divide kidney injury into 3 stages: Risk, Injury, Failure, and 2 outcomes: Loss and End-Stage Kidney Disease (ESKD) (**Fig. 1**). The patient is classified using the worst of the 2 criteria, urine output or serum creatinine. Some of the strengths of the RIFLE criteria were that it considered changes in the creatinine levels from a baseline. If no baseline is known, but baseline function is thought to be normal, then it can be estimated using the Modified Diet in Renal Disease formula and solving for an eGRF of 75 mL/min. Patients can fulfill either creatinine or urine output criteria or both, although the higher stage of either criterion is considered to be the current stage of AKI. Progression along the criteria is associated with higher mortality, increased LOS in ICU, and in hospital. However, concerns are often raised about estimated baseline creatinine for risk that this can lead to the overestimation of AKI in patients with unknown baseline creatinine.[23] In reality though, most healthy individuals with no past medical record of chronic kidney disease (CKD) and no known baseline creatinine actually

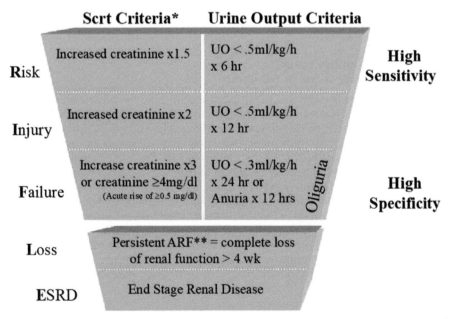

Fig. 1. The RIFLE criteria for staging AKI. UO, urine output. *Alternative measures of glomerular filtration rate may also be used. **Not to be confused with persistent acute kidney injury. Scrt, serum creatinine. (*From* Bellomo R, Ronco C, Kellum JA, Mehta RL, Palevsky P. Acute renal failure - definition, outcome measures, animal models, fluid therapy and information technology needs: The Second International Consensus Conference of the Acute Dialysis Quality Initiative (ADQI) Group. Crit Care. 2004;8(4)).

have estimated GFRs (eGFRs) greater than 75 leading to an underestimate of AKI, not an overestimate.[23] Indeed, in a large multinational study of AKI in the ICU, the rate of AKI increased when patients with estimated baselines were removed.[3]

One of the major limitations of the RIFLE criteria was that the creatinine domain is rather insensitive in patients with underlying CKD. For example, a patient with a baseline creatinine 2.4 mg/dL would need to reach 3.6 mg/dL just to have "Risk." Furthermore, defining AKI by a fixed creatinine percentage increase would take much longer in CKD because of altered creatinine kinetics.[24] For these reasons, a modification to RIFLE was proposed by the Acute Kidney Injury Network (AKIN) in which a small increase in creatinine (0.3 mg/dL or greater) would also meet criteria for AKI if it was documented to occur within a short period of time (48 hours or less).[21] The AKIN modification improves sensitivity of AKI diagnosis as compared with RIFLE criteria[25]; however, it comes with its own limitations. A change in creatinine by 0.3 mg/dL approaches expected variation (due to diet, exercise, and hydration status) for patients with advanced CKD. Thus, specificity of AKI using a 0.3 mg/dL change is reduced. Despite their limitations, both RIFLE and AKIN staging show very strong correlations with mortality and use of dialysis[26,27] and have now been validated in thousands of patients. In 2012, KDIGO developed a clinical practice guideline for AKI[14] that was based on a unified version of RIFLE[20] and AKIN[21] criteria (**Table 1**). The KDIGO definition provided a unified system to maintain consistency in the definition and has become a standard for defining AKI in research and in clinical practice.

Importantly, although these criteria provide guidance, the diagnosis of AKI is a clinical one. As discussed in the KDIGO guideline,[14] patients may meet criteria for AKI but not have the diagnosis (eg, drug-induced inhibition of tubular secretion of creatinine) or not meet the criteria but have the diagnosis (eg, dilution of creatinine with fluid resuscitation). Hydration status, urinary tract patency, and laboratory error are all considerations that the clinician should consider in assessing the likelihood that a patient has AKI. One particularly common source of error comes for a fall in serum creatinine shortly after hospital admission, presumably related to volume expansion, fasting, and bedrest. If the serum creatinine then increases back to the baseline in the next 48 hours, the patient could meet criteria for AKI if the change is 0.3 mg/dL or more. Clinical judgment is therefore always needed.

Table 1
The Kidney Disease Improving Global Outcomes classification of acute kidney injury

Stage	Serum Creatinine	Urine Output
1	15–1.9 times baseline OR $\geq$0.3 mg/dL ($\geq$26.5 μmol/L) increase	<0.5 mL/kg/h for 6–12 h
2	2.0–2.9 times baseline	<0.5 mL/kg/h for $\geq$12 h
3	3.0 times baseline OR Increase in serum creatinine to $\geq$4.0 mg/dL ($\geq$353.6 μmol/l OR Initiation of renal replacement therapy OR, In patients <18 y, decrease in eGFR to <35 mL/min per 1.73 m^2	<0.3 mL/kg/h for $\geq$24 h OR Anuria for $\geq$12 h

From Kellum JA, Lameire N, Aspelin P, Barsoum RS, Burdmann EA, Goldstein SL, et al. Kidney disease: Improving global outcomes (KDIGO) acute kidney injury work group. KDIGO clinical practice guideline for acute kidney injury. Kidney Int Suppl. 2012;2(1):1–138.

RELATIONSHIP TO CLINICAL OUTCOMES

In a study of more than 520,000 patients assessing the influence of a clinical decision support system on patient outcomes using KDIGO criteria, showed that implementing the alert system resulted in small but sustained decreases in-hospital mortality, LOS, and dialysis rates for patients with AKI, whereas there was no such effect on outcomes of patients without AKI.[28] A large systematic meta-analysis included 1,057,332 patients using 92 studies, including both developed and developing countries, out of which 78% of the studies used the RIFLE, KDIGO, or AKIN criteria for defining AKI. This study showed a similar AKI incidence within both developing and developed countries, although the need for dialysis, length of ICU stay, and mortality were higher in developing countries. It was noted that there were several challenges, including a lack of standardization of reference serum creatinine, oliguria, and the timeframe for AKI assessment while comparing different countries.[29] In a recent study of cardiac surgery patients, in-hospital mortality and renal replacement therapy (RRT) rates increased from 4.3% and 0%, respectively, for no AKI to 51.1% and 55.3%, respectively, when serum creatinine level and urine output both met criteria for AKI.[30] Patients meeting both creatinine and urine output criteria for AKI have been shown to have worse outcomes compared with patients who satisfied only 1 criterion.[22]

Short-Term Outcomes

Some short-term outcomes include fluid overload, which has been known to be an independent risk factor for mortality in patients with AKI. Patients with fluid overload who were oliguric or required dialysis had worse outcomes compared with nonoliguric patients who did not require dialysis.[31] A study using data from the FACTT trial also demonstrated that 60-day nonsurvivors were more likely to have a higher stage of AKI.[32] Electrolyte imbalances are also known to increase both mortality and morbidity in patients with AKI.[33] Across multiple studies, hospital LOS doubles with AKI. Mortality increases nearly 10-fold for hospitalized patients with AKI,[28] and for patients with septic shock, 60-day mortality is only 6% for patients without AKI, whereas those with stage 1 had a 17% mortality and those with stage 2 to 3 had a 28% mortality.[34]

Long-Term Outcomes

Although in the past, AKI was often considered to be a self-limiting condition, its association with several long-term outcomes has now been recognized. Specific phenotypes and reversal patterns have been associated with long-term outcomes, which helps in stratification of these patients based on their prognosis. One study showed that the survival in the early reversal group was more than 90% at 1 year, whereas it was less than 40% in the nonreversal group. Relapses were associated with a fivefold increase in risk of death at 1 year.[35] Another study of more than 11,000 patients showed that approximately a quarter of them were rehospitalized with recurrent AKI within 12 months of discharge.[36] AKI also has been shown to be associated with long-term cardiovascular events as demonstrated in a study of 146,941 patients, in which 20% of the 31,245 patients who experienced AKI experienced a cardiovascular event in the year after hospital discharge.[37] Another study of 43,611 patients found that AKI was independently associated with increased odds of developing hypertension over a 2-year follow-up period after hospital discharge.[38] To assess long-term mortality, a large cohort study showed that approximately 28% of the patients with AKI who survived the initial hospitalization, died in the subsequent year after discharge.[39] Several studies have shown an increased incidence of CKD in patients who have suffered an initial episode of AKI, which culminated in a systematic review of 19 cohort studies, showing a threefold increase in the incidence of CKD.[40] Patients who were hospitalized with AKI have been found to have almost a fivefold increase in ESKD.[41] Following AKI in the critical care setting, patients were also found to have an increase in frailty at 12 months, using Clinical Frailty Scale compared with the reference group, with outcomes worsening with increased AKI severity.[42]

ELECTRONIC ALERTS

Delay in the diagnosis and therapy of AKI constitutes an independent risk factor for higher in-hospital mortality. AKI also has been shown to be associated with substantial underdiagnosis and undertreatment.[43] Progression to a higher stage of AKI and case-fatality has been shown to be reduced by optimizing therapy and the use of care bundles.[44] However, care for AKI has been shown to be suboptimal, especially in smaller hospitals over weekends. One study observed an increased risk of death with weekend admission for patients with AKI.[45] Even with the advent of new biomarkers, diagnosis of AKI still relies primarily on serum creatinine and urine output.

Electronic alerts (e-alerts) have been used in thromboembolism prophylaxis,[46] sepsis detection,[47] medication safety,[48] detection of lung injury, optimization of glycemic control, and drug-to-drug interactions,[49] among others, with varying degrees of success. E-alerts have been found to hold promise to dramatically change the rates of nephrotoxin exposure and modestly improve clinical outcomes in patients with AKI, although there was a concern for potential alert fatigue.[50]

The implementation of e-alerts to improve outcomes has had variable results. The first study on the effect of computer-based alerts on treatment and outcomes of hospitalized patients in 1994 showed that computer-based alerts for patients with rising creatinine levels affected physician behavior, prevented serious kidney impairment, and were accepted by clinicians.[51] A systematic review of nonrandomized trials of e-alerts for AKI that were coupled with treatment recommendations showed improved care processes and treatment outcomes for patients with AKI.[52]

However, poorly designed electronic alert systems can hamper patient safety. There is a considerable overlap of overriding appropriate alerts with the occurrence of associated adverse events.[53] Furthermore, even well-designed alerts may not alter clinical practice. A single-blind randomized controlled trial showed that the use of an e-alert system for AKI did not alter clinical practice or improve clinical outcomes among patients in the hospital.[54] A second systematic review demonstrated that the e-alerts for AKI do not improve survival or reduce RRT utilization, with a variable process of care.[55] Both the previously mentioned systematic reviews have been limited by a lack of a substantial number of randomized trials, variable and infrequent description of e-alert implementation, and an overall heterogeneity among studies with a wide variety of endpoints.[52,55] One study by Colpaert and colleagues[56] showed an increase in the proportion of patients receiving fluids, diuretics, and vasopressors with the time to receive any intervention was significantly shorter during the intervention phase after the implementation of e-alerts. One issue may simply be that effect size for e-alert systems may simply be quite small. We recently showed that implementation of an e-alert system could reduce mortality, LOS, and use of dialysis across a 14-hospital medical system.[28] However, the absolute effect sizes were small: crude mortality rate fell from 10.2% before to 9.4% ($P<.001$) and mean hospital duration decreased from 9.3 to 9.0 days ($P<.001$) for patients with AKI. None of the randomized controlled trials conducted to date were powered to detect these differences.

BIOMARKERS IN ACUTE KIDNEY INJURY

Although changes in serum creatinine and urine output have been used to define AKI, these are markers of kidney function not injury per se. They are also late, nonspecific markers; creatinine can be affected by age, sex, hydration status, protein intake, muscularity, and medication. There is a need for identifying AKI phenotypes to improve risk assessment, early detection, differential diagnosis, and prognosis of AKI.[57] Changes in creatinine are not sensitive for the detection of histologic injury in preclinical toxicity studies.[58] Furthermore, creatinine levels are also influenced by active tubular secretion, which can lead to an overestimation of GFR.[23]

A biomarker can be defined as an objective indicator of the medical state of a patient observed from outside, which can be measured accurately and reproducibly.[59] Ideally, biomarkers should be able to predict and diagnose AKI; identify the location, type, and etiology of injury; and predict outcomes.[57] Of course, no single marker would be able to fulfill all these roles. However, several existing biomarkers have found utility for one or more of these indications.

Second-Generation Functional Markers

Cystatin C

Cystatin C acts as a biomarker of glomerular filtration. Its molecular weight is 19 KDa.[60] As GFR falls, an increase in cystatin C levels in the serum will occur. Serum levels of cystatin C are independent of age, sex, and muscle mass. Studies have shown cystatin C to have a higher sensitivity and specificity as compared with serum creatinine[61] and to be a more useful estimate of GFR in mild reductions in kidney function. It is freely filtered at the glomerulus and not reabsorbed or secreted in the tubules. Addition of cystatin C as a supplement to serum creatinine or using it as a replacement for serum creatinine has shown to improve the ability to predict adverse patient outcomes, which was reflected in the meta-analysis that showed that the area under the curve was higher for cystatin C compared with creatinine.[62] Using cystatin C to estimate renal function may sometimes be inaccurate in the setting of sepsis, as the production is increased and its nonrenal clearance is decreased.[63]

Proencephalin

PENK (Proencephalin) is a peptide that is cleaved from the precursor peptide pre-proenkephalin A. Its molecular weight is 4.5 KDa and it is freely filtered at the glomerulus. The rise in creatinine was preceded by PENK elevations by as much as 24 hours in one study.[64] PENK levels have been associated with longer-term outcomes concerning AKI and cardiac disease.[64] It also shows an association with the need for RRT. One study showed a correlation between increased baseline PENK concentrations with a more pronounced annual decline of GFR and increased incidence of CKD.[65]

Biomarkers of Damage

Kidney injury molecule -1

KIM-1 (kidney injury molecule 1) was first reported in 1997. It is a type-1 transmembrane glycoprotein that weighs approximately 90 KDa. It is expressed in proximal tubular epithelial cells in human kidney biopsy specimens of kidneys that underwent an episode of ATN. KIM-1 was initially cloned from murine models after it was found to be markedly upregulated in postischemic rat kidneys.[66] It is also known as hepatitis A virus cellular receptor 1 (HAVcr-1). Elevated concentrations of KIM-1 occur within 12 hours of initial ischemic insult and persists over several hours.[66] Urinary concentrations of KIM-1 protein have been shown to be significantly higher in samples from patients with ischemic ATN as compared with other forms of acute or chronic renal failure. Elevated blood levels of KIM-1 have also shown to be strongly correlated with post cardiopulmonary bypass patients who develop AKI, in patients with CKD, and have shown to have a strong association with GFR loss and progression to end-stage renal disease in diabetic patients with proteinuria.[67] Although in AKI, KIM-1 facilitates repair by anti-inflammatory effects and nuclear factor-κB suppression, in the CKD population, prolonged KIM-1 expression stimulates inflammation and fibrosis.[68] The TRIBE AKI study demonstrated that the combination of urinary KIM-1, plasma neutrophil gelatinase-associated lipocalin (NGAL), and urinary interleukin-8 yielded an area under the curve (AUC) of 0.78, which was the highest for the prediction of AKI.[69]

Neutrophil gelatinase-associated lipocalin

NGAL is a small secreted glycoprotein of 25 kD,[70] which was initially identified in mature neutrophil granules in 1992.[71] It is expressed not only in renal cells, but also liver, muscle cells, neurons, and immune cells.[70] NGAL is involved in antibacterial defense through iron sequestration.[70] Ischemia/reperfusion injury induces a significant increase in renal NGAL levels within 3 hours. Elevation in serum NGAL concentrations precede any increase in serum creatinine by 1 to 3 days. Serum NGAL levels in patients with AKI correlate with the severity of renal damage and an increased risk of mortality.[72] Its levels have also been shown to be highly predictive of AKI in emergency room patients and cardiac surgery patients. NGAL levels continue to increase or remain elevated for a while after initial insult, making it useful for a long time to allow diagnosis. NGAL is protective in AKI, but has pro-fibrotic effects that can prove to be harmful in long-standing CKD. NGAL also has been known to show increased levels in the setting of inflammatory and infectious conditions.

Second-Generation Acute Kidney Injury Biomarkers; Kidney Stress

TIMP-2*IGFB7. Tissue inhibitor of metalloproteinases (TIMP-2) is a tumor suppressor and member of the TIMP family. It belongs to a class of proteins that are natural inhibitors of matrix metalloproteinase. It is combined with insulinlike growth factor binding protein (IGFBP7) to form the Nephrocheck test (Astute Medical, Sand Diego CA).[73] Like other epithelia, renal tubular cells enter a period of G1 cell-cycle arrest after being exposed to a variety of insults (eg, inflammation, oxidative stress, toxins). IGFBP7 and TIMP-2 are both mediators of G1 cell-cycle arrest during the early phase of cellular injury. These markers are the first modern, or "second-generation" biomarkers since they were discovered and validated using KDIGO criteria. The Sapphire study showed that the AUC values to predict the development of AKIN Stage 2 and 3 AKI in critically ill patients within 12 hours were 0.76 and 0.79, respectively, for IGFBP7 and TIMP-2.[74] However, the product of these 2 markers [TIMP-2]*[IGFBP7] resulted in an AUC of 0.80, which was superior to previously described markers of AKI. [TIMP-2]*[IGFBP7] concentration in the urine of patients undergoing cardiac surgery has shown to have both a high sensitivity and specificity in predicting AKI after cardiac surgery.[75]

PERSISTENT ACUTE KIDNEY INJURY AND ACUTE KIDNEY DISEASE
Conceptional Framework

AKI and CKD are now recognized to represent a continuum of closely interconnected syndromes (**Fig. 2**), with patients who have sustained an episode of AKI having an increased risk of developing new-onset CKD or worsening of underlying CKD, and patients with CKD being at an increased risk of AKI.[5,76] To improve patient care, research, and public health, classifications for these various trajectories are needed.

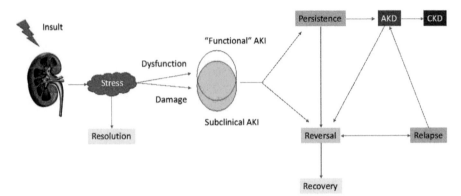

Fig. 2. Clinical course following a potentially injurious exposure to the kidney. Depicted are different clinical courses that the kidney may take after an initial insult. An insult will produce stress that can either resolve without injury or lead to damage and/or dysfunction. Damage and dysfunction usually overlap but damage may be subclinical (GFR >90 mL/min, renal functional reserve [RFR] <30 mL/min), and dysfunction may be without damage. AKI can either continue as persistent AKI (defined temporally as AKI lasting more than 72 hours) or might undergo a reversal of damage and recover, either completely or partially. Both persistent AKI and AKD can act as a continuum to CKD, at which point the kidney is considered to have lost its ability to recover from the damage completely. Persistent AKI is defined as AKI lasting greater than 72 hrs. AKD can be defined as the period of persistent dysfunction between day 7 and day 90. CKD is a steady-state condition defined by the Kidney Disease Global Initiative criteria into 5 stages that can be defined as dysfunction that lasts for more than 90 days.

There are a substantial number of risk factors that have a significant overlap between both AKI and CKD, and AKI that is severe enough and does not resolve, will become CKD. It is challenging to determine which trajectory a patient's kidney dysfunction will take while initially evaluating a patient, and furthermore, there is concern that return of renal function can belie ongoing injury in the kidney, as seen in animal models.[77] Noninjurious physiologic perturbations like dehydration will alter kidney function and yet, can be reversed rapidly with fluids. However, kidney dysfunction also may resolve rapidly after injury and the 2 scenarios can be difficult to distinguish clinically. As the standardization of the definitions and staging of AKI became clearer, the duration of AKI also came into question, particularly with its association to long-term outcomes and mortality. Complete and sustained reversal of dysfunction within 48 to 72 hours after an AKI episode has been found to be associated with significantly better outcomes compared with dysfunction that persists for longer.[35] Duration of AKI based on creatinine following surgery was shown to be independently associated with subsequent outcomes. It was seen that 4 days at stage 3 AKI resulted in an approximately 30% rate of death or dialysis at 1 year. To reach similar outcomes at stage 1 required more than a week.

Persistent Acute Kidney Injury

Persistent AKI is characterized by the continuance of AKI by serum creatinine or urine output criteria (as defined by KDIGO) beyond 48 to 72 hours from AKI onset.[78] Complete reversal of AKI by KDIGO criteria within 48 hours of AKI onset characterizes rapid reversal of AKI.[79] Perinel and colleagues[80] demonstrated that patients with persistent AKI were more severe and more likely to die before hospital discharge even after adjusting for severity of illness. The RUBY study[81] identified a new biomarker, urinary C–C motif chemokine ligand 14 (CCL14) as predictive of persistent stage 3 AKI (lasting for 72 hours or more), as defined by the KDIGO criteria with an AUC (95% CI) of 0.83 (0.78–0.87). Interestingly, CCL14 appears to regulate macrophage infiltration and may signal a shift toward fibrosis.

Acute Kidney Disease

Given that CKD cannot be diagnosed before 90 days, everything before 90 days is, by definition, "acute kidney disease" (AKD), whether or not a patient ever meets criteria for AKI. Thus, the KDIDO guideline proposed a definition of AKD that was equivalent to CKD, only before 90 days.[14] This definition is pragmatic and has high construct validity as a "pre-CKD" state. However, as the preceding discussion of persistent AKI illustrates, AKD can arise from AKI and there may be reasons to classify it differently under these circumstances. For example, if a patient with an eGFR of 130 mL/min per 1.73 m^2 loses half their renal function (and has no albuminuria) they will not fulfill these criteria for AKD, yet they will have persistent (stage 2) AKI with significant long-term risks for reduced survival. Thus, ADQI has proposed to define AKD in the post-AKI setting according to creatinine criteria for AKI and representing the period of day 7 to day 90, when medical interventions might be appropriate and possibly effective in altering the course of the disease.[81] AKI (whether persistent or not) can be considered a subset of AKD, which can occur with or without progression to CKD or disorders (see **Fig. 2**). Thus, AKD is both a "pre-CKD" and "post-AKI" syndrome. When AKI is observed, it may be best to classify it according to AKI staging, as this stratifies risk, although when it occurs outside the context of AKI, it may be best to classify it according to AKD. Biomarkers and imaging may help differentiate AKD versus CKD, especially if the duration of abnormality is known. For example, cortical thinning is considered to be a specific finding in CKD, which tends to be absent in AKD.

Recovery from AKD can be operationally defined as a reduction in peak AKI stage (based on KDIGO criteria) and can be further refined by change in serum creatinine level, GFR, biomarkers of injury or repair, and/or return of renal reserve. The long-term outcomes among patients with AKD are not predetermined and might be influenced by care during transition from the acute care setting.

CLINICS CARE POINTS

- Electronic alert systems implemented for AKI based on standardized definitions have shown variable effects on patient outcomes: the largest studies have shown small but consistent benefit.
- AKI biomarkers including NGAL and TIMP2*IGFB7 can detect AKI before a rise in serum creatinine.
- Oliguria is part of the definition of AKI and the combination of urine output and creatinine provide better discrimination of AKI severity than either parameter alone.

ACKNOWLEDGMENTS

The authors thank Ms Karen Nieri for her editorial assistance with this article.

DISCLOSURE

J.A. Kellum discloses consulting fees and grant support from Astute Medical/Bio-Merieux; S. Verma has no disclosures.

REFERENCES

1. Ostermann M, Joannidis M. Acute kidney injury 2016: diagnosis and diagnostic workup. Crit Care 2016;20(1):1–13 [Internet].
2. Wang HE, Muntner P, Chertow GM, et al. Acute kidney injury and mortality in hospitalized patients. Am J Nephrol 2012;35(4):349–55.
3. Hoste EAJ, Bagshaw SM, Bellomo R, et al. Epidemiology of acute kidney injury in critically ill patients: the multinational AKI-EPI study. Intensive Care Med 2015; 41(8):1411–23.
4. Hoste EAJ, Schurgers M. Epidemiology of acute kidney injury: how big is the problem? Crit Care Med 2008;36(SUPPL. 4):S146–51.
5. Ronco C, Bellomo R, Kellum JA. Acute kidney injury. Lancet 2019;394(10212): 1949–64 [Internet].
6. Singbartl K, Bishop JV, Wen X, et al. Differential effects of kidney-lung cross-talk during acute kidney injury and bacterial pneumonia. Kidney Int 2011;80(6): 633–44.
7. Perner A, Haase N, Guttormsen AB, et al. Hydroxyethyl starch 130/0.42 versus Ringer's acetate in severe sepsis. N Engl J Med 2012;367(2):124–34.
8. Mehta RL, Bouchard J, Soroko SB, et al. Sepsis as a cause and consequence of acute kidney injury: program to improve care in acute renal disease. Intensive Care Med 2011;37(2):241–8.
9. Tolpin DA, Collard CD, Lee VV, et al. Subclinical changes in serum creatinine and mortality after coronary artery bypass grafting. J Thorac Cardiovasc Surg 2012; 143(3):682–8.e1 [Internet].
10. Odutayo A, Wong CX, Farkouh M, et al. AKI and long-term risk for cardiovascular events and mortality. J Am Soc Nephrol 2017;28(1):377–87.
11. Zappitelli M, Parikh CR, Akcan-Arikan A, et al. Ascertainment and epidemiology of acute kidney injury varies with definition interpretation. Clin J Am Soc Nephrol 2008;3(4):948–54.
12. Barrantes F, Feng Y, Ivanov O, et al. Acute kidney injury predicts outcomes of non-critically ill patients. Mayo Clin Proc 2009;84(5):410–6.
13. Silver SA, Harel Z, McArthur E, et al. 30-day readmissions after an acute kidney injury hospitalization. Am J Med 2017;130(2):163–72.e4 [Internet].
14. Kellum JA, Lameire N, Aspelin P, et al. Kidney disease: improving global outcomes (KDIGO) acute kidney injury work group. KDIGO clinical practice guideline for acute kidney injury. Kidney Int Suppl 2012;2(1):1–138.
15. Bright R. Reports of medical cases, selected with a view of illustrating the symptoms and cure of diseases by a reference to morbid anatomy, 2. London (United Kingdom): Longmans; 1831.
16. Millard HB. A treatise on Bright's disease of the kidneys [Internet]. Am J Med Sci 1892;104(3):330–4. Available at: https://archive.org/details/treatiseonbright00mill/page/n6/mode/2up.
17. Raw N. Trench nephritis: a record of five cases [Internet]. BMJ 1915;2(2856):468. Available at: http://www.bmj.com/cgi/doi/10.1136/bmj.2.2856.468.
18. Atenstaedt RL. The medical response to trench nephritis in World War One. Kidney Int 2006;70(4):635–40 [Internet].

19. Bywaters EGL, Beall D. Crush injuries with impairment of renal function. Br Med J 1941;1(4185):427.
20. Bellomo R, Ronco C, Kellum JA, et al. Acute renal failure - definition, outcome measures, animal models, fluid therapy and information technology needs: the second international consensus conference of the acute dialysis quality initiative (ADQI) group. Crit Care 2004;8(4):R204–12.
21. Mehta RL, Kellum JA, Shah SV, et al. Acute kidney injury network: report of an initiative to improve outcomes in acute kidney injury. Crit Care 2007;11(2):1–8.
22. Kellum JA, Sileanu FE, Murugan R, et al. Classifying AKI by urine output versus serum creatinine level. J Am Soc Nephrol 2015;26(9):2231–8.
23. Bagshaw SM, Uchino S, Cruz D, et al. A comparison of observed versus estimated baseline creatinine for determination of RIFLE class in patients with acute kidney injury. Nephrol Dial Transplant 2009;24(9):2739–44.
24. Waikar SS, Bonventre JV. Creatinine kinetics and the definition of acute kidney injury. J Am Soc Nephrol 2009;20(3):672–9.
25. Lopes JA, Fernandes P, Jorge S, et al. Acute kidney injury in intensive care unit patients: a comparison between the RIFLE and the acute kidney injury network classifications. Crit Care 2008;12(4):1–8.
26. Hoste EAJ, Clermont G, Kersten A, et al. RIFLE criteria for acute kidney injury are associated with hospital mortality in critically ill patients: a cohort analysis. Crit Care 2006;10(3):1–10.
27. Cruz DN, Bolgan I, Perazella MA, et al. North east Italian prospective hospital renal outcome survey on acute kidney injury (NEiPHROS-AKI): targeting the problem with the RIFLE criteria. Clin J Am Soc Nephrol 2007;2(3):418–25.
28. Al-Jaghbeer M, Dealmeida D, Bilderback A, et al. Clinical decision support for in-hospital AKI. J Am Soc Nephrol 2018;29(2):654–60.
29. Melo FDAF, Macedo E, Bezerra ACF, et al. A systematic review and meta-analysis of acute kidney injury in the intensive care units of developed and developing countries. PLoS One 2020;15(1):1–26.
30. Priyanka P, Zarbock A, Izawa J, et al. The impact of acute kidney injury by serum creatinine or urine output criteria on major adverse kidney events in cardiac surgery patients. J Thorac Cardiovasc Surg [Internet] 2020;15213. https://doi.org/10.1016/j.jtcvs.2019.11.137.
31. Payen D, de Pont AC, Sakr Y, et al. A positive fluid balance is associated with a worse outcome in patients with acute renal failure. Crit Care 2008;12(3):1–7.
32. Grams ME, Estrella MM, Coresh J, et al. Fluid balance, diuretic use, and mortality in acute kidney injury. Clin J Am Soc Nephrol 2011;6(5):966–73.
33. Statland HA. Fluid and electrolyte balance service for clinical use [Internet]. JAMA 1952;150(8):771. Available at: http://jama.jamanetwork.com/article.aspx?doi=10.1001/jama.1952.03680080033007.
34. Kellum JA, Chawla LS, Keener C, et al. The effects of alternative resuscitation strategies on acute kidney injury in patients with septic shock. Am J Respir Crit Care Med 2016;193(3):281–7.
35. Kellum JA, Sileanu FE, Bihorac A, et al. Recovery after acute kidney injury. Am J Respir Crit Care Med 2017;195(6):784–91.
36. Siew ED, Parr SK, Abdel-Kader K, et al. Predictors of recurrent AKI. J Am Soc Nephrol 2016;27(4):1190–200.
37. Go AS, Hsu CY, Yang J, et al. Acute kidney injury and risk of heart failure and atherosclerotic events. Clin J Am Soc Nephrol 2018;13(6):833–41.
38. Hsu CY, Hsu RK, Yang J, et al. Elevated BP after AKI. J Am Soc Nephrol 2016;27(3):914–23.

39. Silver SA, Harel Z, McArthur E, et al. Causes of death after a hospitalization with AKI. J Am Soc Nephrol 2018;29(3):1001–10.

40. See EJ, Jayasinghe K, Glassford N, et al. Long-term risk of adverse outcomes after acute kidney injury: a systematic review and meta-analysis of cohort studies using consensus definitions of exposure. Kidney Int [Internet] 2019;95(1):160–72.

41. Pannu N, James M, Hemmelgarn B, et al. Association between AKI, recovery of renal function, and long-term outcomes after hospital discharge. Clin J Am Soc Nephrol 2013;8(2):194–202.

42. Abdel-Kader K, Girard TD, Brummel NE, et al. Acute kidney injury and subsequent frailty status in survivors of critical illness: a secondary analysis. Crit Care Med 2018;46(5):e380–8.

43. Yang L, Xing G, Wang L, et al. Acute kidney injury in China: a cross-sectional survey. Lancet 2015;386(10002):1465–71.

44. Kolhe NV, Staples D, Reilly T, et al. Impact of compliance with a care bundle on acute kidney injury outcomes: a prospective observational study. PLoS One 2015;10(7):1–12.

45. James MT, Wald R, Bell CM, et al. Weekend hospital admission, acute kidney injury, and mortality. J Am Soc Nephrol 2010;21(5):845–51.

46. Spirk D, Stuck AK, Hager A, et al. Electronic alert system for improving appropriate thromboprophylaxis in hospitalized medical patients: a randomized controlled trial. J Thromb Haemost 2017;15(11):2138–46.

47. Nguyen SQ, Mwakalindile E, Booth JS, et al. Automated electronic medical record sepsis detection in the emergency department. PeerJ 2014;2014(1):1–10.

48. Weingart SN, Simchowitz B, Shiman L, et al. Clinicians' assessments of electronic medication safety alerts in ambulatory care. Arch Intern Med 2009;169(17):1627–32.

49. Phansalkar S, Zachariah M, Seidling HM, et al. Evaluation of medication alerts in electronic health records for compliance with human factors principles. J Am Med Inform Assoc 2014;21(e2):332–40.

50. Martin M, Wilson FP. Utility of electronic medical record alerts to prevent drug nephrotoxicity. Clin J Am Soc Nephrol 2019;14(1):115–23.

51. Rind DM. Effect of computer-based alerts on the treatment and outcomes of hospitalized patients [Internet]. Arch Intern Med 1994;154(13):1511. Available at: http://archinte.jamanetwork.com/article.aspx?doi=10.1001/archinte.1994.00420130107014.

52. Haase M, Kribben A, Zidek W, et al. Electronic alerts for acute kidney injury - a systematic review. Dtsch Arztebl Int 2017;114(1–2):1–8.

53. Van Der Sijs H, Aarts J, Vulto A, et al. Overriding of drug safety alerts in computerized physician order entry. J Am Med Inform Assoc 2006;13(2):138–47.

54. Wilson FP, Shashaty M, Testani J, et al. Automated, electronic alerts for acute kidney injury: a single-blind, parallel-group, randomised controlled trial [Internet]. Lancet 2015;385(9981):1966–74. Available at: https://linkinghub.elsevier.com/retrieve/pii/S0140673615602665.

55. Lachance P, Villeneuve PM, Rewa OG, et al. Association between e-alert implementation for detection of acute kidney injury and outcomes: a systematic review. Nephrol Dial Transplant 2017;32(2):265–72.

56. Colpaert K, Hoste EA, Steurbaut K, et al. Impact of real-time electronic alerting of acute kidney injury on therapeutic intervention and progression of RIFLE class. Crit Care Med 2012;40(4):1164–70.

57. Westhuyzen J, Endre ZH, Reece G, et al. Measurement of tubular enzymuria facilitates early detection of acute renal impairment in the intensive care unit. Nephrol Dial Transplant 2003;18(3):543–51.
58. Vaidya VS, Ferguson MA, Bonventre JV. Biomarkers of acute kidney. Annu Rev Pharmacol Toxicol 2009;48:1–29.
59. Strimbu K, Tavel JA. What are biomarkers? [Internet]. Curr Opin HIV AIDS 2010; 5(6):463–6. Available at: http://journals.lww.com/01222929-201011000-00003.
60. Ferguson TW, Komenda P, Tangri N. Cystatin C as a biomarker for estimating glomerular filtration rate. Curr Opin Nephrol Hypertens 2015;24(3):295–300.
61. Coll E, Botey A, Alvarez L, et al. Serum cystatin C as a new marker for noninvasive estimation of glomerular filtration rate and as a marker for early renal impairment. Am J Kidney Dis 2000;36(1):29–34.
62. Dharnidharka VR, Kwon C, Stevens G. Serum cystatin C is superior to serum creatinine as a marker of kidney function: a meta-analysis. Am J Kidney Dis 2002;40(2):221–6 [Internet].
63. Doi K, Yuen PST, Eisner C, et al. Reduced production of creatinine limits its use as marker of kidney injury in sepsis. J Am Soc Nephrol 2009;20(6):1217–21.
64. Matsue Y, ter Maaten JM, Struck J, et al. Clinical correlates and prognostic value of proenkephalin in acute and chronic heart failure. J Card Fail 2017;23(3):231–9 [Internet].
65. Schulz CA, Christensson A, Ericson U, et al. High level of fasting plasma proenkephalin-a predicts deterioration of kidney function and incidence of CKD. J Am Soc Nephrol 2017;28(1):291–303.
66. Ichimura T, Bonventre JV, Bailly V, et al. Kidney injury molecule-1 (KIM-1), a putative epithelial cell adhesion molecule containing a novel immunoglobulin domain, is up-regulated in renal cells after injury. J Biol Chem 1998;273(7): 4135–42.
67. Sabbisetti VS, Waikar SS, Antoine DJ, et al. Blood kidney injury molecule-1 is a biomarker of acute and chronic kidney injury and predicts progression to ESRD in type I diabetes. J Am Soc Nephrol 2014;25(10):2177–86.
68. Brooks CR, Bonventre JV. KIM-1/TIM-1 in proximal tubular cell immune response. Oncotarget 2015;6(42):44059–60.
69. Jha P, Wang X, Auwerx J. Analysis of mitochondrial respiratory chain supercomplexes using blue native polyacrylamide gel electrophoresis (BN-PAGE) [Internet]. Curr Protoc Mouse Biol 2016;6(1):1–14. Available at: http://www.ncbi.nlm.nih.gov/pubmed/26928661.
70. Buonafine M, Martinez-Martinez E, ric JF. More than a simple biomarker: the role of NGAL in cardiovascular and renal diseases. Clin Sci 2018;132(9):909–23.
71. Kjeldsen L, Johnsen AH, Sengelov H, et al. Isolation and primary structure of NGAL, a novel protein associated with human neutrophil gelatinase. J Biol Chem 1993;268(14):10425–32.
72. Kümpers P, Hafer C, Lukasz A, et al. Serum neutrophil gelatinase-associated lipocalin at inception of renal replacement therapy predicts survival in critically ill patients with acute kidney injury. Crit Care 2010;14(1):1–9.
73. Dusse F, Edayadiyil-Dudásova M, Thielmann M, et al. Early prediction of acute kidney injury after transapical and transaortic aortic valve implantation with urinary G1 cell cycle arrest biomarkers. BMC Anesthesiol 2016;16(1):1–12 [Internet].
74. Kashani K, Al-Khafaji A, Ardiles T, et al. Discovery and validation of cell cycle arrest biomarkers in human acute kidney injury [Internet]. Crit Care 2013;17(1):R25. Available at: http://ccforum.com/content/17/1/R25.

75. Meersch M, Schmidt C, Van Aken H, et al. Urinary TIMP-2 and IGFBP7 as early biomarkers of acute kidney injury and renal recovery following cardiac surgery. PLoS One 2014;9(3):1–9.
76. Chawla LS, Eggers PW, Star RA, et al. Acute kidney injury and chronic kidney disease as interconnected syndromes. N Engl J Med 2014;371(1):58–66.
77. Wen X, Li S, Frank A, et al. Time-dependent effects of histone deacetylase inhibition in sepsis-associated acute kidney injury. Intensive Care Med Exp 2020; 8(1):9.
78. Kellum JA. Persistent acute kidney injury* [Internet]. Crit Care Med 2015;43(8): 1785–6. Available at: http://journals.lww.com/00003246-201508000-00034.
79. Chawla LS, Bellomo R, Bihorac A, et al. Acute kidney disease and renal recovery: consensus report of the acute disease quality initiative (ADQI) 16 workgroup. Nat Rev Nephrol 2017;13(4):241–57.
80. Perinel S, Vincent F, Lautrette A, et al. Transient and persistent acute kidney injury and the risk of hospital mortality in critically ill patients: results of a multicenter cohort study. Crit Care Med 2015;43(8):e269–75.
81. Hoste E, Bihorac A, Al-Khafaji A, et al. Identification and validation of biomarkers of persistent acute kidney injury: the RUBY study. Intensive Care Med 2020;46(5): 943–53.

Acute Kidney Injury in Cardiac Surgery

Christina Massoth, MD, Alexander Zarbock, MD, Melanie Meersch, MD*

KEYWORDS

- Acute kidney injury • Cardiac surgery • Cardiopulmonary bypass
- Ischemia-reperfusion injury

KEY POINTS

- Incidence of cardiac surgery–associated acute kidney injury is still high and has a detrimental impact on adverse short- and long-term outcomes.
- Recognition of kidney stress before clinical manifestation of kidney injury by biomarker-complemented risk stratification provides better guidance of preventive options.
- The implementation of the Kidney Disease: Improving Global Outcomes care bundle in high-risk patients reduces the incidence of cardiac surgery–associated acute kidney injury.

INTRODUCTION

The demand for cardiac surgery is constantly growing worldwide for reasons of increasing incidence of degenerative and lifestyle diseases, and rheumatic heart conditions. Presently, levels of cardiac surgical procedures range from 0.5 to 500 per million in low-middle to upper-middle-income countries, and estimated needs range from 200 to greater than 1000 procedures per million in low-income and high-income countries, respectively.[1]

Cardiac and vascular procedures are well-known risk factors for the postoperative development of acute kidney injury (AKI). Incidence of cardiac surgery–associated AKI (CSA-AKI) is as high as 40%, with about 3% of patients requiring renal replacement therapy at least temporarily.[2,3] According to the Kidney Disease: Improving Global Outcomes (KDIGO) criteria, AKI is defined as a sudden deterioration of renal function, developing within a period of hours to days. Based on either a decrease of urine output or an increase of serum creatinine, AKI is classified in 3 stages with increasing severity (**Table 1**).

Although the fatality of severe AKI seems to be obvious: newly required renal replacement therapy is associated with in-hospital mortalities as high as 60% and

Department of Anesthesiology, Intensive Care, and Pain Medicine, University Hospital Münster, Albert-Schweitzer-Campus 1, A1, Münster 48149, Germany
* Corresponding author.
E-mail address: meersch@uni-muenster.de

Crit Care Clin 37 (2021) 267–278
https://doi.org/10.1016/j.ccc.2020.11.009
0749-0704/21/© 2020 Elsevier Inc. All rights reserved.

Table 1
Kidney disease: improving global outcomes criteria for acute kidney injury

Stage	Serum Creatinine	Urine Output
1	≥0.3 mg/dL in 48 h or 1.5–1.9 times baseline within the last 7 d	<0.5 mL/kg/h for ≥6 h
2	2.0–2.9 times baseline	<0.5 mL/kg/h for ≥12 h
3	≥3 times baseline or ≥4.0 mg/dL or initiation of renal replacement therapy	<0.3 mL/kg/h for ≥24 h or anuria for ≥12 h

persistent dialysis dependency affecting about 14% of survivors, consequences of mild or transient AKI stages are still underestimated.[4] Nevertheless, these patients present mortalities of 10% to 20% and a significantly increased risk for disease progression: about 25% of patients with an event of AKI will suffer from chronic kidney disease (CKD) after a 3-year period.[5] Apart from the substantial contribution to the development of chronic diseases (eg, CKD, chronic heart disease), the role of AKI as an economic cost factor is also alarming. This finding elucidates the need for strategies of AKI prevention.

Pathophysiology and Role of Cardiopulmonary Bypass

The pathophysiology of CSA-AKI is multifactorial and not entirely understood so far. Mechanisms of ischemia-reperfusion injury, activation of proinflammatory cascades, hemodynamic determinants, microemboli, oxidative stress, and nephrotoxins are some of the factors resulting in renal impairment.

The use of cardiopulmonary bypass (CPB) is associated with profoundly altered hemodynamics, but although maintenance of defined mean arterial blood pressure was identified as a mainstay of intraoperative renal protection in noncardiac surgery,[6] effects of nonpulsatile flow and hemodynamic goals for CPB are less clear. A recent randomized controlled trial enrolled 90 patients undergoing on-pump cardiac surgery in a high arterial pressure group (mean arterial pressure [MAP] >60 mm Hg) and a control group.[7] Although the overall postoperative incidence of AKI was 41%, no significant differences between the control group (MAP 47 ± 5 mm Hg) and the high pressure group (mean MAP 61 ± 4 mm Hg) assessed by risk injury failure loss end-stage criteria and a renal biomarker (urinary neutrophil gelatinase-associated lipocalin [NGAL]) were detectable (control: 38% vs high pressure: 46%; $P = .447$).

Besides arterial perfusion pressure, venous congestion was discussed as another hemodynamic determinant for renal dysfunction in cardiac surgery. Detrimental effects of perioperative high central venous pressure (CVP) and the significance of active treatment of acute increases may be underestimated in patients undergoing cardiac surgery.[8] A prospective observational trial classified 1941 patients undergoing cardiac surgery with CPB to a high (>10 mm Hg) and a low CVP (<10 mm Hg) group. Incidence of AKI was found to be significantly higher in the high CVP group (43.3% vs 7.5% [CVP > 10 mm Hg vs CVP < 10 mm Hg]; $P<.001$), and high CVP was identified as an independent risk factor for increased mortality after cardiac surgery.[9]

Further detrimental consequences of CPB result from contact activation by bypass circuit materials, which provides a significant stimulus for proinflammatory pathways, activation of the complement system, and hemolysis.[10] Reperfusion to hypoxic tissues following aortic cross-clamping and cardiac arrest generates reactive oxygen species, causing oxidative stress, endothelial damage, and damage-associated molecular pattern (DAMP) -induced inflammation and cell death.[11] A mathematical animal model simulating medullary hypoxic injury suggested the phase of rewarming of CPB may be the most vulnerable for renal injury, because of the most distinct mismatch between oxygen demand and supply.[12]

DISCUSSION
Off-Pump versus On-Pump Surgery

Despite the major contribution of CBP to systemic inflammatory response, evidence for an inferiority of on-pump surgery with regard to renal outcomes is still inconclusive. The latest Cochrane Analysis included 86 trials with 10,716 enrolled patients and reported higher mortalities associated with off-pump surgery, but no significant differences in renal insufficiency (risk ratio [RR] 0.86; 95% cardiac index [CI] 0.62–1.20; P = .38).[13] The GOPCABE (German Off-Pump Coronary Artery Bypass Grafting in Elderly Patients) study randomly assigned 2539 patients beyond the age of 75 to either off-pump or on-pump cardiopulmonary bypass grafting (CABG).[14] Neither incidence nor severity of AKI differed significantly between the groups (on-pump vs off-pump: acute kidney injury network [AKIN] 1: 37% vs 42%, AKIN 2: 5% vs 5%, AKIN 3: 6% vs 6%; P = .174). Also, incidences of new renal replacement therapy at 12 months, which were 13.1% and 14.0%, respectively, were comparable (hazard ratio, 0.93; 95% CI, 0.76–1.16; P = .48).[15]

These findings were however contrasted by the previous results of the CORONARY study, a large multinational multicenter randomized controlled trial that enrolled 4752 patients at 79 sites in 19 countries as well for primary isolated CABG with comparable patient characteristics except for an 11-years-younger age on average and a 10% lower proportion of women. Patients undergoing surgery without CPB were found to have a significantly reduced incidence of AKI within 30 days after surgery (28.0% vs 32.1%; RR, 0.87; 95% CI, 0.80–0.96; P = .01).[16] However, the 1-year follow-up revealed no differences between both groups in loss of kidney function (off-pump: 17.1% vs on-pump 15.3%, respectively; RR, 1.10; 95% CI, 0.95–1.29, P = .23)[17] Thus, off-pump surgery seems to be advantageous in younger patients undergoing primary CABG with regard to postoperative kidney function. Because this is not associated with an improved long-term renal outcome however, its initial benefits on renal outcomes must be outweighed against potential disadvantages of this procedure, as higher early revascularization rates.[16]

RISK ASSESSMENT
Risk Scores

Because therapeutic approaches for impaired renal function are still lacking, strategies to prevent AKI remain paramount. Although exposure to cardiac surgery poses a risk per se, several scores have been developed to further identify patients at high risk in this specific setting, as the Cleveland Clinic Score (CCS), the Ng Score, the Mehta Score, and the Birnie Score.[18–21] Although the Birnie Score predicts any stage of AKI, the main outcome of the other scores prognosticates the probability of AKI requiring dialysis. Among these, the CCS is probably the best known and most widely used. Developed from a single-center data set of 15,838 patients and validated in a training set of another 17,379 patients undergoing cardiac surgery, the area under the receiver operating curve (AUROC) was 0.82 (95% CI, 0.80–0.85). It provides 13 items of predisposing conditions and exposure with different weighting, indicating an increased likelihood to require new renal replacement therapy from a score of 6 and up.[18]

Although age and chronic comorbidities, such as diabetes and heart and lung diseases, have been identified as independent risk factors, CKD was recognized as the most important contributor to AKI, being associated with odds ratios of 6.5 (95% CI, 5.6–7.7), 28.5 (95% CI, 24.5–33.1), and 40 (95% CI, 33.8–47.6) in patients with a baseline glomerular filtration rate of 30 to 45 mL/min, 15 to 30 mL/min, and less than 15 mL/min, respectively.[22] Gender was identified as another risk factor, but remarkably, it depends on the analyzed population, whether men or women are more at risk.[18,21] However, few data are available whether these risk scores are regularly used in clinical routine beyond research and clinical trials.

Biomarkers

Because management of patients at high risk offers better chances to improve patient outcomes than treatment of already established AKI, risk stratification and early recognition before clinical manifestation are mandatory. However, the current diagnostic criteria are not appropriate for a timely diagnosis of AKI, as neither the decrease in urine output nor the increase in serum creatinine is eligible for early recognition. Although oliguria is an unspecific marker, occurring from various clinical conditions, serum creatinine levels require a 50% loss of excretory function to increase, thus being especially inaccurate in subjects with formerly unrestricted organ function and elderly and frail patients. Research efforts have been attempted to find an indicator of incipient renal damage, allowing for a rapid determination with a high specificity and sensitivity, irrespective of potentially interfering conditions. On this account, several biomarkers, such as cystatin C, tissue inhibitor of metalloproteinases 2 (TIMP-2), insulin-like growth factor-binding protein 7 (IGFBP7), neutrophil gelatinase-associated lipocalin (NGAL), kidney injury molecule 1 (KIM-1), or interleukin-18 (IL-18), have been, among others, identified, validated, and discussed.

Currently, available commercial tests are limited to measurements of [TIMP-2]•[IGFBP7] (NephroCheck Test, Astute Medical), which has an AUROC of 0.88 and NGAL (NGAL Test BioPorto A/S), for which a composite AUROC of 0.72 was determined.[23] Recently, the enhanced recovery after surgery society recommendations included the measurement of renal biomarkers to the current Guidelines for Perioperative Care in Cardiac Surgery.[24] However, testing for biomarkers is only complementing overall risk stratification: the concept of renal angina proposes to consider the use of renal biomarkers in analogy to troponin for cardiac risk assessment not as a screening tool, but, in selected high-risk-patients, to avoid a decrease in specificity.[25]

INTERVENTIONS
The Kidney Disease: Improving Global Outcomes Care Bundle

Considering AKI as multifactorial condition resulting from the sum of several injuries, avoidance of further insults beyond the inevitable sequelae of the surgical trauma may prevent or at least attenuate its manifestation. Hence, completion of risk stratification provides the basis to initiate basic treatment measures, with the KDIGO guidelines recommending a care bundle for patients at high risk. The concept of bundled interventions is not new and emerged previously in sepsis therapy as a package of key elements of care, extracted from current evidence intended to reduce mortality.[26] The KDIGO bundle includes the discontinuation of all nephrotoxic agents when possible, the consideration of alternatives to radio contrast procedures, tight glycemic control, close monitoring of urine output and serum creatinine, maintenance of adequate perfusion pressure and volume status, and the consideration of a functional hemodynamic monitoring (**Fig. 1**).[27]

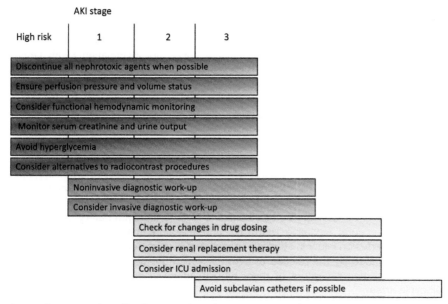

Fig. 1. The KDIGO bundles for stage-based management of AKI. ICU, intensive care unit. (*Modified from* KDIGO AKI Work Group. KDIGO Clinical Practice Guideline for Acute Kidney Injury. 2012;2(1). https://doi.org/10.1038/kisup.2012.1.)

However, comparable to the setting of sepsis treatment, whereby compliance to current recommendations and intervention bundles was found to be low,[28] a recent multinational observational study to assess the adherence to the KDIGO recommendations in patients undergoing cardiac surgery reported similar results. On average, only 3.4 (standard deviation 1.1) of 5 components of the bundle were applied, and merely 5.3% of patients were treated in full compliance with all 6 measures.[29] The low compliance rate is of critical importance, as there is some evidence for a beneficial impact of a strict implementation on patient outcomes.

In a prospective observational study including 2297 patients with AKI, Kolhe and colleagues[30] found the KDIGO bundles to be associated with lower progression to higher AKI stages (3.9% vs 8.1%, P = .01), lower in-hospital fatality (18% vs 23.1%, P = .046), and lower short- and long-term mortality. Also, 2 randomized controlled trials assessed the effectiveness of the KDIGO recommendations on renal outcomes in comparison to standard care: the PrevAKI trial used a biomarker-guided strategy to identify patients at high risk for AKI after CPB ([TIMP-2]•[IGFBP7]) and randomized 276 patients to receive either the standard care or a rigorous implementation of the KDIGO bundle. The incidence of AKI within 72 hours after cardiac surgery was not only significantly decreased in the intervention group (55.1 vs 71.7%; absolute risk reduction [ARR] 16.6% [95 CI, 5.5%–27.9%]; P = .004) but also the occurrence of moderate and severe AKI was significantly lower compared with the standard group (29.7% vs 44.9%; P = .009; odds ratio [OR], 0.52 [95% CI, 0.32–0.85]; ARR, 15.2% [95% CI, 4.0%–26.5%]).[31] The BigpAK study used a similar biomarker-guided approach in patients after major noncardiac surgery. Comparably, the intervention was associated with a reduction of AKI (27.1% vs 48%; P = .03), a decreased incidence of moderate and severe AKI (6.7% vs 19.7%, P = .04; OR, 3.43 [95% CI, 1.04–11.32]), and shorter lengths of intensive care unit and hospital stay.[32] However, both studies might overestimate the effect size of the intervention because of their single-center design.

Recently, a quality improvement initiative in patients undergoing cardiac surgery demonstrated a biomarker-triggered activation of a multidisciplinary acute kidney response team and implementation of therapeutic measures to effectively decrease the incidence of postoperative moderate and severe AKI (2.3% vs 0.24%, $P = .01$)[33]

Soon more evidence will be provided from a multinational multicenter trial: the PrevAKI2 trial (#NCT03244514), conducted at 12 participating sites, which lately completed recruitment; results are pending.[34]

Remote Ischemic Preconditioning

Remote ischemic preconditioning (RIPC) is a technique of repetitive short cycles of limb ischemia performed by inflating a blood pressure cuff for several minutes followed by deflation and reperfusion. Although the mechanism of action is not entirely understood, RIPC is considered to stimulate several anti-inflammatory, neural autonomic, and humoral signaling pathways and therefore mitigate the sequelae of ischemia-reperfusion injury in sensitive organs and tissues. A potential renoprotective effect is mediated by the release of DAMPs, which are assumed to take effect at pattern recognition receptors of renal tubular epithelial cells, inducing temporary cell-cycle arrest.[35]

The use of RIPC in comparison to sham RIPC in patients undergoing surgery is controversial however, and data on beneficial effects are inconclusive so far: The REPAIR trial found RIPC before induction of anesthesia for living-donor kidney transplantation to be associated with improved postoperative renal function and even sustained in the 5-year follow-up.[36] Consistently, the multicenter RenalRIPC trial assessing the effect of RIPC in patients at high risk for AKI undergoing cardiac surgery reported a significantly reduced incidence of postoperative AKI (RIPC 37.5% vs control 52.5%; ARR, 15%; 95% CI, 2.56% to 27.44%; $P = .02$) and decreased need for renal replacement therapy.[37] However, the ERICCA trial and the RIPHeart trial, the 2 largest multicenter studies, including together about 3000 patients undergoing cardiac surgery, failed to show a beneficial effect with regard to renal outcomes (ERICCA: incidence of AKI 38.0% vs 38.3% [control vs RIPC]; $P = .98$; RIPHeart: incidence of acute renal failure: 6.1% vs 5.1% [RIPC vs control]; $P = .45$).[38,39] Because of differing study designs, varying primary and secondary endpoints, and different or inconsistent anesthetic management, the comparability of these trials is limited though. The differing anesthetic approaches, especially, offer a great potential to affect the preconditioning effects, as it has been demonstrated that propofol may reverse the protective effects of RIPC.[40,41] This finding has recently been confirmed in a secondary analysis of the RIPHeart trial, whereby an activation of known RIPC-associated mediators and pathways or an impact on the inflammatory response in propofol-anesthetized patients could not be demonstrated.[42]

Thus, as the mechanism of action and its potential interferences have not been fully understood so far, further research is warranted to identify specific patients and conditions with a clear benefit from this intervention.

Transfusion of Packed Red Blood Cells

Patients undergoing cardiac surgery are at high risk for intraoperative hemodynamic dysfunction and hemorrhage and are highly susceptible to the sequelae of hypoxia. Thus, restrictive transfusion thresholds have been critically discussed in this cohort. Transfusion regimens are a particularly difficult balancing act, as both transfusion of packed red blood cells and anemia-induced tissue hypoxia are associated with an increased probability for AKI.[43,44] Determination of transfusion thresholds by 2 large randomized controlled trials resulted in a noninferiority of restrictive regimens for morbidity and mortality: neither the Transfusion Indication Threshold Reduction trial, which compared transfusions at hemoglobin concentrations of less than 7.5 g/dL versus less than 9 g/dL in 2007 participants, reported any differences with regard to AKI in both groups,[45] nor did the larger Transfusion Requirements in Cardiac Surgery III trial. This study enrolled 5243 participants to be treated with a restrictive transfusion threshold at less than 7.5 g/dL or a liberal threshold at less than 9.5 g/dL. Of patients, 52.3% in the restrictive group received a transfusion with a median of 2 units, as compared with 72.6% of patients in the liberal group, who received a median of 3 units. Incidence of AKI (34% vs 33.9%; OR, 1.0, 95% CI, 0.89–1.13) and new required renal replacement therapy (2.5% vs 3.0%; OR, 0.5; 95% CI, 0.6–1.19) were comparable though.[46] Also, the storage duration of packed red blood cells seems to be insignificant for the incidence of CSA-AKI. A randomized controlled trial comparing storage times of 7 days with 28 days reported no difference between the treatment arms with regard to renal outcomes ($P = .76$).[47]

Pharmacologic Treatment Strategies

Several pharmacologic strategies for the prevention or treatment of CSA-AKI were introduced, assessed, and abandoned again. The latest, more extensively investigated approaches evaluated the efficacy of the following drugs.

Statins

3-Hydroxy-3-methylglutaryl coenzyme A reductase inhibitors (statins) were considered potentially renoprotective substances because of their attenuation of inflammation and oxidative stress. A large retrospective data analysis of 17,077 patients who underwent cardiac surgery indicated a beneficial effect of statins on postoperative incidence of AKI (RR, 0.78; 95% CI, 0.63–0.96).[48] However, although the randomized controlled trial by Park and colleagues[49] with 200 enrolled patients undergoing cardiac surgery reported similar results for the incidence of postoperative AKI and level of the renal biomarkers NGAL and IL-1 in the atorvastatin as well as in the placebo group, 2 larger randomized controlled trials in a similar cohort indicated even detrimental effects associated with perioperative statin treatment.

Billings and colleagues[50] enrolled 615 participants and assessed patients with and without previous statin treatment. Although patients with previous statin treatment who received either perioperative high-dose statin therapy or placebo were found to have a comparable risk for postoperative AKI in both groups (RR, 1.06; 95% CI, 0.78–1.46; $P = .75$), in statin-naïve patients AKI, and increased levels of serum creatinine were more common in the intervention group (21.6% atorvastatin group vs 13.4% placebo group; RR, 1.61; 95% CI, 0.8–3.01; $P = .15$). The STICS (Statin Therapy In Cardiac Surgery) trial enrolled 1922 patients to receive either perioperative rosuvastatin or placebo and reported even significantly higher incidence of AKI (absolute [$\pm$ standard error] excess, 5.4 $\pm$ 1.9 percentage points; $P = .005$) in the intervention group,[51] leading to the assumption that perioperative high-dose and new-onset statin treatment should be avoided in patients undergoing cardiac surgery to prevent adverse renal events.

Levosimendan

Levosimendan is a calcium sensitizing inotropic and vasodilating agent, used in low-cardiac output states and perioperative cardiovascular dysfunction after cardiac surgery. It is considered to have antioxidant, anti-inflammatory, and antiapoptotic properties and was found to significantly attenuate ischemia-reperfusion injury in the renal tubules in animal models.[52]

A metaanalysis of small randomized controlled trials assessing the effect of levosimendan in cardiac surgical patients reported reduced incidence of postoperative AKI (OR, 0.51; 95% CI, 0.34–0.76; P = .001; I^2 = 0.0%) and renal replacement therapy (OR, 0.43; 95% CI, 0.25–0.76; P = .002; I^2 = 0.0%)[53] However, because of a wide variety of treatment regimens, differing anesthetic management, and incomplete reporting, comparability and quality of data are limited and conflict with the results of 2 larger randomized controlled trials.

In the multicenter LEVO-CTS trial with a total of 882 enrolled patients, application of levosimendan was not associated with lower requirement of renal replacement therapy at day 30 (2.1% vs 3.8%; OR 0.54; 95% CI, 0.24–1.24; P = .15)[54] Comparably, the CHEETAH trial with 506 included patients at 14 sites reported no differences with regard to incidence of AKI or renal replacement therapy (9.7% vs 12.8%, absolute difference −3.1; 95% CI, −8.6–2.4; P = .27).[55]

Other agents with vasodilating properties, such as natriuretic peptides or nitric oxide, have been assessed with regard to beneficial effects on CSA-AKI, but currently limited data from only few small randomized controlled trials allow no reliable conclusions so far.

Dexmedetomidine

The alpha-2-adrenoceptor agonist dexmedetomidine offers a multitude of beneficial effects for surgical patients as sedation, analgesia, sympatholysis, and sparing effects of anesthetics and analgesics. It is currently under review for the perioperative management of delirium, pain, organ protection, and overall improvement of morbidity and mortality.[56]

Data from animal models suggested renoprotective effects of dexmedetomidine pretreatment before ischemia-reperfusion injury by attenuated levels of inflammatory cytokines and DAMPs, leading to reduced cell death and toll-like receptor 4 expression in tubular cells following renal ischemia.[57] These results are also reflected by data from clinical research: a current metaanalysis assessed 9 randomized controlled trials with 1308 included patients and reported a significantly reduced incidence of CSA-AKI (RR = 0.60; 95% CI, 0.41–0.87; P = .008, I^2 = 30%). Moreover, patients older than 60 years of age who received dexmedetomidine preoperatively and intraoperatively were most likely to benefit.[58] These results warrant further investigation in high-quality trials to reach a high recommendation grading.

SUMMARY

An increasing number of cardiac surgery procedures along with unaltered high incidence of postoperative AKI and its drastic effects on patient outcomes is an alarming development. These negative effects emphasize that the continuation of research efforts on preventing CSA-AKI is paramount. A biomarker-guided risk stratification allows for early identification of kidney stress before full establishment of renal damage and enables the implementation of an early targeted care that may alter the course of AKI and attenuate its consequences. Several approaches focusing on the systemic inflammatory response of ischemia-reperfusion injury and CPB have been investigated extensively, but neither the use of off-pump surgery nor most numerous pharmacologic interventions were associated with improved renal outcomes. The perioperative administration of dexmedetomidine seems to have attenuating effects on CSA-AKI, but further high-quality multicenter trials are required to implement its use in clinical routine. Data supporting the use of nonpharmacologic interventions as RIPC are controversial, and more differentiated investigations with regard to study design and anesthetic type are needed. Its routine use may be considered in high-risk patients with regard to the absence of side effects and its nature as a simple, noninvasive measure. Postoperative implementation of the KDIGO care bundle, including the cessation of nephrotoxic drugs, the avoidance of radiocontrast agents, close monitoring of serum creatinine and urine output, avoidance of hyperglycemia, ensuring of perfusion pressure and adequate volume status, and the consideration of a functional hemodynamic monitoring, was found to reduce the postoperative incidence and severity of AKI in high-risk patients.

CLINICS CARE POINTS

- Risk assessment is pivotal and should be complemented by renal biomarkers for improving timely detection of acute kidney injury and the early implementation of a targeted therapy.
- Despite the potential renal implications of cardiopulmonary bypass, off-pump surgery was not found to be advantageous with regard to renal outcomes.
- Data on beneficial effects of remote ischemic preconditioning are controversial but, as a low-cost noninvasive intervention without known adverse effects, its use may be considered in high-risk patients.
- Postoperative implementation of the Kidney Disease: Improving Global Outcomes care bundle is associated with lower incidence and reduced severity of acute kidney injury and is recommendable in high-risk patients.

DISCLOSURE

A. Zarbock and M. Meersch have received lecture fess from Astute Medical, FMC, and Baxter. C. Massoth declares no conflicts of interest.

REFERENCES

1. Zilla P, Yacoub M, Zühlke L, et al. Global unmet needs in cardiac surgery. Glob Heart 2018;13(4):293–303.
2. Vandenberghe W, Gevaert S, Kellum JA, et al. Acute kidney injury in cardiorenal syndrome type 1 patients: a systematic review and meta-analysis. Cardiorenal Med 2016;6(2):116–28.
3. Machado MN, Nakazone MA, Maia LN. Prognostic value of acute kidney injury after cardiac surgery according to Kidney Disease: Improving Global Outcomes definition and staging (KDIGO) criteria. PLoS One 2014;9(5):e98028. Landoni G, ed.
4. Uchino S, Kellum JA, Bellomo R, et al. Acute renal failure in critically ill patients: a multinational, multicenter study. JAMA 2005;294(7):813–8.
5. Horne KL, Packington R, Monaghan J, et al. Three-year outcomes after acute kidney injury: results of a prospective parallel group cohort study. BMJ Open 2017; 7(3):e015316.
6. Sun LY, Wijeysundera DN, Tait GA, et al. Association of intraoperative hypotension with acute kidney injury after elective noncardiac surgery. Anesthesiology 2015; 123(3):515–23.

7. Kandler K, Nilsson JC, Oturai P, et al. Higher arterial pressure during cardiopulmonary bypass may not reduce the risk of acute kidney injury. J Cardiothorac Surg 2019;14(1):107.

8. Gambardella I, Gaudino M, Ronco C, et al. Congestive kidney failure in cardiac surgery: the relationship between central venous pressure and acute kidney injury. Interact Cardiovasc Thorac Surg 2016;23(5):800–5.

9. Yang Y, Ma J, Zhao L. High central venous pressure is associated with acute kidney injury and mortality in patients underwent cardiopulmonary bypass surgery. J Crit Care 2018;48:211–5.

10. Kirklin JK, Westaby S, Blackstone EH, et al. Complement and the damaging effects of cardiopulmonary bypass. J Thorac Cardiovasc Surg 1983;86(6): 845–57. Available at: http://www.ncbi.nlm.nih.gov/pubmed/6606084. Accessed November 10, 2019.

11. Wu M-Y, Yiang G-T, Liao W-T, et al. Current mechanistic concepts in ischemia and reperfusion injury. Cell Physiol Biochem 2018;46(4):1650–67.

12. Sgouralis I, Evans RG, Layton AT. Renal medullary and urinary oxygen tension during cardiopulmonary bypass in the rat. Math Med Biol 2016;34(3):dqw010.

13. Møller CH, Penninga L, Wetterslev J, et al. Off-pump versus on-pump coronary artery bypass grafting for ischaemic heart disease. Cochrane Database Syst Rev 2012;(3):CD007224.

14. Reents W, Hilker M, Börgermann J, et al. Acute kidney injury after on-pump or off-pump coronary artery bypass grafting in elderly patients. Ann Thorac Surg 2014; 98(1):9–15.

15. Diegeler A, Börgermann J, Kappert U, et al. Off-pump versus on-pump coronary-artery bypass grafting in elderly patients. N Engl J Med 2013;368(13):1189–98.

16. Lamy A, Devereaux PJ, Prabhakaran D, et al. Off-pump or on-pump coronary-artery bypass grafting at 30 days. N Engl J Med 2012;366(16):1489–97.

17. Garg AX, Devereaux PJ, Yusuf S, et al. Kidney function after off-pump or on-pump coronary artery bypass graft surgery. JAMA 2014;311(21):2191.

18. Thakar CV, Arrigain S, Worley S, et al. A clinical score to predict acute renal failure after cardiac surgery. J Am Soc Nephrol 2004;16(1):162–8.

19. Ng SY, Sanagou M, Wolfe R, et al. Prediction of acute kidney injury within 30 days of cardiac surgery. J Thorac Cardiovasc Surg 2014;147(6):1875–83.e1.

20. Mehta RH, Grab JD, O'Brien SM, et al. Bedside tool for predicting the risk of postoperative dialysis in patients undergoing cardiac surgery. Circulation 2006; 114(21):2208–16.

21. Birnie K, Verheyden V, Pagano D, et al. Predictive models for Kidney Disease: Improving Global Outcomes (KDIGO) defined acute kidney injury in UK cardiac surgery. Crit Care 2014;18(6):606.

22. Hsu CY, Ordoñez JD, Chertow GM, et al. The risk of acute renal failure in patients with chronic kidney disease. Kidney Int 2008;74(1):101–7.

23. Ho J, Tangri N, Komenda P, et al. Urinary, plasma, and serum biomarkers' utility for predicting acute kidney injury associated with cardiac surgery in adults: a meta-analysis. Am J Kidney Dis 2015;66(6):993–1005.

24. Engelman DT, Ben Ali W, Williams JB, et al. Guidelines for perioperative care in cardiac surgery: enhanced recovery after surgery society recommendations. JAMA Surg 2019. https://doi.org/10.1001/jamasurg.2019.1153.

25. Goldstein SL, Chawla LS. Renal angina. Clin J Am Soc Nephrol 2010;5(5):943–9.

26. Levy MM, Pronovost PJ, Dellinger RP, et al. Sepsis change bundles: converting guidelines into meaningful change in behavior and clinical outcome. Crit Care

Med 2004;32(11 Suppl):S595–7. Available at: http://www.ncbi.nlm.nih.gov/pubmed/15542969. Accessed May 14, 2019.

27. KDIGO AKI Work Group. KDIGO clinical practice guideline for acute kidney injury. Kidney Int Suppl 2012;2(1). https://doi.org/10.1038/kisup.2012.1.

28. Leone M, Ragonnet B, Alonso S, et al. Variable compliance with clinical practice guidelines identified in a 1-day audit at 66 French adult intensive care units. Crit Care Med 2012;40(12):3189–95.

29. Küllmar M, Weiß R, Ostermann M, et al. A multinational observational study exploring adherence with the kidney disease. Anesth Analg 2020;1. https://doi.org/10.1213/ane.0000000000004642.

30. Kolhe NV, Staples D, Reilly T, et al. Impact of compliance with a care bundle on acute kidney injury outcomes: a prospective observational study. PLoS One 2015;10(7):e0132279. James LR, ed.

31. Meersch M, Schmidt C, Hoffmeier A, et al. Prevention of cardiac surgery-associated AKI by implementing the KDIGO guidelines in high risk patients identified by biomarkers: the PrevAKI randomized controlled trial. Intensive Care Med 2017;43(11):1551–61.

32. Göcze I, Jauch D, Götz M, et al. Biomarker-guided intervention to prevent acute kidney injury after major surgery: the prospective randomized BigpAK study. Ann Surg 2018;267(6):1013–20.

33. Engelman DT, Crisafi C, Germain M, et al. Using urinary biomarkers to reduce acute kidney injury following cardiac surgery. J Thorac Cardiovasc Surg 2019. https://doi.org/10.1016/j.jtcvs.2019.10.034.

34. Küllmar M, Massoth C, Ostermann M, et al. Biomarker-guided implementation of the KDIGO guidelines to reduce the occurrence of acute kidney injury in patients after cardiac surgery (PrevAKI-multicentre): protocol for a multicentre, observational study followed by randomised controlled feasibility trial. BMJ Open 2020;10(4):e034201.

35. Zarbock A, Kellum JA. Remote ischemic preconditioning and protection of the kidney—a novel therapeutic option. Crit Care Med 2016;44(3):607–16.

36. Veighey KV, Nicholas JM, Clayton T, et al. Early remote ischaemic preconditioning leads to sustained improvement in allograft function after live donor kidney transplantation: long-term outcomes in the REnal Protection against Ischaemia–Reperfusion in transplantation (REPAIR) randomised trial. Br J Anaesth 2019;123(5):584–91.

37. Zarbock A, Schmidt C, Van Aken H, et al. Effect of remote ischemic preconditioning on kidney injury among high-risk patients undergoing cardiac surgery. JAMA 2015;313(21):2133.

38. Hausenloy DJ, Candilio L, Evans R, et al. Remote ischemic preconditioning and outcomes of cardiac surgery. N Engl J Med 2015;373(15):1408–17.

39. Meybohm P, Bein B, Brosteanu O, et al. A multicenter trial of remote ischemic preconditioning for heart surgery. N Engl J Med 2015;373(15):1397–407.

40. Behmenburg F, van Caster P, Bunte S, et al. Impact of anesthetic regimen on remote ischemic preconditioning in the rat heart in vivo. Anesth Analg 2018;126(4):1377–80.

41. Kottenberg E, Musiolik J, Thielmann M, et al. Interference of propofol with signal transducer and activator of transcription 5 activation and cardioprotection by remote ischemic preconditioning during coronary artery bypass grafting. J Thorac Cardiovasc Surg 2014;147(1):376–82.

42. Ney J, Hoffmann K, Meybohm P, et al. Remote ischemic preconditioning does not affect the release of humoral factors in propofol-anesthetized cardiac surgery patients: a secondary analysis of the RIPHeart study. Int J Mol Sci 2018;19(4):1094.

43. Loor G, Li L, Sabik JF, et al. Nadir hematocrit during cardiopulmonary bypass: end-organ dysfunction and mortality. J Thorac Cardiovasc Surg 2012;144(3): 654–62.e4.

44. Khan UA, Coca SG, Hong K, et al. Blood transfusions are associated with urinary biomarkers of kidney injury in cardiac surgery. J Thorac Cardiovasc Surg 2014; 148(2):726–32.

45. Murphy GJ, Pike K, Rogers CA, et al. Liberal or restrictive transfusion after cardiac surgery. N Engl J Med 2015;372(11):997–1008.

46. Mazer CD, Whitlock RP, Fergusson DA, et al. Restrictive or liberal red-cell transfusion for cardiac surgery. N Engl J Med 2017;377(22):2133–44.

47. Steiner ME, Ness PM, Assmann SF, et al. Effects of red-cell storage duration on patients undergoing cardiac surgery. N Engl J Med 2015;372(15):1419–29.

48. Layton JB, Kshirsagar AV, Simpson RJ, et al. Effect of statin use on acute kidney injury risk following coronary artery bypass grafting. Am J Cardiol 2013;111(6): 823–8.

49. Park JH, Shim J-K, Song J-W, et al. Effect of atorvastatin on the incidence of acute kidney injury following valvular heart surgery: a randomized, placebo-controlled trial. Intensive Care Med 2016;42(9):1398–407.

50. Billings FT, Hendricks PA, Schildcrout JS, et al. High-dose perioperative atorvastatin and acute kidney injury following cardiac surgery. JAMA 2016;315(9):877.

51. Zheng Z, Jayaram R, Jiang L, et al. Perioperative rosuvastatin in cardiac surgery. N Engl J Med 2016;374(18):1744–53.

52. Yakut N, Yasa H, Bahriye Lafci B, et al. The influence of levosimendan and iloprost on renal ischemia-reperfusion: an experimental study. Interact Cardiovasc Thorac Surg 2008;7(2):235–9.

53. Zhou C, Gong J, Chen D, et al. Levosimendan for prevention of acute kidney injury after cardiac surgery: a meta-analysis of randomized controlled trials. Am J Kidney Dis 2016;67(3):408–16.

54. Mehta RH, Leimberger JD, van Diepen S, et al. Levosimendan in patients with left ventricular dysfunction undergoing cardiac surgery. N Engl J Med 2017;376(21): 2032–42.

55. Landoni G, Lomivorotov VV, Alvaro G, et al. Levosimendan for hemodynamic support after cardiac surgery. N Engl J Med 2017;376(21):2021–31.

56. Giovannitti JA, Thoms SM, Crawford JJ. Alpha-2 adrenergic receptor agonists: a review of current clinical applications. Anesth Prog 2015;62(1):31–8.

57. Gu J, Sun P, Zhao H, et al. Dexmedetomidine provides renoprotection against ischemia-reperfusion injury in mice. Crit Care 2011;15(3):R153.

58. Peng K, Li D, Applegate RL, et al. Effect of dexmedetomidine on cardiac surgery-associated acute kidney injury: a meta-analysis with trial sequential analysis of randomized controlled trials. J Cardiothorac Vasc Anesth 2019. https://doi.org/10.1053/j.jvca.2019.09.011.

Sepsis-Associated Acute Kidney Injury

Carlos L. Manrique-Caballero, MD[a,b,1], Gaspar Del Rio-Pertuz, MD[a,b,c,1], Hernando Gomez, MD, MPH[a,b,*]

KEYWORDS

- Sepsis • AKI • Microcirculation • Metabolic reprogramming • Biomarkers
- Inflammation

KEY POINTS

- Sepsis-associated acute kidney injury (S-AKI) is a life-threatening complication characterized by an abrupt deterioration of renal function, manifested by increased serum creatinine level, oliguria, or both, associated with infection or sepsis.
- Sepsis is the most common cause of AKI, and AKI is a sepsis-defining event by virtue of being one of the earliest manifestations of sepsis.
- Although the pathophysiology of S-AKI remains incompletely understood, the interplay of microcirculatory dysfunction, dysregulated inflammation, and metabolic reprogramming in the context of tubular dysfunction are important contributors to S-AKI.
- Novel biomarkers of tubular stress and damage recently validated for risk prediction and early diagnosis of AKI promise to provide the next step in the evolution of strategies to diagnose and monitor therapy.
- Recovery from S-AKI is possible, and it is associated with a decline in mortality. Thus, unraveling mechanisms that promote renal recovery and restore function should be a priority in developing treatment strategies for S-AKI.

Funding: This work was supported in part by National Institutes of Health (NIH) grant 1K08GM117310-01 and the University of Pittsburgh School of Medicine Dean's Faculty Advancement Award.
^a Department of Critical Care Medicine, Center for Critical Care Nephrology, University of Pittsburgh School of Medicine, 3347 Forbes Avenue, Suite 220, Room 207, Pittsburgh, PA 15213, USA; ^b Department of Critical Care Medicine, The CRISMA (Clinical Research, Investigation and Systems Modeling of Acute Illness) Center, University of Pittsburgh School of Medicine, 3347 Forbes Avenue, Suite 220, Room 207, Pittsburgh, PA 15213, USA; ^c Department of Internal Medicine, Texas Tech University Health Sciences Center, 3601 4th Street, Lubbock, TX 79430, USA
¹ Both authors contributed equally in the writing of this article.
* Corresponding author. Department of Critical Care Medicine, Center for Critical Care Nephrology, University of Pittsburgh School of Medicine, 3347 Forbes Avenue, Suite 220, Pittsburgh, PA 15213.
E-mail address: gomezh@upmc.edu

Crit Care Clin 37 (2021) 279–301
https://doi.org/10.1016/j.ccc.2020.11.010
0749-0704/21/© 2020 Elsevier Inc. All rights reserved.

INTRODUCTION

Sepsis-associated acute kidney injury (S-AKI) is a common, life-threatening complication in hospitalized and critically ill patients. S-AKI increases in-hospital mortality 6-fold to 8-fold,[1] and the risk of developing chronic kidney disease (CKD) 3-fold.[2,3] Furthermore, up to a quarter of patients with S-AKI require renal replacement therapy (RRT).[4]

The kidney is one of the earliest injured organs during sepsis. Acute kidney injury (AKI) develops in about two-thirds of patients with septic shock,[5,6] and, in half of them, AKI develops before presenting to the emergency department.[1] Therefore, it is reasonable to consider AKI as an early sign of sepsis. Importantly, patients who recover from S-AKI have similar 1-year mortality to patients with sepsis who never developed AKI in the first place, suggesting that the pathophysiologic processes leading to S-AKI are reversible to a certain extent.

The early presentation of S-AKI limits the impact of preventive interventions but opens the door to the development of therapeutic strategies focusing on reversing cell injury and promoting adaptive repair. To embrace this change in paradigm, the mechanisms by which renal tubular epithelial cells (TECs) are injured during sepsis, the defense strategies that TECs use to defend from such injury, and the mechanisms by which defense strategies may become maladaptive need to be better understood.

This issue provides an overview of the current understanding of S-AKI, with emphasis on pathophysiology and biomarker development, and concludes with remarks on current preventive and therapeutic approaches.

DEFINITIONS

In 2016, sepsis was redefined as a "life-threatening organ dysfunction caused by a dysregulated host immune response to infection."[7] This new definition emphasizes the importance of organ dysfunction in the pathophysiology of sepsis, and underscores the preponderant role that organ dysfunction plays in mortality by sepsis. Despite broad tools to assess organ dysfunction, such as the sequential organ failure assessment (SOFA) score,[8,9] or more precise tools such as the Kidney Disease: Improving Global Outcomes (KDIGO) criteria for AKI, sepsis remains a clinical diagnosis, one that relies heavily on the experience of the clinician.

Similar to sepsis, ongoing efforts to unify the definition of AKI have yielded the 3 largest classification systems developed in the last 2 decades: the Risk, Injury, Failure, Loss of kidney function, and End-stage Kidney Disease (RIFLE) criteria proposed by the Acute Dialysis Quality Initiative (ADQI),[10] the Acute Kidney Injury Network (AKIN) criteria, and the most recent KDIGO criteria (**Table 1**).[11] All 3 classification systems rely on an increase in serum creatinine (sCr) level and/or a decrease in urinary output (UO) to establish the diagnosis of AKI.[11] Despite this, current sepsis guidelines still recommend the use of the SOFA score to define AKI, which is problematic because SOFA neither distinguishes between chronic and acute kidney disease nor considers demographic differences in baseline sCr level.

In the absence of a consensus definition and based on current clinical and pathophysiologic understanding, it is reasonable to define S-AKI as a clinical syndrome characterized by an abrupt deterioration of renal function manifested by an increase in sCr level, oliguria, or both, in the presence of sepsis without other meaningful explaining factors.[4,12]

EPIDEMIOLOGY

Current estimates show that S-AKI affects 10% to 67% of septic patients.[13,14] More specifically, up to two-thirds of patients with sepsis or septic shock develop S-AKI.[1,6]

Table 1 Kidney disease: improving global outcomes criteria for acute kidney injury		
Stage	**sCr**	**Urine Output**
1	1.5–1.9× baseline Or ≥0.3 mg/dL (>26.5 µmol/L) increase	<0.5 mL/kg/h for 6–12 h
2	2.0–2.9× baseline	<0.5 mL/kg/h for 12 h
3	3× baseline Or Increase in SCr ≥4.0 mg/dL (353.6 µmol/L) Or Initiation of RRT Or In patients <18 y old, decrease in eGFR to <35 mL/min per 1.73 m²	<0.3 mL/kg/h for ≥24 h Or Anuria for ≥12 h

Abbreviations: SCr, serum creatinine; eGFR, estimated glomerular filtration rate.
Adopted and adapted from: Khwaja, A. KDIGO clinical practice guidelines for acute kidney injury. Nephron. Clinical practice 120, c179-184, https://doi.org/10.1159/000339789 (2012).[11]

With approximately 19 million cases of sepsis occurring globally every year,[15] it is reasonable to estimate that up to 11 million patients develop S-AKI every year. In addition, compared with AKI of other causes in critically ill patients, S-AKI carries an increased risk of death, fewer ventilator-free days, and longer hospital stays.[16,17] An important feature is that S-AKI is an early event in the progression of sepsis. Half of the patients with septic shock develop AKI before presenting to the emergency department.[1] In this context, AKI can play a fundamental role as a sepsis-defining event. Analogous to the canaries that alert coal miners about the presence of lethal toxins in the air, AKI may be an early sign alerting to the presence of sepsis.

PATHOPHYSIOLOGY OF SEPSIS-ASSOCIATED ACUTE KIDNEY INJURY
Limitations to a Better Understanding of the Pathophysiology of Sepsis-Associated Acute Kidney Injury (S-AKI)

Advancing the understanding of S-AKI pathophysiology faces multiple limitations. The first limitation is establishing temporality in human S-AKI. Because more than 50% of patients with septic shock develop AKI before receiving medical attention,[1] it is difficult to establish which one came first.[18] This problem not only detracts from developing effective preventive therapies but hinders the possibility of establishing temporality as a scientific principle of causality. Second, because patients with sepsis, and more so with S-AKI, are often in critical condition, the risk of obtaining tissue biopsies largely outweighs the benefit of establishing a pathologic diagnosis, and therefore data on the pathologic evolution of S-AKI are lacking. Furthermore, although some real-time monitoring techniques have been proposed, applicability remains limited.[19] Third, despite recent progress made to unify the diagnosis of S-AKI, reliance on sCr and UO poses significant limitations to the timely diagnosis of AKI and provides no information about the specific cause of injury. The discovery of novel biomarkers of tubular injury[20] and noninvasive techniques to assess renal blood flow (RBF)[19] bear the promise of improving the diagnosis of S-AKI and provide hints to possible causal mechanisms.

Because of these limitations, progress in understanding the mechanisms leading to S-AKI has relied largely on translational in vitro and in vivo animal models. Although these studies have and continue to provide valuable mechanistic insight, there is a translational barrier that prevents direct extrapolation to human sepsis. Studies using postmortem biopsies of patients dying with S-AKI have helped overcome this barrier and have revolutionized the understanding of the pathophysiology of S-AKI, as described later. However, these studies focus on very late stages, and provide no insight into earlier stages of the disease. The Kidney Precision Medicine Project (KPMP) may offer a solution to further the understanding of human S-AKI and other forms of AKI. KPMP is a project created by The National Institutes of Health in the United States that aims to ethically obtain and evaluate kidney biopsies from patients with AKI and CKD, therefore providing an unprecedented opportunity to investigate the evolution of human S-AKI. It is clear that a combination of research strategies that can move knowledge between the bench (in vitro and in vivo models) and the bedside (ie, KPMP, observational and clinical trials) will be the most efficient approach to understand the mechanisms by which sepsis induces AKI.

Disruptive Notions that Have Challenged Existing Paradigms

Although sublethal hypoperfusion may still play a role in certain cases of S-AKI, the concept that lethal cellular hypoxia leading to necrosis (ie, acute tubular necrosis [ATN]), such as during ischemia reperfusion injury animal models or after aortic cross-clamping during an abdominal aneurysm repair, causes S-AKI has been challenged. In an ovine model of gram-negative septic shock, Langenberg and colleagues[21] showed that S-AKI can occur in the setting of normal or increased RBF, suggesting that decreased global perfusion to the kidney was not necessary for S-AKI to occur. In a similar model, Meiden and colleagues[22] confirmed this finding, showing that S-AKI occurred without changes in RBF, oxygen delivery, or renal histology. This finding is relevant to human sepsis because Prowle and colleagues[19] showed that patients with septic shock with preserved RBF still developed S-AKI, and Murugan and colleagues[23] showed that a quarter of septic patients who never presented signs of hemodynamic instability still developed AKI. Importantly, Takasu and Hotchkiss[24] showed in postmortem biopsies of patients dying with sepsis that S-AKI develops in the absence of overt TEC necrosis or apoptosis (<5% of renal tubules examined). Based on this, it is clear that S-AKI can occur in the absence of overt signs of global renal hypoperfusion and/or macrohemodynamic instability,[25] that S-AKI is not equivalent to ATN,[18,22,26] and that mechanisms other than hypoperfusion must be at play.

Microcirculatory dysfunction

Sepsis causes alterations in regional microcirculatory flow characterized by an increase in heterogeneity of blood flow, a decrease in the proportion of capillaries carrying stopped or intermittent (nonnurturing) blood flow, and a decrease in the proportion of capillaries carrying sluggish and continuous (nurturing) flow.[25,27–29] This pattern of microcirculatory dysfunction is present in septic humans and in animal models across every vital organ, is independent of changes in macrohemodynamic parameters,[27–33] and is associated with the development of organ dysfunction and worse outcome. Based on this, microcirculatory dysfunction has been proposed to be a key mechanism in the causal pathway of organ injury.[25]

Multiple mechanisms have been proposed that may lead to microcirculatory dysfunction. Endothelial injury, autonomic dysfunction, shedding of the glycocalyx, and activation of the coagulation cascade result in increased leukocyte and platelet rolling and adhesion, reduction in blood flow velocity, and microthrombi formation, ultimately disrupting microvascular flow (**Fig. 1**).[16,28,34] As a consequence of altered

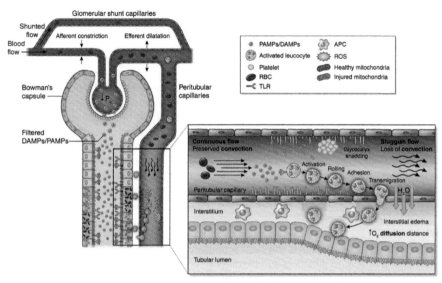

Fig. 1. Inflammatory response and microcirculatory dysfunction. Pathogen-associated molecular patterns (PAMPs) and damage-associated molecular patterns (DAMPs) are inflammatory mediators derived from bacteria and host immune cells, respectively. These inflammatory mediators bind to pattern recognition receptors (PRRs) expressed on the surface of innate immune cells, endothelial cells, and renal TECs initiating a downstream cascade of signals. This cascade increases the synthesis of proinflammatory cytokines, reactive oxygen species (ROS), oxidative stress, and endothelial activation by nitric oxide and nitric oxide synthase (iNOS) upregulation. During inflammation, DAMPs and PAMPs are filtered in the glomeruli. Once in the tubule, these bind the Toll-like receptor (TLRs) present in the apical membrane of the TEC. In addition, some evidence suggests that TECs are also exposed to the inflammatory mediators present in the peritubular circulation, creating a double-hit effect. Moreover, the inflammatory response can also injure the TECs by increasing the oxidative stress and producing ROS. Microcirculatory dysfunction is the result of a series of events that lead to an impaired delivery of oxygen and nutrients to the tissue. Endothelial activation provoked by the inflammatory response results in a cascade of events that lead to shedding of the glycocalyx, increased leukocyte migration, and endothelial permeability. In addition, microcirculatory dysfunction is characterized by a heterogeneous flow, reduced number of capillaries with continuous flow, with an associated increase of capillaries with sluggish or no flow. Sluggish and no flow, a result of the increased expression of adhesion molecules on the inflammatory and endothelial cells, facilitate the migration of neutrophils and macrophage to the interstitial space. Furthermore, the areas with sluggish flow have increased production of ROS and oxidative stress, manifested by TEC apical vacuolization.[16,35,49] APC, antigen-presenting cell; RBC, red blood cell. (*Adapted from*: Peerapornratana, S., Manrique-Caballero, C. L., Gómez, H. & Kellum, J. A. Acute kidney injury from sepsis: current concepts, epidemiology, pathophysiology, prevention and treatment. Kidney international 96, 1083-1099, https://doi.org/10.1016/j.kint.2019.05.026 (2019).)

renal peritubular capillary flow, the release damage-associated molecular patterns (DAMPs) and pathogen-associated molecular patterns (PAMPs) in the vicinity of TECs by slow-moving leukocytes and platelets may induce significant tubular injury.[35] Furthermore, microcirculatory dysfunction can lead to altered regional blood flow distribution, potentially resulting in patchy areas of ischemia and loss of autoregulation, aggravating TEC injury and dysfunction.[25,36–38] In the kidney, peritubular capillary dysfunction can result in direct tubular epithelial injury. Tubular epithelial dysfunction can result in the loss of glomerular filtration rate (GFR) through the activation of the tubuloglomerular feedback by increasing nonreabsorbed chloride concentration to the macula densa. In this way, peritubular capillary dysfunction leading to renal tubular injury can result in decreased GFR and UO, and in increased sCr level.

Loss of GFR during sepsis can also occur as a consequence of impaired microcirculatory hemodynamics at the glomerular level. Under normal physiologic states, GFR is tightly regulated to maintain a constant filtration rate over a wide blood pressure range, through dilation and contraction of the afferent and efferent arterioles. However, during sepsis, GFR control is impaired by at least 2 mechanisms. First, simultaneous constriction of the afferent arteriole and dilation of the efferent arteriole decreases glomerular hydrostatic pressure, and thereby GFR. Second, constriction of the afferent arteriole results in intrarenal shunting through extraglomerular capillaries, which bypass the glomerulus altogether and result in decreased GFR.[19,25,39–41]

Inflammatory response

The inflammatory response is the host's primary defense mechanism against infections, and is critical to initiating and mediating repair processes necessary to recover function after injury. However, a dysregulated inflammatory response may cause further injury and result in maladaptive repair. During sepsis, the recognition of released PAMPs and DAMPs[42] by pattern recognition receptors (ie, Toll-like receptors [TLRs]) expressed on the surface of immune cells and renal TECs initiate intracellular molecular cascades that manifest phenotypically as the inflammatory response to infection.[43] In TECS, binding of DAMPs/PAMPs to TLRs (ie, TLR2 and TLR4) triggers a downstream signaling cascade that activates nuclear factor kappa-light-chain-enhancer of activated B cells (NF-κB), which upregulates the gene expression of inflammatory cytokines and is necessary for immune cell recruitment to the site of injury and bacterial clearance.[44] However, the exposure to these inflammatory mediators and the activation of innate immunity in TECS results in increased oxidative stress, reactive oxygen species production and mitochondrial injury, all of which exacerbate the TEC injury.[43,45–47] Released blood-borne PAMPs and DAMPs in renal peritubular capillaries can gain access to the interstitial space and the vicinity of the basolateral membrane of TECs. In addition, PAMPs/DAMPs can be filtered through the glomerulus, and can be recognized by TLR4 receptors in the apical membrane of TECs, initiating inflammatory responses and inducing inflammatory and oxidative injury (see **Fig. 1**). This double-hit mechanism makes proximal TECs especially susceptible to injury. A critical question that remains unanswered is whether the shutdown of tubular function is an adaptive mechanism of the kidney to avoid further injury and cell death or just an epiphenomenon of TEC injury.

Metabolic reprogramming

Metabolic reprograming is a conserved defense mechanism that cells use to optimize and reprioritize energy expenditure,[16,48,49] and adapt to environmental or intracellular danger signals while preventing cell death.[24,49–51] In sepsis, this has been better characterized in T cells and monocytes. In response to inflammatory signals, monocytes and T cells characteristically shift metabolism from oxidative phosphorylation (OXPHOS) toward aerobic glycolysis during the acute phase of the syndrome, reminiscent of the switch toward Warburg metabolism in cancer cells.[49] Importantly, this metabolic shift is necessary for T cells and monocytes to differentiate into proinflammatory phenotypes such as T-helper (Th)-17 and M1 macrophages, respectively, and to mount an appropriate inflammatory response (**Fig. 2**).[52] Inflammatory

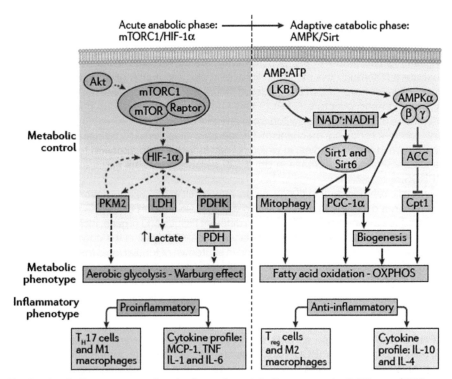

Fig. 2. Metabolic reprogramming. In the early metabolic response to S-AKI, renal TECs undergo a proinflammatory phase (acute anabolic phase) metabolism in which the Akt/mammalian target of rapamycin complex 1 (mTORC1)/hypoxia inducible factor (HIF)-1α complex drives the induction of aerobic glycolysis by increasing the expression of glycolytic enzymes (eg, lactate dehydrogenase [LDH], PKM2 and pyruvate dehydrogenase kinase [PDHK]). HIF-1α promotes the conversion of pyruvate to lactate and, along with PDHK, inhibits the conversion of lactate into acetyl coenzyme A, hindering the induction of the Krebs cycle and decreasing OXPHOS. In the late antiinflammatory (adaptive catabolic phase) OXPHOS, metabolic pathways are reestablished. This process is driven by AMP-activated protein kinase (AMPK) activation, Sirtuin 1 (Sirt 1) and Sirtuin 6 (Sirt 6). AMPK activates Sirt1 and Sirt6. Sirt6 blocks the activity of HIF-1α, switching back from aerobic glycolysis to OXPHOS. This process is induced by the decrease in ATP levels. AMPK activates peroxisome proliferator-activated receptor (PPAR) γ coactivator-1α (PGC)-1α and, with CPT-1, stimulates fatty acid oxidation and oxidative metabolism. Furthermore, PGC1α along with AMPK induces mitochondrial biogenesis.[16,35,49] ACC, acetyl co-enzyme A carboxylase; AMP, adenosine monophosphate; ATP, adenosine triphosphate; LKB-1, Liver kinase B1; MCP-1, monocyte chemoattractant molecule 1; NAD+, nicotinamide adenine dinucleotide (oxidized); NADH, nicotinamide adenine dinucleotide (reduced form); TH17, type 17 T-helper cell; TNF, tumor necrosis factor; Treg, regulatory T-cell. (*Adopted and adapted from*: Gómez, H., Kellum, J. A. & Ronco, C. Metabolic reprogramming and tolerance during sepsis-induced AKI. Nature Reviews Nephrology 13, 143, https://doi.org/10.1038/nrneph.2016.186 (2017).)

cells shift back to OXPHOS in order to turn off inflammation, and return to an antiinflammatory phenotype.[53,54] This switch back to OXPHOS is also necessary for animals to survive sepsis and recover organ function, because persistence of glycolysis results in increased death and, in survivors, in chronic inflammation, fibrotic repair, and CKD.[55,56]

Experimental data suggest that a similar reprioritization of metabolism may occur in TECs during S-AKI.[48,57] Furthermore, this reprioritization might be the explanation of the dissociation that exists between function deterioration and structural changes. Using gas chromatography/mass spectrometry, the authors showed a decrease in the substrate flux through the tricarboxylic acid cycle, and a shift of metabolism toward glycolysis in kidneys of C57BL/6 mice 8 hours after inducing sepsis by performing cecal ligation and puncture (CLP).[48] This finding supports the idea that, during the early phase of sepsis, TECs switch from a highly efficient (ie, OXPHOS) to a less efficient energy-producing mechanism (ie, aerobic glycolysis).[49] Similar results have been shown in in vitro studies, in which human kidney 2 cells exposed to lipopolysaccharide show an early increase in drivers of aerobic glycolysis and a switch back to OXPHOS.[58]

Metabolic reprogramming during sepsis may result in the reprioritization of TEC functions and in a decrease in ATP synthetic capacity. In support of this, CLP and human sepsis induce a decrease in ATP levels in different tissues and organs, including the kidney.[59–61] Inflammatory stimuli from cytokines or PAMPs result in the downregulation of the expression of TEC ion transporters and in shutdown of tubular ionic transport,[16,62–66] thereby sacrificing nonvital functions for cell survival (**Fig. 3**). Pharmacologic manipulation of metabolic reprogramming affects renal function and survival during sepsis in experimental models. For instance, stimulation of OXPHOS through pharmacologic activation of the metabolic master regulator AMP-activated protein kinase (AMPK) results in prevention of AKI and increased survival after CLP.[58] Stimulation of other OXPHOS regulators, such as Sirt1 or the peroxisome proliferator-activated receptor (PPAR)-γ coactivator-1α (PGC-1α),[67] also decreases mortality, supporting the notion of a protective effect of OXPHOS during sepsis.[68–70] In contrast, pharmacologic inhibition of AMPK during experimental sepsis increases mortality and may impair metabolic flexibility by limiting the capacity of TECs to recruit OXPHOS and glycolysis (ie, metabolic fitness).[58] Whether protection is a direct consequence of restoring OXPHOS or other effects of these regulators on mitochondrial quality control processes, such as mitophagy (recycling of dysfunctional mitochondria) or biogenesis (synthesis of new mitochondria), or on interference of cell signaling pathways such as the mammalian target of rapamycin complex 1 (mTORC1)/hypoxia inducible factor (HIF)-1α pathway, is still unclear.[71] Regardless, the availability of functional mitochondria is an essential component of cell metabolism, OXPHOS, and metabolic reprogramming,[71] and therefore it is possible that the benefits of promoting OXPHOS may be secondary to the effects of OXPHOS regulators on mitochondrial function.

DIAGNOSIS

The diagnosis of S-AKI is based on sCr levels and UO in the framework of the KDIGO criteria in patients with sepsis (see **Table 1**).[11] However, the definition of sepsis is based on SOFA score, which is problematic when evaluating AKI. First, the renal SOFA score does not account for underlying CKD and, thus, cannot differentiate between new-onset AKI, underlying CKD, or acute or chronic AKI. Second, SOFA relies on a discrete data point of creatinine, which is a delayed marker of renal dysfunction and provides no information about course. The assessment of renal function using the KDIGO criteria overcomes some of these limitations by detecting AKI earlier using urine output criteria, and by discriminating AKI from CKD by using the change in creatinine level from baseline.[11] For instance, UO may be more sensitive than spot sCr levels in detecting changes in renal function during sepsis, because changes in UO can be detected as early as every 3 to 5 hours.[72,73] Furthermore, changes in UO

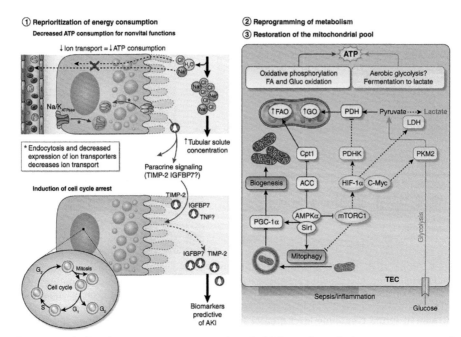

Fig. 3. Metabolic adaptive response to sepsis: prioritizing cell survival. As consequence of the early metabolic reprogramming that TEC undergoes during sepsis, nonvital functions such as cell replication, protein synthesis, and ion transportation are put in stand-by, and the limited amount of ATP available is redirected toward vital functions, prioritizing cell survival at the expense of cell function. Active transport pumps, such as Na$^+$/K$^+$ ATPase, are engulfed by the cell to limit the consumption of ATP. In addition, one of the most cell energy–consuming processes is cell replication. TECs have intrinsic mechanisms that allow them to detect when the cell possesses enough ATP to undergo a complete cell cycle. If this is not the case, it shuts down cell replication, resulting in increased levels of cycle arrest biomarkers (ie, IGFBP7 and TIMP2). In addition, to restore TEC oxidative metabolism and normal TEC metabolism, a healthy pool of mitochondria is required. During sepsis, the mitochondrial population is severely injured. As a protective mechanism, mitochondrial quality control processes, such as mitophagy and biogenesis, are activated as a mechanism to restore the mitochondrial pool and switch back to OXPHOS. ACC, acetyl coenzyme A carboxylase α; AMPKα, adenosine monophosphate kinase α; C-Myc, cell Myc gen; Cpt1, carnitine palmitoyltransferase 1; FA, frataxin; FAO, fatty acid oxidation; Gluc, glucose; GO, golgin; HIF-1α, hypoxia-inducible factor-1α; IGFBP7, insulin-like growth factor binding protein 7; LDH, lactic acid dehydrogenase; mTORC1, mammalian target of rapamycin complex 1; PDH, pyruvate dehydrogenase; PDHK, pyruvate dehydrogenase kinase; PGC-1α, peroxisome proliferator-activated receptor gamma coactivator-1α; PKM2, pyruvate kinase isozyme M2, Sirt, sirtuins; TIMP-2, tissue inhibitor of metalloproteinase-2; TNF, tumor necrosis factor. (*Adopted and adapted from*: Peerapornratana, S., Manrique-Caballero, C. L., Gómez, H. & Kellum, J. A. Acute kidney injury from sepsis: current concepts, epidemiology, pathophysiology, prevention and treatment. Kidney international 96, 1083-1099, https://doi.org/10.1016/j.kint.2019.05.026 (2019).)

and sCr level are associated with the severity of injury and with short-term and long-term outcomes such as the need for dialysis and mortality,[74] and rigorous monitoring of UO is associated with an improved survival.[75] Therefore, the authors propose an evaluation of renal function in patients with suspected or documented infection based on KDIGO criteria and not SOFA (**Fig. 4**).

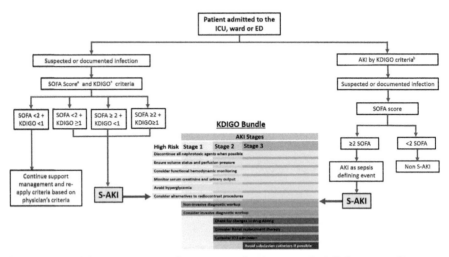

Fig. 4. Proposed diagnostic approach to S-AKI and AKI as a sepsis-defining event. [a]Sequenctial Organ Failure Assessment (SOFA) score in the context of Sepsis 3 criteria[7]: patient with suspected or documented infection who has a total SOFA score greater than or equal to 2. [b]KDIGO criteria.[11] Stage 1 AKI: increase in serum creatinine level 1.5 to 1.9 times baseline or increase in serum creatinine level greater than or equal to 0.3 mg/dL within 48 hours or urine output less than 0.5 mL/kg/h for 6 to 12 hours. Stage 2 AKI: increase in serum creatinine level 2.0 to 2.9 times baseline or urine output less than 0.5 mL/kg/h for greater than or equal to 12 hours. Stage 3 AKI: increase in serum creatinine level greater than or equal to 3.0 times baseline, or increase in serum creatinine level greater than or equal to 4.0 mg/dL, or urine output less than 0.3 mL/kg/h for greater than or equal to 24 hours, or anuria for greater than or equal to 12 hours, or need for initiation of RRT. ED, emergency department; ICU, intensive care unit.

However, even with KDIGO criteria, the reliance on sCr and UO is problematic because of their lack of sensitivity and specificity and other several limitations.[76] For instance, UO is difficult to track outside of the intensive care unit (ICU), where a significant proportion of patients with early sepsis are usually admitted.[77] In addition, aggressive fluid resuscitation of septic patients may result in dilution of sCr, resulting in the underdiagnosis of S-AKI. Furthermore, decreased skeletal muscle perfusion during sepsis results in decreased creatinine production, leading once again to an underrepresentation of the alterations in glomerular filtration and tubular injury by sCr.[78] In addition, ascertaining baseline sCr values is sometimes difficult, making it challenging to define real changes from baseline and determining the presence of chronic renal injury before the septic insult. In contrast, diagnosing AKI may not be sufficient, because treatment options depend on defining and identifying the mechanisms leading to AKI. For instance, differentiating contrast-induced AKI from S-AKI is important and influences therapeutic decision making as well as prognostication of outcome. Several techniques have been put forth to address the origin of renal injury. The score based on the number of renal tubular cells and casts found in the urinary sediment has been suggested to differentiate S-AKI from other causes of AKI. Using RIFLE criteria and the need for RRT as reference standards, a score greater than or equal to 3 was associated with higher urine neutrophil gelatinase-associated lipocalin (NGAL) levels and with increased severity of S-AKI with a sensitivity and specificity of 67.0% and 95.0%.[79] Another example is the presence of de novo dipstick albuminuria within the first 24 hours of hospital admission, which has been associated with the development of S-AKI after adjusting for comorbidities, critical illness parameters, baseline renal function, demographics, and exposure to nephrotoxins (odds ratio [OR],1.87; 95% confidence interval [CI], 1.21–2.89; $P<.01$).[80]

A promising strategy to improve the diagnosis of S-AKI is the development of better kidney injury biomarkers. The ideal S-AKI biomarker should predict or diagnose S-AKI early in the disease course, provide information about the mechanism and location of renal injury, serve as a monitor for progression and recovery, and predict outcome. Although it is unlikely that a single biomarker will fit this profile, it is plausible that a combination of injury and functional biomarkers could fulfill these characteristics.[81] The most relevant available biomarkers, their physiologic function, and their performance in the diagnosis of S-AKI are summarized in **Table 2** and are described later.

Neutrophil Gelatinase-Associated Lipocalin

Neutrophil Gelatinase-Associated Lipocalin (NGAL) is expressed in many cell types, including prostate, uterus, salivary gland, lung, trachea, stomach, colon, and kidney.[82] NGAL functions as an iron transporter into the renal tubular cells, and it is released in the serum primarily by TECs in the presence of ischemia.[83,84] Bagshaw and colleagues,[85] showed that plasma and urinary NGAL levels are higher in S-AKI than in other AKI causes; however, despite similar sensitivity (plasma NGAL, 83.0%, and urinary NGAL, 80.0%), urine NGAL has higher specificity than plasma NGAL for S-AKI (80.0% vs 57.0%).[86]

Kidney Injury Molecule-1

Kidney injury molecule-1 (KIM-1) is a type 1 glycoprotein expressed in the membrane of proximal renal tubules on ischemic or inflammatory injury. A meta-analysis of 11 clinical studies suggested that urinary KIM-1 had a sensitivity of 74.0% (95% CI, 61.0%–84.0%), a specificity of 86.0% (95% CI, 74.0%–93.0%), and an area under the curve (AUC) of 0.86 (95% CI, 0.83–0.89) for the diagnosis of AKI.[87] Despite its good performance in AKI, the evidence supporting its role specifically in S-AKI is scarce. A sepsis model in zebrafish found higher transcriptional levels of KIM-1 on the nephritic tubule at 24 hours in septic compared with nonseptic fish.[88] In a cross-sectional study of 102 patients with different AKI causes, including contrast induced and nephrotoxins, urinary KIM-1 levels were higher in S-AKI.[89] The performance of urinary KIM-1 in S-AKI has been evaluated in 1 prospective study in 150 patients with sepsis, which showed that urinary KIM-1 measured within the first 24 hours of admission had an AUC of 0.91 for the diagnosis of S-AKI.[90]

Liver-Type Fatty Acid–Binding Protein

Liver-type fatty acid–binding protein (L-FABP) is a part of the lipocalin protein family and is in charge of binding free fatty acids on the cytoplasm and transporting them to the mitochondria and peroxisomes for their metabolism.[91] Data on the performance of L-FABP in S-AKI are limited, in part because L-FABP is not expressed in mice, but it has shown promise in predicting the severity of S-AKI. One study including 145 septic patients showed that a high urinary L-FABP level at admission to the ICU was associated with higher mortality, with higher AUC for predicting mortality than APACHE (Acute Physiologic Assessment and Chronic Health Evaluation) II or SOFA (0.99 vs 0.92 and vs 0.81, respectively).[92]

Table 2
Biomarkers for sepsis-associated acute kidney injury

Biomarker	Sample Source	Primary Tubular Release Location	Physiologic Function	Use in S-AKI
NGAL	Plasma/urine	Thick ascending limb and collecting duct	Antiinflammatory and antiapoptotic protein that is involved in the synthesis and transport of iron into the renal tubular epithelium.[20,125,126] NGAL confers a bacteriostatic effect limiting bacterial iron uptake[126]	Urine NGAL is more specific than plasma NGAL.[86,127] However, plasma NGAL has been shown to predict S-AKI recovery[128]
KIM-1	Plasma/urine	Proximal tubules	Type 1 transmembrane glycoprotein that has an antiinflammatory effect on the kidney. Participates in renal recovery and tubular regeneration[20]	In 1 prospective study, KIM-1 in the first 24 h after admission had an AUC of 0.91 for the diagnosis of S-AKI. Nonsurvivors had higher level of urinary KIM-1 at 24 and 48 h than survivors[90]
L-FABP	Urine	Proximal tubules	From the lipocalin family, involved in binding and transportation of long-chain fatty acids to the peroxisome and mitochondria to be metabolized. Plays a role as antioxidant reducing cellular oxidative stress caused by the binding of fatty acid oxidation products[91]	In a cohort of 145 patients with S-AKI, urinary levels of L-FABP at admission were higher in nonsurvivors with S-AKI and had a higher AUC score than APACHE II and SOFA score.[92] It has also been shown to be a predictor of mortality in septic children[129]

(continued on next page)

	Sample	Primary Tubular		
Biomarker	**Source**	**Release Location**	**Physiologic Function**	**Use in S-AKI**
TIMP2-IGFBP7	Urine	Proximal tubules	Both proteins regulate cell growth and apoptosis. In the presence of cell injury, TIMP2 and IGFBP7 are upregulated and may lead to G1 cell cycle arrest through the induction of p27 and p21, respectively[20,93,94]	FDA-approved biomarker for risk assessment tool of AKI in sepsis. Urine TIMP2/IGFBP7 has the highest specificity for renal injury, because there is minimal increase in the presence of other organ injury.[96] High TIMP2 and IGFBP7 levels in the early phase of septic shock are independent risk factors for progression to severe AKI in the next 24 h[97]

Table 2
(continued)

Abbreviations: APACHE, Acute Physiology and Chronic Health Evaluation; AUC, area under the curve; FDA, US Food and Drug Administration; IGFBP7, insulinlike growth factor binding protein 7; KIM-1, kidney injury molecule-1; L-FABP, liver-type fatty acid-binding protein; TIMP2, tissue inhibitor of metalloproteinase 2.

Tissue Inhibitor of Metalloproteinase 2 and Insulinlike Growth Factor–binding Protein 7

Tissue inhibitor of metalloproteinase 2 (TIMP2) and insulinlike growth factor–binding protein 7 (IGFBP7) are proteins involved in the induction of G1 cell cycle arrest, and the regulation of cell growth and apoptosis.[20,93,94] In the discovery and validation studies for TIMP2 and IGFBP7, which included 522 and 744 critically ill patients respectively, the combination of urine TIMP2 and IGFBP7 had the highest sensitivity and specificity for the prediction of AKI compared with any other biomarker, including urine KIM-1, NGAL, L-FABP, and interleukin (IL)-18.[93,95] Importantly, the diagnostic performance of TIMP2/IGFBP7 was better in septic patients (AUC for any AKI, 0.80 vs S-AKI, 0.84) and increased minimally in the presence of other causes of organ dysfunction.[93,96] In addition, an increase in TIMP2 and IGFBP7 levels early in the course of septic shock was an independent predictor of the progression from mild/moderate (KDIGO stage 1 or 2) to severe AKI (KDIGO stage 3) over the next 24 hours.[97]

RECOVERY FROM SEPSIS-ASSOCIATED ACUTE KIDNEY INJURY AND LONG-TERM FOLLOW-UP

The recognition that cell death alone is insufficient to explain the profound loss of renal function during S-AKI,[24] and that organ dysfunction may be a manifestation of cellular adaptive defense strategies,[58] has led to the consideration that S-AKI may be reversible. The progression of renal dysfunction and failure to recover have been attributed to maladaptive repair. Disordered regeneration in the tubular, vascular, and interstitial compartments of the kidney in response to AKI results in vascular insufficiency, glomerular hypertension, and interstitial fibrosis leading to progression to CKD.[98,99] The evaluation of renal recovery after AKI has many pitfalls,[100] the most significant of which is the lack of a definition of recovery, until recently. The ADQI 16 consensus group recently defined AKI recovery as the absence of sCr and UO criteria (by KDIGO) within 7 days of AKI diagnosis.[101]

A prospective observational study including 1753 patients found that S-AKI is associated with higher risk of death and longer hospital stay than nonseptic AKI.[17] However, this study also showed that patients with S-AKI had lower sCr levels at hospital discharge compared with patients with nonseptic AKI (median, 1.2 mg/dL; interquartile range [IQR], 0.83–1.79 mg/dL; versus 1.37 mg/dL; IQR, 1–2.08 mg/dL ; $P = .01$), suggesting that patients with S-AKI may have higher rates of recovery. Importantly, recovery from S-AKI improves short-term and long-term survival of patients with sepsis. Kellum and colleagues[102] and Fiorentino and colleagues[103] showed that patients who recover from S-AKI have similar 1-year and 3-year mortalities as patients who never developed AKI in the first place,[1] supporting the theory that organ dysfunction during sepsis is not permanent.

Because of the importance to long-term outcomes and the association with the development of life-threatening complications such as CKD, cardiovascular disease, bone fractures, and proteinuria,[104,105] it is recommended that recovery from S-AKI is monitored during the hospital stay and beyond discharge if absent.[4,11,106]

PREVENTION AND TREATMENT OF SEPSIS-ASSOCIATED ACUTE KIDNEY INJURY

Most therapies for S-AKI remain reactive and nonspecific, focusing on preventing secondary sources of injury such as prerenal injury, venous congestion, and the use of nephrotoxins, and rely on the ability of clinicians to approach each individual case. Furthermore, because of the difficulties of establishing the precise timing of injury, it has been challenging to develop preventive therapies for patients admitted with new-onset sepsis. However, preventive strategies may still prove useful for hospitalized patients in whom timely diagnosis can be established.

The Kidney Disease: Improving Global Outcomes (KDIGO) Bundle

The KDIGO guidelines have suggested a bundle of selected supportive strategies to prevent AKI (see **Fig. 4**). This strategy, despite not being specific to any mechanism, seems promising, because the application of the KDIGO bundle in patients undergoing cardiothoracic surgery has already shown benefit in reducing the frequency and severity of AKI.[107] To our knowledge, the only randomized clinical trial addressing the effectiveness of the KDIGO bundle in patients with sepsis is underway in Alicante, Spain, and started recruitment in January 2020 (ClinicalTrials.gov, NCT04222361). This study will specifically assess whether the implementation of the KDIGO bundle can reduce the occurrence and severity of AKI in high-risk abdominal postsurgical septic patients.

Antibiotics, Source Control, and Nephrotoxins

Whether infection is suspected, or sepsis is diagnosed, early and appropriate initiation of antibiotic treatment and identification of septic source is crucial to prevent AKI and reduce mortality. Delays in initiating appropriate antimicrobial therapy from the time of onset of hypotension in septic shock are associated with early AKI development.[108,109] However, caution should be used when prescribing and monitoring antibiotic therapy, because many of the antibiotics used to treat the infection leading to sepsis are also nephrotoxic. Medications such as vancomycin, particularly in combination with other antimicrobials such as piperacillin-tazobactam, aminoglycosides, or amphotericin B, or with other nephrotoxins such as intravenous radiocontrast media, should be used with caution.[11]

Types of Intravenous Fluids

The evidence is now clear that in critically ill patients, and especially in septic patients, the use of hydroxyethyl starch and gelatin-based solutions increases the risk of AKI and mortality,[110,111] and that balanced crystalloids are the fluid of choice.[112,113] Furthermore, the use of saline should be abandoned based on large randomized controlled trials (RCTs) that have now confirmed the findings of observational[114,115] studies showing that the use of fluids with high chloride concentration increases the risk of AKI.

The most recent SALT-ED[116] and SMART[112] trials were performed to compare balanced crystalloids against 0.9% saline on different clinical outcomes in noncritically and critically ill patients, respectively. Both studies favored the use of balanced crystalloids, showing a protective effect on major kidney adverse events at 30 days. Furthermore, the SMART trial showed a larger protective effect of balanced crystalloids in septic patients than in the general population (OR 0.8, 95% CI 0.67-0.97 vs. OR 0.8, 95% CI 0.82-0.99).[113]

Although albumin-based solutions have been shown to be safe in recent multicenter RCTs,[117,118] dissipating concerns about renal toxicity, albumin has not been found to be superior to balanced crystalloids,[117] and thus current recommendations still favor the use of balanced crystalloids for the resuscitation of patients with sepsis.

Hemodynamic Support

Fluid resuscitation followed by vasopressor agents is the cornerstone treatment in septic shock. In 2001, Rivers and colleagues[119] published a landmark study showing that early goal-directed therapy (EGDT) decreased mortality in patients with septic shock. Although this was a single-center trial and had limitations that have been eagerly criticized throughout the past 2 decades, this study changed the approach to the resuscitation of septic patients, setting a new standard of care and probably saving many lives. This finding may be one of the reasons why more recent trials analyzing the effect of EGDT have shown no benefit in terms of S-AKI, use of RRT, or mortality.[120]

The SEPSISPAM multicenter RCT showed that the mean arterial pressure (MAP) target in sepsis must be 65 to 70 mm Hg, because, except for patients with underlying hypertension, a higher MAP (80–85 mm Hg) did not improve survival.[121] At present, norepinephrine is the recommended first-line agent for treatment of septic shock,[122] whereas the use of vasopressin has been discouraged based on its cost and the confirmation in a multicenter RCT and patient-level meta-analysis that, although safe, vasopressin does not improve survival compared with norepinephrine.[123,124]

SUMMARY

S-AKI, defined as abrupt renal function deterioration in the presence of sepsis, is an early, common, life-threatening complication and an independent risk factor for mortality. The early presentation of renal dysfunction in the course of sepsis suggests that AKI may well be one of the earliest markers of the presence of sepsis and, in the context of the new definition of sepsis, a sepsis-defining event. Although the pathophysiology of S-AKI remains incompletely understood, it is clear that S-AKI is not equivalent to ATN, and that, in addition to hypoperfusion, other mechanisms are at play. The interplay between microcirculatory dysfunction, inflammation, and metabolic reprogramming of the TECs in response to sepsis are candidate mechanisms that, if better understood, could open doors to specific therapies to prevent or reverse S-AKI. In parallel to understanding specific mechanisms, the identification of better biomarkers to enhance early and mechanism-sensitive detection of S-AKI remains a critical step in improving outcomes.

CLINICS CARE POINTS

- Diagnosis and definition of S-AKI primarily rely on the KDIGO criteria and SOFA score; however, these tools present many limitations and pitfalls. Therefore, a high clinical suspicion of S-AKI is needed for early diagnosis and treatment initiation.
- Newer kidney injury biomarkers, with higher sensitivity and specificity, are necessary for the early diagnosis and prevention of S-AKI.
- S-AKI is considered a sepsis-defining event and AKI may be one of the earliest complications of sepsis. Therefore, sepsis must be suspected in AKI with unknown origin.
- Therapies for S-AKI remain reactive and nonspecific. Early initiation of antibiotics, adequate hemodynamic support, and avoidance of nephrotoxins remain the pillars of therapy.

ACKNOWLEDGMENTS

The authors thank Dr John A. Kellum for the many insightful, enriching, and foresightful discussions about sepsis and AKI, and the role of AKI as a sepsis-defining event.

DISCLOSURE

H. Gomez received a research grant from TES pharma to study mechanisms of AKI in sepsis, and is site principal investigator of an industry-sponsored grant (AM Pharma) to study the effect of recombinant alkaline phosphatase in sepsis-induced AKI.

REFERENCES

1. Kellum JA, Chawla LS, Keener C, et al. The effects of alternative resuscitation strategies on acute kidney injury in patients with septic shock. Am J Respir Crit Care Med 2016;193(3):281–7.
2. Wald R, Quinn RR, Luo J, et al. Chronic dialysis and death among survivors of acute kidney injury requiring dialysis. JAMA 2009;302(11):1179–85.
3. Coca SG, Yusuf B, Shlipak MG, et al. Long-term risk of mortality and other adverse outcomes after acute kidney injury: a systematic review and meta-analysis. Am J Kidney Dis 2009;53(6):961–73.
4. Godin M, Murray P, Mehta RL. Clinical approach to the patient with AKI and sepsis. Semin Nephrol 2015;35(1):12–22.
5. Hoste EA, Bagshaw SM, Bellomo R, et al. Epidemiology of acute kidney injury in critically ill patients: the multinational AKI-EPI study. Intensive Care Med 2015; 41(8):1411–23.
6. Uchino S, Kellum JA, Bellomo R, et al. Acute renal failure in critically ill patients: a multinational, multicenter study. JAMA 2005;294(7):813–8.

7. Singer M, Deutschman CS, Seymour CW, et al. The third international consensus definitions for sepsis and septic shock (Sepsis-3). JAMA 2016; 315(8):801–10.
8. Churpek MM, Snyder A, Han X, et al. Quick sepsis-related organ failure assessment, systemic inflammatory response syndrome, and early warning scores for detecting clinical deterioration in infected patients outside the intensive care unit. Am J Respir Crit Care Med 2017;195(7):906–11.
9. Mao Q, Jay M, Hoffman JL, et al. Multicentre validation of a sepsis prediction algorithm using only vital sign data in the emergency department, general ward and ICU. BMJ Open 2018;8(1):e017833.
10. Bellomo R, Ronco C, Kellum JA, et al. Acute renal failure - definition, outcome measures, animal models, fluid therapy and information technology needs: the Second International Consensus Conference of the Acute Dialysis Quality Initiative (ADQI) Group. Crit Care 2004;8(4):R204–12.
11. Khwaja A. KDIGO clinical practice guidelines for acute kidney injury. Nephron Clin Pract 2012;120(4):c179–84.
12. Bellomo R, Kellum JA, Ronco C, et al. Acute kidney injury in sepsis. Intensive Care Med 2017;43(6):816–28.
13. White LE, Hassoun HT, Bihorac A, et al. Acute kidney injury is surprisingly common and a powerful predictor of mortality in surgical sepsis. J Trauma Acute Care Surg 2013;75(3):432–8.
14. Bagshaw SM, George C, Bellomo R. Early acute kidney injury and sepsis: a multicentre evaluation. Crit Care 2008;12(2):R47.
15. Adhikari NK, Fowler RA, Bhagwanjee S, et al. Critical care and the global burden of critical illness in adults. Lancet 2010;376(9749):1339–46.
16. Peerapornratana S, Manrique-Caballero CL, Gómez H, et al. Acute kidney injury from sepsis: current concepts, epidemiology, pathophysiology, prevention and treatment. Kidney Int 2019;96(5):1083–99.
17. Bagshaw SM, Uchino S, Bellomo R, et al. Septic acute kidney injury in critically ill patients: clinical characteristics and outcomes. Clin J Am Soc Nephrol 2007; 2(3):431–9.
18. Rosen S, Heyman SN. Difficulties in understanding human "acute tubular necrosis": limited data and flawed animal models. Kidney Int 2001;60(4):1220–4.
19. Prowle JR, Molan MP, Hornsey E, et al. Measurement of renal blood flow by phase-contrast magnetic resonance imaging during septic acute kidney injury: a pilot investigation. Crit Care Med 2012;40(6):1768–76.
20. Srisawat N, Kellum JA. The role of biomarkers in acute kidney injury. Crit Care Clin 2020;36(1):125–40.
21. Langenberg C, Wan L, Egi M, et al. Renal blood flow in experimental septic acute renal failure. Kidney Int 2006;69(11):1996–2002.
22. Maiden MJ, Otto S, Brealey JK, et al. Structure and function of the kidney in septic shock. A prospective controlled experimental study. Am J Respir Crit Care Med 2016;194(6):692–700.
23. Murugan R, Karajala-Subramanyam V, Lee M, et al. Acute kidney injury in non-severe pneumonia is associated with an increased immune response and lower survival. Kidney Int 2010;77(6):527–35.
24. Takasu O, Gaut JP, Watanabe E, et al. Mechanisms of cardiac and renal dysfunction in patients dying of sepsis. Am J Respir Crit Care Med 2013; 187(5):509–17.
25. Post EH, Kellum JA, Bellomo R, et al. Renal perfusion in sepsis: from macro- to microcirculation. Kidney Int 2017;91(1):45–60.

26. Kosaka J, Lankadeva YR, May CN, et al. Histopathology of septic acute kidney injury: a systematic review of experimental data. Crit Care Med 2016;44(9): e897–903.

27. Seely KA, Holthoff JH, Burns ST, et al. Hemodynamic changes in the kidney in a pediatric rat model of sepsis-induced acute kidney injury. Am J Physiol Renal Physiol 2011;301(1):F209–17.

28. De Backer D, Donadello K, Taccone FS, et al. Microcirculatory alterations: potential mechanisms and implications for therapy. Ann Intensive Care 2011; 1(1):27.

29. Verdant CL, De Backer D, Bruhn A, et al. Evaluation of sublingual and gut mucosal microcirculation in sepsis: a quantitative analysis. Crit Care Med 2009;37(11):2875–81.

30. De Backer D, Creteur J, Preiser JC, et al. Microvascular blood flow is altered in patients with sepsis. Am J Respir Crit Care Med 2002;166(1):98–104.

31. Tiwari MM, Brock RW, Megyesi JK, et al. Disruption of renal peritubular blood flow in lipopolysaccharide-induced renal failure: role of nitric oxide and caspases. Am J Physiol Renal Physiol 2005;289(6):F1324–32.

32. Holthoff JH, Wang Z, Seely KA, et al. Resveratrol improves renal microcirculation, protects the tubular epithelium, and prolongs survival in a mouse model of sepsis-induced acute kidney injury. Kidney Int 2012;81(4):370–8.

33. Ince C. Hemodynamic coherence and the rationale for monitoring the microcirculation. Crit Care 2015;19(Suppl 3):S8.

34. Verma SK, Molitoris BA. Renal endothelial injury and microvascular dysfunction in acute kidney injury. Semin Nephrol 2015;35(1):96–107.

35. Gomez H, Ince C, De Backer D, et al. A unified theory of sepsis-induced acute kidney injury: inflammation, microcirculatory dysfunction, bioenergetics, and the tubular cell adaptation to injury. Shock 2014;41(1):3–11.

36. Dyson A, Bezemer R, Legrand M, et al. Microvascular and interstitial oxygen tension in the renal cortex and medulla studied in a 4-h rat model of LPS-induced endotoxemia. Shock 2011;36(1):83–9.

37. Almac E, Siegemund M, Demirci C, et al. Microcirculatory recruitment maneuvers correct tissue CO2 abnormalities in sepsis. Minerva Anestesiol 2006; 72(6):507–19.

38. Rajendram R, Prowle JR. Venous congestion: are we adding insult to kidney injury in sepsis? Crit Care 2014;18(1):104.

39. Martensson J, Bellomo R. Sepsis-induced acute kidney injury. Crit Care Clin 2015;31(4):649–60.

40. Singh P, Okusa MD. The role of tubuloglomerular feedback in the pathogenesis of acute kidney injury. Contrib Nephrol 2011;174:12–21.

41. Calzavacca P, Evans RG, Bailey M, et al. Cortical and medullary tissue perfusion and oxygenation in experimental septic acute kidney injury. Crit Care Med 2015; 43(10):e431–9.

42. Jang HR, Rabb H. Immune cells in experimental acute kidney injury. Nat Rev Nephrol 2015;11(2):88–101.

43. Fry DE. Sepsis, systemic inflammatory response, and multiple organ dysfunction: the mystery continues. Am Surg 2012;78(1):1–8.

44. Novak ML, Koh TJ. Macrophage phenotypes during tissue repair. J Leukoc Biol 2013;93(6):875–81.

45. Hotchkiss RS, Karl IE. The pathophysiology and treatment of sepsis. N Engl J Med 2003;348(2):138–50.

46. Kalakeche R, Hato T, Rhodes G, et al. Endotoxin uptake by S1 proximal tubular segment causes oxidative stress in the downstream S2 segment. J Am Soc Nephrol 2011;22(8):1505–16.
47. Dellepiane S, Marengo M, Cantaluppi V. Detrimental cross-talk between sepsis and acute kidney injury: new pathogenic mechanisms, early biomarkers and targeted therapies. Crit Care 2016;20:61.
48. Waltz P, Carchman E, Gomez H, et al. Sepsis results in an altered renal metabolic and osmolyte profile. J Surg Res 2016;202(1):8–12.
49. Gómez H, Kellum JA, Ronco C. Metabolic reprogramming and tolerance during sepsis-induced AKI. Nat Rev Nephrol 2017;13(3):143.
50. Hotchkiss RS, Swanson PE, Freeman BD, et al. Apoptotic cell death in patients with sepsis, shock, and multiple organ dysfunction. Crit Care Med 1999;27(7): 1230–51.
51. Singer M, De Santis V, Vitale D, et al. Multiorgan failure is an adaptive, endocrine-mediated, metabolic response to overwhelming systemic inflammation. Lancet 2004;364(9433):545–8.
52. Frauwirth KA, Riley JL, Harris MH, et al. The CD28 signaling pathway regulates glucose metabolism. Immunity 2002;16(6):769–77.
53. Cheng SC, Scicluna BP, Arts RJ, et al. Broad defects in the energy metabolism of leukocytes underlie immunoparalysis in sepsis. Nat Immunol 2016;17(4): 406–13.
54. Cheng SC, Quintin J, Cramer RA, et al. mTOR- and HIF-1α-mediated aerobic glycolysis as metabolic basis for trained immunity. Science 2014;345(6204): 1250684.
55. Bataille A, Galichon P, Chelghoum N, et al. Increased fatty acid oxidation in differentiated proximal tubular cells surviving a reversible episode of acute kidney injury. Cell Physiol Biochem 2018;47(4):1338–51.
56. Lan R, Geng H, Singha PK, et al. Mitochondrial pathology and glycolytic shift during proximal tubule atrophy after ischemic AKI. J Am Soc Nephrol 2016; 27(11):3356–67.
57. Smith JA, Stallons LJ, Schnellmann RG. Renal cortical hexokinase and pentose phosphate pathway activation through the EGFR/Akt signaling pathway in endotoxin-induced acute kidney injury. Am J Physiol Renal Physiol 2014; 307(4):F435–44.
58. Jin K, Ma Y, Manrique-Caballero CL, et al. Activation of AMP-activated protein kinase during sepsis/inflammation improves survival by preserving cellular metabolic fitness. FASEB j. 2020;34(5):7036.
59. Brealey D, Brand M, Hargreaves I, et al. Association between mitochondrial dysfunction and severity and outcome of septic shock. Lancet 2002; 360(9328):219–23.
60. Brealey D, Karyampudi S, Jacques TS, et al. Mitochondrial dysfunction in a long-term rodent model of sepsis and organ failure. Am J Physiol Regul Integr Comp Physiol 2004;286(3):R491–7.
61. Patil NK, Parajuli N, MacMillan-Crow LA, et al. Inactivation of renal mitochondrial respiratory complexes and manganese superoxide dismutase during sepsis: mitochondria-targeted antioxidant mitigates injury. Am J Physiol Renal Physiol 2014;306(7):F734–43.
62. Mandel LJ, Balaban RS. Stoichiometry and coupling of active transport to oxidative metabolism in epithelial tissues. Am J Physiol 1981;240(5):F357–71.
63. Bhargava P, Schnellmann RG. Mitochondrial energetics in the kidney. Nat Rev Nephrol 2017;13(10):629.

64. Schmidt C, Hocherl K, Schweda F, et al. Proinflammatory cytokines cause down-regulation of renal chloride entry pathways during sepsis. Crit Care Med 2007; 35(9):2110–9.

65. Good DW, George T, Watts BA, et al. Lipopolysaccharide directly alters renal tubule transport through distinct TLR4-dependent pathways in basolateral and apical membranes. Am J Physiol Renal Physiol 2009;297(4):F866–74.

66. Hsiao HW, Tsai KL, Wang LF, et al. The decline of autophagy contributes to proximal tubular dysfunction during sepsis. Shock 2012;37(3):289–96.

67. Haden DW, Suliman HB, Carraway MS, et al. Mitochondrial biogenesis restores oxidative metabolism during Staphylococcus aureus sepsis. Am J Respir Crit Care Med 2007;176(8):768–77.

68. Yang L, Xie M, Yang M, et al. PKM2 regulates the Warburg effect and promotes HMGB1 release in sepsis. Nat Commun 2014;5:4436.

69. Escobar DA, Botero-Quintero AM, Kautza BC, et al. Adenosine monophosphate-activated protein kinase activation protects against sepsis-induced organ injury and inflammation. J Surg Res 2015;194(1):262–72.

70. Opal SM, Ellis JL, Suri V, et al. Pharmacological sirt1 activation improves mortality and markedly alters transcriptional profiles that accompany experimental sepsis. Shock 2016;45(4):411–8.

71. Sun J, Zhang J, Tian J, et al. Mitochondria in sepsis-induced AKI. J Am Soc Nephrol 2019;30(7):1151–61.

72. Leedahl DD, Frazee EN, Schramm GE, et al. Derivation of urine output thresholds that identify a very high risk of AKI in patients with septic shock. Clin J Am Soc Nephrol 2014;9(7):1168–74.

73. Prowle JR, Liu YL, Licari E, et al. Oliguria as predictive biomarker of acute kidney injury in critically ill patients. Crit Care 2011;15(4):R172.

74. Kellum JA, Sileanu FE, Murugan R, et al. Classifying AKI by urine output versus serum creatinine level. J Am Soc Nephrol 2015;26(9):2231–8.

75. Jin K, Murugan R, Sileanu FE, et al. Intensive monitoring of urine output is associated with increased detection of acute kidney injury and improved outcomes. Chest 2017;152(5):972–9.

76. Waikar SS, Betensky RA, Emerson SC, et al. Imperfect gold standards for kidney injury biomarker evaluation. J Am Soc Nephrol 2012;23(1):13–21.

77. Szakmany T, Lundin RM, Sharif B, et al. Sepsis prevalence and outcome on the general wards and emergency departments in wales: results of a multi-centre, observational, point prevalence study. PLoS One 2016;11(12):e0167230.

78. Doi K, Yuen PS, Eisner C, et al. Reduced production of creatinine limits its use as marker of kidney injury in sepsis. J Am Soc Nephrol 2009;20(6):1217–21.

79. Bagshaw SM, Haase M, Haase-Fielitz A, et al. A prospective evaluation of urine microscopy in septic and non-septic acute kidney injury. Nephrol Dial Transpl 2012;27(2):582–8.

80. Neyra JA, Manllo J, Li X, et al. Association of de novo dipstick albuminuria with severe acute kidney injury in critically ill septic patients. Nephron Clin Pract 2014;128(3–4):373–80.

81. Murray PT, Mehta RL, Shaw A, et al. Potential use of biomarkers in acute kidney injury: report and summary of recommendations from the 10th Acute Dialysis Quality Initiative consensus conference. Kidney Int 2014;85(3):513–21.

82. Friedl A, Stoesz SP, Buckley P, et al. Neutrophil gelatinase-associated lipocalin in normal and neoplastic human tissues. Cell type-specific pattern of expression. Histochem J 1999;31(7):433–41.

83. Wang K, Xie S, Xiao K, et al. Biomarkers of sepsis-induced acute kidney injury. Biomed Res Int 2018;2018:6937947.
84. Charlton JR, Portilla D, Okusa MD. A basic science view of acute kidney injury biomarkers. Nephrol Dial Transpl 2014;29(7):1301–11.
85. Bagshaw SM, Bennett M, Haase M, et al. Plasma and urine neutrophil gelatinase-associated lipocalin in septic versus non-septic acute kidney injury in critical illness. Intensive Care Med 2010;36(3):452–61.
86. Zhang A, Cai Y, Wang PF, et al. Diagnosis and prognosis of neutrophil gelatinase-associated lipocalin for acute kidney injury with sepsis: a systematic review and meta-analysis. Crit Care 2016;20:41.
87. Shao X, Tian L, Xu W, et al. Diagnostic value of urinary kidney injury molecule 1 for acute kidney injury: a meta-analysis. PLoS One 2014;9(1):e84131.
88. Wen X, Cui L, Morrisroe S, et al. A zebrafish model of infection-associated acute kidney injury. Am J Physiol Renal Physiol 2018;315(2):F291–9.
89. Vaidya VS, Waikar SS, Ferguson MA, et al. Urinary biomarkers for sensitive and specific detection of acute kidney injury in humans. Clin Transl Sci 2008;1(3): 200–8.
90. Tu Y, Wang H, Sun R, et al. Urinary netrin-1 and KIM-1 as early biomarkers for septic acute kidney injury. Ren Fail 2014;36(10):1559–63.
91. Pelsers MM, Hermens WT, Glatz JF. Fatty acid-binding proteins as plasma markers of tissue injury. Clin Chim Acta 2005;352(1–2):15–35.
92. Doi K, Noiri E, Maeda-Mamiya R, et al. Urinary L-type fatty acid-binding protein as a new biomarker of sepsis complicated with acute kidney injury. Crit Care Med 2010;38(10):2037–42.
93. Kashani K, Al-Khafaji A, Ardiles T, et al. Discovery and validation of cell cycle arrest biomarkers in human acute kidney injury. Crit Care 2013;17(1):R25.
94. Vijayan A, Faubel S, Askenazi DJ, et al. Clinical use of the urine biomarker [TIMP-2] × [IGFBP7] for acute kidney injury risk assessment. Am J Kidney Dis 2016;68(1):19–28.
95. Zhang D, Yuan Y, Guo L, et al. Comparison of urinary TIMP-2 and IGFBP7 cut-offs to predict acute kidney injury in critically ill patients. Medicine 2019;98(26): e16232.
96. Honore PM, Nguyen HB, Gong M, et al. Urinary tissue inhibitor of metalloproteinase-2 and insulin-like growth factor-binding protein 7 for risk stratification of acute kidney injury in patients with sepsis. Crit Care Med 2016; 44(10):1851–60.
97. Maizel J, Daubin D, Vong LV, et al. Urinary TIMP2 and IGFBP7 identifies high risk patients of short-term progression from mild and moderate to severe acute kidney injury during septic shock: a prospective cohort study. Dis Markers 2019; 2019:3471215.
98. Basile DP, Bonventre JV, Mehta R, et al. Progression after AKI: understanding maladaptive repair processes to predict and identify therapeutic treatments. J Am Soc Nephrol 2016;27(3):687–97.
99. Chawla LS, Eggers PW, Star RA, et al. Acute kidney injury and chronic kidney disease as interconnected syndromes. N Engl J Med 2014;371(1):58–66.
100. Forni LG, Darmon M, Ostermann M, et al. Renal recovery after acute kidney injury. Intensive Care Med 2017;43(6):855–66.
101. Chawla LS, Bellomo R, Bihorac A, et al. Acute kidney disease and renal recovery: consensus report of the Acute Disease Quality Initiative (ADQI) 16 Workgroup. Nat Rev Nephrol 2017;13(4):241–57.

102. Kellum JA, Sileanu FE, Bihorac A, et al. Recovery after Acute Kidney Injury. Am J Respir Crit Care Med 2017;195(6):784–91.
103. Fiorentino M, Tohme FA, Wang S, et al. Long-term survival in patients with septic acute kidney injury is strongly influenced by renal recovery. PLoS One 2018; 13(6):e0198269.
104. Noble RA, Lucas BJ, Selby NM. Long-term outcomes in patients with acute kidney injury. Clin J Am Soc Nephrol 2020;15(3):423–9.
105. See EJ, Jayasinghe K, Glassford N, et al. Long-term risk of adverse outcomes after acute kidney injury: a systematic review and meta-analysis of cohort studies using consensus definitions of exposure. Kidney Int 2019;95(1):160–72.
106. Odutayo A, Wong CX, Farkouh M, et al. AKI and long-term risk for cardiovascular events and mortality. J Am Soc Nephrol 2017;28(1):377–87.
107. Meersch M, Schmidt C, Hoffmeier A, et al. Erratum to: prevention of cardiac surgery-associated AKI by implementing the KDIGO guidelines in high risk patients identified by biomarkers: the PrevAKI randomized controlled trial. Intensive Care Med 2017;43(11):1749–61.
108. Kumar A, Roberts D, Wood KE, et al. Duration of hypotension before initiation of effective antimicrobial therapy is the critical determinant of survival in human septic shock. Crit Care Med 2006;34(6):1589–96.
109. Kumar A. Optimizing antimicrobial therapy in sepsis and septic shock. Crit Care Clin 2009;25(4):733–viii, viii.
110. Perner A, Haase N, Guttormsen AB, et al. Hydroxyethyl starch 130/0.42 versus Ringer's acetate in severe sepsis. N Engl J Med 2012;367(2):124–34.
111. Pisano A, Landoni G, Bellomo R. The risk of infusing gelatin? Die-hard misconceptions and forgotten (or ignored) truths. Minerva Anestesiol 2016;82(10):1107–14.
112. Semler MW, Self WH, Wanderer JP, et al. Balanced crystalloids versus saline in critically ill adults. N Engl J Med 2018;378(9):829–39.
113. Semler MW, Wanderer JP, Ehrenfeld JM, et al. Balanced crystalloids versus saline in the intensive care unit. The SALT randomized trial. Am J Respir Crit Care Med 2017;195(10):1362–72.
114. Yunos NM, Bellomo R, Glassford N, et al. Chloride-liberal vs. chloride-restrictive intravenous fluid administration and acute kidney injury: an extended analysis. Intensive Care Med 2015;41(2):257–64.
115. Yunos NM, Bellomo R, Hegarty C, et al. Association between a chloride-liberal vs chloride-restrictive intravenous fluid administration strategy and kidney injury in critically ill adults. JAMA 2012;308(15):1566–72.
116. Self WH, Semler MW, Wanderer JP, et al. Balanced crystalloids versus saline in noncritically ill adults. N Engl J Med 2018;378(9):819–28.
117. Caironi P, Tognoni G, Masson S, et al. Albumin replacement in patients with severe sepsis or septic shock. N Engl J Med 2014;370(15):1412–21.
118. Finfer S, Finfer S, McEvoy S, et al. Impact of albumin compared to saline on organ function and mortality of patients with severe sepsis. Intensive Care Med 2011;37(1):86–96.
119. Rivers E, Nguyen B, Havstad S, et al. Early goal-directed therapy in the treatment of severe sepsis and septic shock. N Engl J Med 2001;345(19):1368–77.
120. Angus DC, Barnato AE, Bell D, et al. A systematic review and meta-analysis of early goal-directed therapy for septic shock: the ARISE, ProCESS and ProMISe Investigators. Intensive Care Med 2015;41(9):1549–60.
121. Asfar P, Meziani F, Hamel JF, et al. High versus low blood-pressure target in patients with septic shock. N Engl J Med 2014;370(17):1583–93.

122. Rhodes A, Evans LE, Alhazzani W, et al. Surviving sepsis campaign: international guidelines for management of sepsis and septic shock: 2016. Intensive Care Med 2017;43:304–77. https://doi.org/10.1007/s00134-017-4683-6.
123. Gordon AC, Mason AJ, Thirunavukkarasu N, et al. Effect of early vasopressin vs norepinephrine on kidney failure in patients with septic shock: the VANISH randomized clinical trial. JAMA 2016;316(5):509–18.
124. Nagendran M, Russell JA, Walley KR, et al. Vasopressin in septic shock: an individual patient data meta-analysis of randomised controlled trials. Intensive Care Med 2019;45(6):844–55.
125. Li JY, Ram G, Gast K, et al. Detection of intracellular iron by its regulatory effect. Am J Physiol Cell Physiol 2004;287(6):C1547–59.
126. Mori K, Lee HT, Rapoport D, et al. Endocytic delivery of lipocalin-siderophore-iron complex rescues the kidney from ischemia-reperfusion injury. J Clin Invest 2005;115(3):610–21.
127. Mårtensson J, Bell M, Oldner A, et al. Neutrophil gelatinase-associated lipocalin in adult septic patients with and without acute kidney injury. Intensive Care Med 2010;36(8):1333–40.
128. Srisawat N, Murugan R, Lee M, et al. Plasma neutrophil gelatinase-associated lipocalin predicts recovery from acute kidney injury following community-acquired pneumonia. Kidney Int 2011;80(5):545–52.
129. Yoshimatsu S, Sugaya T, Hossain MI, et al. Urinary L-FABP as a mortality predictor in <5-year-old children with sepsis in Bangladesh. Pediatr Int 2016;58(3):185–91.

Nephrotoxin Stewardship

Sandra L. Kane-Gill, PharmD, MSc, FCCM, FCCP

KEYWORDS

- Acute kidney injury • Nephrotoxin stewardship • Adverse drug event • Critically ill
- Intensive care unit • Medication error

KEY POINTS

- This article provides a definition and patient care goals for nephrotoxin stewardship.
- Coordinated patient care strategies to ensure medication safety by preventing adverse drug events and promoting kidney health through prevention of drug associated acute kidney injury are discussed.
- Hypervigilance of patients' risk and use of early warning biomarkers are currently the best strategies to the prevention of acute kidney injury, thus applications to drug associated acute kidney injury are reviewed.

INTRODUCTION AND NEPHROTOXIN STEWARDSHIP DEFINITION

The United States has the most critical care beds per capita at 34.7 per 100,000 inhabitants.[1] There were 5256 community hospitals registered with the American Hospital Association in 2015 with approximately 100,000 intensive care unit (ICU) beds including adults and pediatrics.[2] Patients receive a maximum of 17 medications per day and 34 during their ICU stay, and approximately 10 of the medications are considered high risk, presenting a potential for harm if used inappropriately.[3] Critical care clinicians are entrusted with the care of patients in the ICUs. This requires individualized care and broad stewardship. Stewardship according to the Webster dictionary is "the conducting, supervising or managing of something; especially the careful and responsible management of something entrusted to one's care."[4]

The common stewardship activity that is labeled in the hospital and critical care and familiar to most clinicians is antibiotic stewardship. Antibiotic stewardship is "a set of coordinated strategies to improve the use of antimicrobial medications with the goal of enhancing patient health outcomes, reducing resistance to antibiotics, and decreasing unnecessary costs" per the Society of Healthcare Epidemiology of America.[5] Antibiotic stewardship is a priority at many institutions with more than half of the hospitals in the United States reporting infrastructure for a program.[6] Positive

Department of Pharmacy and Therapeutics, School of Pharmacy, Center for Critical Care Nephrology, School of Medicine, University of Pittsburgh, PRESBY/SHY Pharmacy Administration Building, 3507 Victoria Street, Mailcode PFG-01-01-01, Pittsburgh, PA 15213, USA
E-mail address: Kane-Gill@Pitt.edu

Crit Care Clin 37 (2021) 303–320
https://doi.org/10.1016/j.ccc.2020.11.002
0749-0704/21/© 2020 Elsevier Inc. All rights reserved.

criticalcare.theclinics.com

outcomes with antibiotic stewardship include reducing inappropriate antimicrobial use, slowing microbial resistance, and minimizing secondary infections.[7,8]

Some antibiotic stewardship programs have suggested broader targeted outcomes including a reduction in nephrotoxicity,[9] although a stewardship program adding prospective audit and feedback to preauthorization restrictions and therapeutic drug monitoring for vancomycin did not yield a reduction in acute kidney injury (AKI).[10] Another antibiotic stewardship program focused on better vancomycin use with reauthorization restrictions, therapeutic drug monitoring, and monthly education to medical staff indicated that mortality was increased in patients with nephrotoxicity.[11,12] Simply incorporating nephrotoxin surveillance into an antibiotic stewardship program seems like a limited approach to reducing drug-associated AKI (D-AKI) because so many nephrotoxins are not antibiotics.

AKI occurs in up to 22% of hospitalized patients and 65% of critically ill patients.[13,14] Drugs contribute to approximately 30% of AKI cases in hospitalized patients.[15] Drugs commonly associated with AKI include nonsteroidal anti-inflammatories, immunotherapies, and chemotherapeutic agents, in addition to antibiotics.[16] Irrational prescribing of nephrotoxic drugs has contributed to an increase in mortality in critically ill patients.[17] Also, patients with unstable kidney function require medication dosing management for renally cleared drugs because overdosing occurs in up to 67% of patients and underdosing occurs in at least 7.3% of patients.[18,19] There is a need for better medication management in hospitalized patients to prevent D-AKI and harm related to medication errors from inappropriate dosing.

A comprehensive definition of nephrotoxin stewardship is unavailable in the literature and has not been outlined with detailed patient care strategies so this article fills the current gap.[20,21] After careful consideration to the previous definitions for stewardship provided previously, the definition created for *nephrotoxin stewardship* is a set of coordinated patient care management strategies for safe medication use, and ensuring kidney health and avoiding unnecessary costs to improve the use of nephrotoxins, renally eliminated drugs, and kidney disease treatments with the goal of enhancing patient outcomes. Renal dosing is included because of the medication safety concerns, including inappropriate dosing in patients with unstable kidney function, and the need for heightened surveillance to address these preventable medication errors. The goals to enhance patient outcomes through nephrotoxin stewardship are further delineated in the following 3 items:

1. Medication safety is appropriate drug dosing (avoid overdosing or underdosing) and preventing/ameliorating adverse drug events (ADEs).
2. Ensure kidney health by preventing and ameliorating D-AKI, AKI to chronic kidney disease (CKD) transition, or worsening of CKD.
3. Avoid unnecessary costs by choosing tests and treatments wisely and implement coordinated patient care management strategies efficiently so excessive costs are reduced.

Each goal is addressed in detail to provide a plan for coordinated patient care strategies.

GOAL 1: MEDICATION SAFETY

Medication errors occur at any stage during the medication use process, including prescribing, dispensing, administration, and monitoring.[22] Medication errors are preventable. Unfortunately, inappropriate prescribing with overdosing/underdosing of renally eliminated drugs is a common error in patients with kidney disease.[18,19]

Another possible scenario for inappropriate prescribing is drug-drug interactions that can lead to poor clinical outcomes in critically ill patients.[17,23,24] In hospitalized patients, approximately 13% of drug-drug interactions increased the risk for nephrotoxicity, and risk increases in critically ill patients with complex drug regimens.[25] So, a major risk factor for avoidable events in hospitalized patients is kidney insufficiency.[26] These medication errors can lead to patient harm, known as an ADE, from drug accumulation and toxicity or therapeutic failure from underdosing. Critically ill patients with kidney injury are 16 times more likely to have an ADE.[3] Fatality associated with patients hospitalized for ADEs is more common in patients with kidney insufficiency.[27] These medication errors occur due to lack of drug knowledge or lack of monitoring during changing/unstable kidney function. **Table 1** summarizes the coordinated

Table 1		
Goal 1: Coordinated patient care strategies providing actions to enhance medication safety		
Nephrotoxin Stewardship	**Coordinating Patient Care Strategies: Actions Associated with Goals to Enhance Patient Outcomes**	
Safe medication use of nephrotoxins, renally eliminated drugs and kidney disease treatments	*Medication safety (preventing medication errors, ADEs and therapeutic failures)*	*Avoid unnecessary costs*
Renally cleared drug	Standardize a minimum list of renally cleared drugs to target for surveillance and update list at least annually	Automate with accurate and appropriate CDS. Use standardized list for order verification, changes in kidney function, and at discharge
	Recommendations for/or verification of initial and maintenance dose; evaluate functional biomarkers to determine initial and maintenance dose	Automate with accurate and appropriate CDS
	Recheck dosages when kidney function changes (increase or decrease)	Automate with accurate and appropriate CDS
	Recheck maintenance dose at the time of hospital discharge especially in patients with unstable kidney function	Automate with accurate and appropriate CDS (only effective if serum creatinine is checked so protocol for patient care and dedicated clinician at the time of discharge assures appropriate monitoring)
	Appropriate dosing of drugs in patients receiving continuous renal replacement therapy and hemodialysis	Develop institutional drug dosing guidelines for patients receiving dialysis to conserve clinician time in researching appropriate management
	Therapeutic drug monitoring for non-nephrotoxic drugs (eg, digoxin)	Choose appropriate monitoring wisely (eg, time of sample relative to dose; need depending on stability of kidney function)

Abbreviations: ADE, adverse drug event; CDS, clinical decision support.

patient care strategies providing actions associated with goal to enhance medication safety.

Standardized List of Renally Eliminated Drugs

Health care professionals are expected to recall a compendium of drugs that require renal dosage adjustments. This expectation can be even more complex when various drug information sources provide conflicting data.[28] It is this lack of drug knowledge that contributes to excessive dosing in 19% to 67% of drug orders in patients with unstable kidney function.[18] The higher end of this excessive dosing range is more applicable to older patients. Assurance of consistency in patient care calls for standardization. The America Geriatrics Society developed the Beers criteria for potentially inappropriate medication use in older adults and this includes recommendations for medications that require dose adjustments.[29] Hanlon and colleagues[30] used a modified Delphi model to create a standardized list of medications that need to be adjusted in elderly patients. The most recent published, standardized list focused on dosing requirements in primary care practices.[31] Interestingly, all of these standardized lists lack concordance, suggesting that standardization may need to consider specific populations (AKI vs CKD, critically ill vs noncritically ill, children vs adults) and institution specific due to formulary considerations. Most importantly, the list should be reviewed and updated annually because new drugs are continuously available and information on old drugs may become available. The standardized list can be implemented for surveillance of overdosing and underdosing into practice using a manual or automated approach using clinical decision support (CDS) within the electronic health record.

Therapeutic Monitoring of Drugs that Are Renally Cleared or Affected by Kidney Disease

The goal of therapeutic drug monitoring is to provide individualized drug dosing to ensure optimal effectiveness and avoid toxicity or subtherapeutic drug concentrations of drugs with narrow therapeutic ranges or significant pharmacokinetic variability. Critically ill patients receive approximately 2 medications considered to have narrow therapeutic index during their ICU stay.[3] Medications that are cleared by the kidney and require close drug concentration monitoring, especially in patients with unstable kidney function include aminoglycosides, digoxin, lithium, and vancomycin. Digoxin is 1 of 5 drugs that account for 60% of fatal adverse drug reactions that lead to hospitalization, and fatality is more common in patients with kidney failure.[27] Another drug to consider for close therapeutic drug monitoring is phenytoin because of changes in protein binding for critical illness and kidney failure. Computerized advice for drug dosing improves the accuracy of achieving therapeutic drug concentrations.[32]

GOAL 2: KIDNEY HEALTH

Ensuring kidney health is inclusive of many strategies, such as health literacy, patient follow-up after an AKI episode, nutritional considerations, and medication management. Kidney health involving medication management remains a medication safety issue and, in fact, D-AKI is an ADE. In this context, compared with Goal 1, kidney health involves patient care strategies that are centered on prevention and amelioration of D-AKI or preventing CKD progression. This also means optimizing medication management in a patient with AKI who has an ongoing pathophysiologic process, which is known as acute kidney disease (AKD).[33] There is a substantial risk of worsening or developing CKD after an episode of AKI.[34] Nephrotoxin exposure in predialysis patients is common.[35] Following an episode of D-AKI, 70% of patients have residual kidney damage at 6 months.[36]

The concept of medication management for kidney health means performing stewardship tasks that identify potential hazards so that injury can be prevented. This requires surveillance of drug-related hazardous conditions (DRHCs) known as deviations in biochemical, physiologic, or clinical status caused by medications, portending further injury.[37] In addition to DRHCs, this should also consist of risk factor assessment for hazardous conditions before initiating the drug therapy to ensure kidney health. **Table 2** summarizes the coordinated patient care strategies providing actions associated with goals to ensure kidney health.

Standardized List of Nephrotoxins

Again, the expectation for health care professionals to recall the numerous nephrotoxins and to negotiate nephrotoxic potential in each patient is a challenge. Developing a standardized list to target for surveillance ensures consistency and agreement among clinicians. The standardized list should provide consideration to specialized populations including the ICU, where drug use patterns can be different from outside of the ICU. Goswami and colleagues[16] used a structured consensus model to generate a list of 57 nephrotoxins for surveillance intended for a collaborative group of pediatric hospitals. Importantly, the investigators outline a process for developing and updating the standardized list that can be adopted by other institution. A modified illustration of the process is provided in **Fig. 1**. It is important to update the list annually because of the availability of new drugs and new information on old drugs may change the clinician's perspective about nephrotoxicity.[38] Other considerations in prioritizing drugs to include on the list are supporting literature for nephrotoxin potential, severity of nephrotoxicity, affected patient populations, frequency of drug use, and drug cost.[39] The standardized list could be used to surveille duration of exposure and cumulative or total daily dose exposure for acute drugs because these are modifiable drug-specific exposures and when managed appropriately can promote kidney health.[40]

Therapeutic Monitoring of Nephrotoxins

It is known that for drugs such as aminoglycosides, vancomycin and calcineurin inhibitors are associated with nephrotoxicity and monitoring drug concentrations can reduce toxicity.[41–43] A therapeutic drug monitoring (TDM) program with Bayesian forecasting for vancomycin demonstrated the utility of attaining targeted trough concentrations more consistently than no TDM.[44] In addition, there was a reduction in the occurrence of vancomycin-associated nephrotoxicity. A formalized TDM program of nephrotoxins can lead to better patient outcomes.

Although TDM is beneficial, it is important to note that there is still an opportunity to improve estimates of glomerular filtration rate (eGFR) for even more accurate attainment of target drug concentrations. Cystatin C is a functional biomarker that overcomes some of the limitations of serum creatinine because it has less interference from confounders (ie, age, muscle mass).[45] In fact, the $eGFR_{Cr-CysC}$ model better predicted achievement of targeted vancomycin troughs than the $eGFR_{Cr}$ model. Also, consistently cystatin C concentrations and $eGFR_{CysC}$ demonstrated to be as good if not better at predicting elimination of drugs than $eGFR_{Cr}$.[46] In critically ill patients with unstable serum creatinine, eGFR-based creatinine equations are not recommended. Better estimates in this population may occur with the calculation of a kinetic eGFR and result in optimal medication dosing.[47,48]

Another potential advantage to TDM is that aminoglycosides can be used as an estimate of GFR. Aminoglycosides are not secreted or absorbed but are filtered with little

Table 2
Goal 2: coordinated patient care strategies providing actions to ensure kidney health

Nephrotoxin Stewardship	Coordinating Patient Care Strategies: Actions Associated with Goals to Enhance Patient Outcomes	
Safe medication use of nephrotoxins, and kidney disease treatments	*Prevention of AKI/worsening of kidney function*[a]	*Avoid unnecessary costs*
Nephrotoxins	Standardize a minimum list of nephrotoxins to target for surveillance; implement systems for hypervigilance to assess risk with a valid and reliable renal risk assessment tool when a new drug is added[b] *Prevention or worsening*	Automate with accurate and appropriate CDS; use standardized list for alert knowledge
	Evaluate damage biomarkers to determine risk before nephrotoxin administration *Prevention*	Consider if serial monitoring of damage biomarkers is necessary to evoke a clinical decision
	Select evidence-based prevention strategies (eg, hydration for drugs causing crystalluria); use implementation strategies to ensure adoption of prevention strategy *Prevention*	Avoid non–evidence-based approaches that can be costly so efficacy/effectiveness data should guide selection; in addition, economic evaluations will assist with selections
	Therapeutic monitoring of nephrotoxic drugs (eg, calcineurin inhibitors); evaluate functional biomarkers to determine appropriate initial and maintenance drug dosing *Prevention or worsening*	Choose appropriate monitoring wisely (ie, time of sample relative to dose; need depending on stability of kidney function)
	Monitor pharmacokinetic and pharmacodynamic drug-drug interactions specific to the potential for nephrotoxicity	Automate with accurate and appropriate CDS
	Hypervigilance system for nephrotoxin burden assessment with the addition of each new nephrotoxin *Prevention or worsening*	
	Hypervigilance for detection of D-AKI so recommendations for discontinuing, dose adjustment, alternate therapy or alternative therapies occur; use damage and functional biomarkers for surveillance after drug administration *Worsening*	Automate with accurate and appropriate CDS

(continued on next page)

Table 2 (continued)		
Nephrotoxin Stewardship	**Coordinating Patient Care Strategies: Actions Associated with Goals to Enhance Patient Outcomes**	
	Avoid unnecessary nephrotoxins post-AKI (eg, over-the-counter medications such as NSAIDs) Transition of care protocol for patients with *de novo* AKI (especially if at risk for CKD) or CKD at risk for ESRD *Worsening*	Clinician dedicated to patient education and drug monitoring to avoid worsening of kidney function and hospital readmissions; requires close monitoring and coordinated care
	Cautiously start/restart necessary nephrotoxins post-AKI (eg, ACE/ARBs); evaluate risk vs benefit when start/restarting Evaluate functional and damage biomarkers to determine recovery potential *Worsening*	Close monitoring and coordinated care following restarting of nephrotoxin
Kidney Treatments	Select evidence-based treatment strategies for treatment *Worsening*	Avoid non–evidence-based approaches that can be costly, so efficacy/ effectiveness data should guide selection; in addition, economic evaluations will assist with selections

Abbreviations: ACE, angiotensin-converting enzyme; AKI, acute kidney injury; ARB, angiotensin receptor blocker; CDS, clinical decision support; D-AKI, drug-associated acute kidney injury; ESRD, end-stage renal disease; NSAIDs, nonsteroidal anti-inflammatory drugs.

[a] Prevention of AKI could be medication safety because D-AKI is an adverse drug event (ADE) but separated because medication errors and ADEs for the medication safety goal can extend beyond AKI as an ADE.

[b] Hypervigilance of risk when a new drug is added (manual or automated with CDS) includes risk assessment at the time of nephrotoxin initiation (prevention of AKI), includes D-AKI onset (worsening kidney) and new-onset AKI with nephrotoxin ordered (worsening kidney).

nonrenal clearance.[49] In fact, aminoglycoside clearance provides a better estimate of GFR than creatinine-based equations in ICU patients.[50] This may be even more applicable in a patient with a rapidly changing serum creatinine when typical creatinine-based GFR estimates are not useful. So, for kidney health, a decrease in aminoglycoside clearance and increase in drug concentrations may be an early warning marker for AKI. This concept also may be applicable to vancomycin even in non–critically ill patients.[51]

Pharmacokinetic Drug Interactions

The coadministration of 2 drugs that results in the altered absorption, distribution, or elimination of one of the drugs is a pharmacokinetic drug interaction. Critically ill patients receive approximately 1 cytochrome P450 enzyme-inducing drug and 1 cytochrome P450 enzyme-inhibiting drug during their ICU stay.[3] Approximately 60% of critically ill patients experience a potential drug-drug interaction during an admission.[52] Patients have a greater odds of an adverse drug reaction if receiving a drug

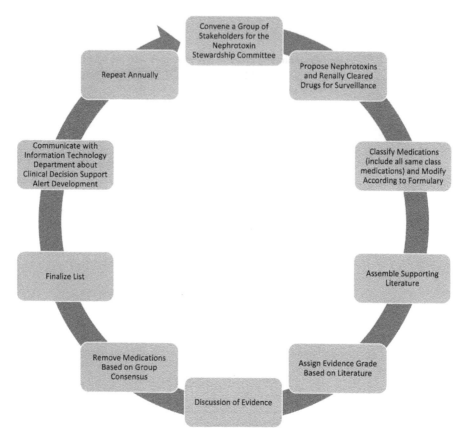

Fig. 1. Process for developing a standardized list of renally cleared drugs and nephrotoxins.

with the potential for an interaction.[3] An example representative of drug combination leading to kidney injury is the combination of clarithromycin with diltiazem. Clarithromycin inhibits the metabolism of diltiazem through the cytochrome P450 isoenzyme 3A4 leading to increased diltiazem concentrations, hypotension, and possibly contributing to ischemic kidney injury.[53] In a large, retrospective cohort study, a statistically significant risk of hospitalization with AKI occurred at 30 days in older patients receiving clarithromycin and amlodipine, felodipine, nifedipine, diltiazem, or verapamil compared with azithromycin (a macrolide that does not inhibit cytochrome P450 isoenzyme 3A4) and a calcium channel blocker. This pharmacokinetic drug interaction leads to the potential of AKI and can be prevented with alternative antibiotic management that does not include clarithromycin for better kidney health. There are other pharmacokinetic drug interactions with some evidence to support a concern for developing AKI, such as simvastatin plus cyclosporin, statins plus macrolides, tacrolimus plus azole antifungals, and cyclosporin plus ciprofloxacin.[23,54]

Pharmacodynamic Drug Interactions

The concomitant administration of 2 or more drugs interact to influence (additive, synergistic, or antagonistic) the body's reaction to the effects from the combination. Nonsteroidal anti-inflammatory drugs (NSAIDs) inhibit prostaglandin synthesis causing vasoconstriction of the afferent arteriole contributing the possibility of developing AKI. Diuretics are associated with AKI because of a decrease in effective blood volume, in particular when other risk factors are present such as dehydration. It is the additive effect of the NSAID and diuretic that can potentiate the occurrence of AKI.[55] This effect is further influenced by the addition of an angiotensin-converting enzyme inhibitor known as the "triple whammy" for the kidney.[56,57] There are other pharmacodynamic interactions to consider such as cisplatin plus aminoglycosides and clindamycin and gentamicin that can add to the possibility of AKI occurring.[23] Monitoring for these interactions and avoidance of pharmacodynamic interactions can avoid the occurrence or reduce the progression of kidney injury.

Nephrotoxin Burden

Building on the idea of pharmacodynamic drug interactions but without regard for specific drug combinations, the additive effect of nephrotoxins can be thought of as the nephrotoxin burden for a patient. Nephrotoxin burden is not previously defined, so the following definition is proposed: *nephrotoxin burden* is the cumulative or aggregate exposure to nephrotoxins, with consideration to nephrotoxin potential for each drug, evaluated at a given time or within a reasonable time frame depending on the half-life of the drug in the body. The duration of drug exposure will contribute to burden on the kidney, hence the need for a cumulative assessment over time.[58] Also, the nephrotoxic potential of the drug will influence the burden and may require a weighting scheme for individual drugs to complete a thorough assessment. For example, acetaminophen is noted as a nephrotoxin in the literature but has low potential, and calcineurin inhibitors have a high potential. Nephrotoxin burden is an important clinical consideration because it will contribute to damaging a patient's kidney health.

Concomitant administration of nephrotoxins is noted as an independent risk factor for predicting AKI occurrence.[59] The risk of AKI increases with the addition of each nephrotoxin (adjusted odds ratio 1.4; 95% confidence interval 1.06–1.85) in pediatric patients and adult patients (odds ratio 1.53; 95% confidence interval 1.09–2.14).[10,60] Using a semiquantitative computation of drug.day burden, the nephrotoxic burden index was associated with the occurrence or worsening of AKI.[58] This index does not weight the degree of nephrotoxicity associated with each drug. Careful selection of nephrotoxins and duration of exposure must be considered along with a risk assessment of non–drug-related factors to reduce the burden and the possibility of AKI occurrence.

Hypervigilance and Early Detection

A formal process for hypervigilance of nephrotoxin burden has been proposed in the form of the Nephrotoxic Injury Negated by Just-in-Time Action (NINJA) program.[61,62] A CDS alert was developed using the following knowledge: (1) greater than or equal to 3 nephrotoxins on the same day; (2) receiving intravenous aminoglycosides for greater than or equal to 3 days; and (3) receiving intravenous vancomycin for greater than or equal to 3 days. The alert was delivered to the pharmacists who notified the patient care team of the nephrotoxin exposure and recommended daily serum creatinine monitoring. After 1 year, NINJA resulted in a 42% reduction in days of AKI per 100 days of nephrotoxin exposure.[61,62] This positive effect of reducing AKI occurrence and severity was sustained after 3 years at a single-center pediatric hospital.[63] When this hypervigilance surveillance program was implemented in 9 sites, the positive impact on patient outcomes was observed with a 24% reduction in AKI prevalence rates and a 37% reduction in AKI rates per exposure.[64]

Stress and Damage Biomarkers for Drug-Associated Acute Kidney Injury

Damage and stress biomarkers such as kidney injury molecule-1 (KIM-1) and N-acetyl-b-D-glucosaminidase (NAG), neutrophil gelatinase-associated lipocalin (NGAL), and tissue inhibitor of metalloproteinase-2 times insulinlike growth factor-binding protein 7 ([TIMP-2]•[IGFBP7]) have predictive value in the early recognition of D-AKI.[65] Urine NGAL effectively identified amphotericin-associated AKI 1.7 to 2.3 days sooner than using the functional biomarker, serum creatinine.[66] Monitoring KIM-1 and NGAL combined provided a better predictive value for vancomycin-associated AKI compared with serum creatine with an area under the receiving operator curve of 0.852 (95% confidence interval 0.754–0.996) versus 0.782 (95% confidence interval 0.582–0.981), respectively.[67] Similar potential was noted for [TIMP-2]•[IGFBP7] as an early predictor of vancomycin-associated AKI.[68] Monitoring damage and stress biomarkers can be used as a way of risk assessment and early detection of AKI to allow for better medication management preventing AKI occurrence and progression.[69] Use of [TIMP-2]•[IGFBP7] in clinical practice in the ICU resulted in 75% of patients having at least 1 component of the Kidney Disease: Improving Global Outcomes (KDIGO) AKI bundle applied for patients at moderate risk for progressing to AKI (ie, [TIMP-2]•[IGFBP7] >0.3). Specifically, avoiding initiation of nephrotoxins was the most common medication management approach, and overall 51% of patients had at least 1 medication management strategy applied. The translation of medication management guided by stress biomarker monitoring on AKI progression is unknown, but use of [TIMP-2]•[IGFBP7] to facilitate KDIGO bundle management has reduced AKI occurrence and intensity.[70,71]

It is possible to use damage and stress biomarkers as hypervigilance tools to facilitate medication management and ensure kidney health.[72] At the University of Florida, a CDS alert was developed for the early identification of sepsis, so after a patient is identified, the pharmacist is expected to order a [TIMP-2]•[IGFBP7] test within 12 hours of the sepsis alert, then make medication adjustments consistent with the risk for AKI progression. At UPMC, alerts were developed similar to the NINJA program but instead of serum creatinine monitoring, a [TIMP-2]•[IGFBP7] test is ordered in the patients at risk for D-AKI (**Fig. 2**). Again, the impact of damage and stress biomarkers in hypervigilance and early detection of D-AKI is uncertain at this point; however, incorporation in clinical practice is ongoing.

Risk Assessment Beyond Drugs

The kidney health stewardship strategies discussed to this point have focused on medication management and assessment of drug-related risk, still a full risk assessment for AKI and D-AKI includes consideration of other susceptibilities and exposures. Per the KDIGO AKI guidelines, susceptibilities include dehydration, advanced age, female gender, black race, CKD, diabetes mellitus, cancer, and anemia.[73] Exposures include sepsis, critical illness, circulatory shock, burns, trauma, cardiac surgery, major noncardiac surgeries, and radiocontrast. For example, a risk prediction score for AKI in the ICU is available that combines chronic comorbidities and acute events.[74] Also incorporating damage biomarkers into the risk assessment, as has been done with the renal angina index, can improve discrimination for severe AKI.[75] These assessment approaches can be made more dynamic with the incorporation of a full array of data from the electronic health record.[76] There are risk assessment tools that aid in identifying patients at risk for AKI that could be considered in the cumulative risk when prescribing nephrotoxins. In other words, nephrotoxin stewardship to ensure kidney health requires a comprehensive patient assessment by a multiprofessional team.

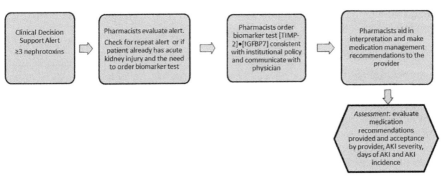

Fig. 2. Surveillance of nephrotoxin burden using a stress biomarker for prevention of D-AKI.

Evidence-Based Prevention Strategies

We need to continue to understand and investigate other prevention strategies for D-AKI. Contrast is often included as a drug-related event. According to a meta-analysis, hemodynamic-guided hydration strategies are effective at preventing contrast-associated AKI and should be considered especially in patients with CKD and cardiac dysfunction.[77] Still, the Prevention of Serious Adverse Events Following Angiography (PRESERVE) trial, a randomized controlled study evaluating prevention strategies for contrast-associated AKI, demonstrated that there was not a clinical benefit with intravenous sodium bicarbonate or intravenous sodium chloride and oral acetylcysteine compared with placebo.[78] Because current prevention strategies for contrast-associated AKI are still uncertain, additional therapies should be evaluated. When evidence becomes available, then implementation in patient care is essential.

Nephrotoxicity occurs in 12% to 48% of patients receiving intravenous acyclovir, especially at high doses.[79] It has low solubility in the urine and can precipitate or crystallize in the renal tubules, leading to obstruction and cellular necrosis. Volume depletion and rapid administration contribute to the occurrence of nephrotoxicity. Nephrotoxicity is reduced with low-dose intravenous and oral acyclovir administration in the presence of euvolemia. Evidence suggests that adequate hydration and slow intravenous infusion are prevention strategies for acyclovir-associated nephrotoxicity that should be implemented in practice.

Similar to standardized lists of nephrotoxins and significant drug interactions, an evidence-based list of prevention strategies should be developed for each institution. This list requires an evaluation and updating process similar to **Fig. 1**. Strategies to ensure evidence-based prevention reaches each patient is an essential component of nephrotoxin stewardship. A regularly scheduled quality assurance assessment of process outcomes and adherence to policy can provide insight into compliance with stewardship practices.

Drug Management During Acute Kidney Disease

The Acute Disease Quality Initiative group recommends continuous medication management throughout the AKD period in all settings (ICU, hospital, and community).[80] Management strategies include adjusting doses of renally cleared drugs, avoiding nephrotoxins, cautiously restarting necessary nephrotoxins, and reaching target treatment goals of chronic medications for diseases such as diabetes and hypertension that contribute to kidney disease.[81] The general thought is that optimizing medication management could prevent progression from AKI to CKD; however, research ensuring improvement in patient outcomes is needed.

Treatment of Acute Kidney Injury

Treatment approaches for AKI have not been successfully developed. The most effective approach has been prevention to reduce nephrotoxin burden and application of the KDIGO bundle to reduce AKI intensity for those patients at risk for AKI.[63,70,71] Many therapies are under investigation for the treatment of AKI according to clinicaltrials.gov (accessed April 2020), such as levosimendan, aminophylline, fenoldopam pirfenidone, pentoxifylline, and various antioxidants. Researchers may have better success at identifying an effective treatment because stress and damage biomarkers are useful in determining who is at risk AKI, so treatment can be initiated early. Previous studies may have lacked success because determining patient candidates in need of treatment was less clear. When a treatment option is available, then stewardship will require that implementation in practice is undertaken as appropriate.

GOAL 3: AVOIDING UNNECESSARY COSTS

Nephrotoxin stewardship must be used in a cost-efficient manner, which is highlighted in **Tables 1** and **2**. First, many of the nephrotoxin stewardship strategies discussed for Goal 1 and Goal 2 can be implemented with the use of automated CDS alerts that will provide resourceful surveillance. For example, alerts for dose adjustments with changing renal function, nephrotoxin burden, drug interactions, and patients at high risk for AKI development require automation for efficiency in management. Alert use in practice does need testing for performance and quality assurance to ensure accurate use and to avoid impending alert fatigue.[82] Second, choosing wisely is a concept introduced by the American Board of Internal Medicine Foundation that supports conversations about avoiding unnecessary medical tests, treatments, and procedures.[83] Choosing wisely is applicable to stewardship when deciding if daily serum creatinine monitoring and serial monitoring of damage biomarkers is necessary to evoke a clinical response. For TDM, recommendations for vancomycin monitoring is needed for patients with a serious methicillin-resistant *Staphylococcus aureus* infection to achieve a targeted area under the curve, patients at high risk for nephrotoxicity, those with unstable kidney function, and those receiving prolonged therapy.[84] Next, once ordering a test is deemed necessary, then it should be done correctly. Approximately 40% vancomycin trough concentrations are obtained too early. An evaluation over 13 months in a 777-bed hospital indicated that there were 2597 vancomycin trough concentrations obtained and 1065 were obtained inappropriately, so using an estimate of $109 for a vancomycin concentration would result in a cost to the institution of $116,085.[85] Last, implementing non–evidence-based practices, such as N-acetylcysteine for prevention of contrast-associated AKI is costly and not beneficial to the patients. These practices can be avoided if surveilling for inappropriate use is completed in this population and education is provided on current and appropriate practices. This same stewardship will be required for kidney treatments when they become available.

Costs can be considered in the overall implementation and evaluation of the nephrotoxin stewardship program. If this comprehensive program were implemented and the improvement in patient care, including outcomes such as AKI incidence, AKI severity, AKI to CKD progression prevention, length of stay, and readmissions, were measured, then the financial impact could be determined. It is important to keep in mind that there is an incremental increase in health care costs as AKI severity increases, even with small changes in serum creatinine.[86] In fact, the incremental increase ranges from \$9400 to \$81,000.[87] It is also noteworthy that these costs are applicable to non-ICU and ICU patients with cost of AKI for an ICU patient being approximately double that of a non-ICU patient. A comprehensive nephrotoxin stewardship program can help contain the financial burden of kidney disease on the national health care system.

SUMMARY

Drugs are estimated to be the third leading cause of AKI in critically ill patients. Clinicians and institutions need to embrace the concept of nephrotoxin stewardship to ensure a structured and consistent approach to the safe use of medications and prevention of patient harm. This is especially important in the ICU where the risk of D-AKI is more substantial. Comprehensive nephrotoxin stewardship requires coordinated patient care management strategies for safe medication use, ensuring kidney health and avoiding unnecessary costs to improve the use of nephrotoxins, renally eliminated drugs, and kidney disease treatments. Implementing a nephrotoxin stewardship program can reduce medication errors and ADEs, prevent D-AKI, reduce D-AKI severity, prevent progression to or worsening of CKD, and alleviate financial burden on the health care system.

CLINICS CARE POINTS

- Drugs are estimated to be the third to fifth leading cause of acute kidney injury in critically ill patients.
- There is a need for better medication management in hospitalized patients to prevent drug associated acute kidney injury and harm related to inappropriate medication prescribing errors in patients with kidney impairment.
- Clinicians and institutions need to embrace the implementation of nephrotoxin stewardship to assure a structured and consistent approach to the safe use of medications and prevention of patient harm.
- As new information about medication dosing in kidney disease, nephrotoxic potential of new and existing medications and pharmacologic treatments for acute kidney disease becomes available then nephrotoxin stewardship efforts should be updated.

DISCLOSURE

The author has nothing to disclose.

REFERENCES

1. McCarthy N. The countries with the most critical care beds per capita. Secondary the countries with the most critical care beds per capita March 12, 2020. Available at: https://www.statista.com/chart/21105/number-of-critical-care-beds-per-100000-inhabitants/. Accessed November 21, 2020.

2. Halpern NA, Tan KS, DeWitt M, et al. Intensivists in U.S. acute care hospitals. Crit Care Med 2019;47(4):517–25.

3. Kane-Gill SL, Kirisci L, Verrico MM, et al. Analysis of risk factors for adverse drug events in critically ill patients*. Crit Care Med 2012;40(3):823–8.

4. Webster's. Secondary. Available at: https://www.merriam-webster.com/dictionary/stewardship. Accessed November 21, 2020.

5. America SoHEo. Secondary. Available at: https://www.shea-online.org/index.php/practice-resources/priority-topics/antimicrobial-stewardship. Accessed November 21, 2020.

6. Pollack LA, van Santen KL, Weiner LM, et al. Antibiotic stewardship programs in U.S. acute care hospitals: findings from the 2014 national healthcare safety network annual hospital survey. Clin Infect Dis 2016;63(4):443–9.

7. Barlam TF, Cosgrove SE, Abbo LM, et al. Implementing an antibiotic stewardship program: guidelines by the infectious diseases society of America and the society for healthcare Epidemiology of America. Clin Infect Dis 2016;62(10):e51–77.

8. Akpan MR, Ahmad R, Shebl NA, et al. A review of quality measures for assessing the impact of antimicrobial stewardship programs in hospitals. Antibiotics (Basel) 2016;5(1). https://doi.org/10.3390/antibiotics5010005.

9. Karino S, Kaye KS, Navalkele B, et al. Epidemiology of acute kidney injury among patients receiving concomitant vancomycin and piperacillin-tazobactam: opportunities for antimicrobial stewardship. Antimicrob Agents Chemother 2016;60(6):3743–50.

10. Hsu AJ, Tamma PD. Impact of an antibiotic stewardship program on the incidence of vancomycin-associated acute kidney injury in hospitalized children. J Pediatr Pharmacol Ther 2019;24(5):416–20.

11. Fodero KE, Horey AL, Krajewski MP, et al. Impact of an antimicrobial stewardship program on patient safety in veterans prescribed vancomycin. Clin Ther 2016;38(3):494–502.

12. Conway EL, Sellick JA, Horey A, et al. Decreased mortality in patients prescribed vancomycin after implementation of antimicrobial stewardship program. Am J Infect Control 2017;45(11):1194–7.

13. Susantitaphong P, Cruz DN, Cerda J, et al. World incidence of AKI: a meta-analysis. Clin J Am Soc Nephrol 2013;8(9):1482–93.

14. Hoste EA, Bagshaw SM, Bellomo R, et al. Epidemiology of acute kidney injury in critically ill patients: the multinational AKI-EPI study. Intensive Care Med 2015;41(8):1411–23.

15. Mehta RL, Awdishu L, Davenport A, et al. Phenotype standardization for drug-induced kidney disease. Kidney Int 2015;88(2):226–34.

16. Goswami E, Ogden RK, Bennett WE, et al. Evidence-based development of a nephrotoxic medication list to screen for acute kidney injury risk in hospitalized children. Am J Health Syst Pharm 2019;76(22):1869–74.

17. Ali M, Naureen H, Tariq MH, et al. Rational use of antibiotics in an intensive care unit: a retrospective study of the impact on clinical outcomes and mortality rate. Infect Drug Resist 2019;12:493–9.

18. Long CL, Raebel MA, Price DW, et al. Compliance with dosing guidelines in patients with chronic kidney disease. Ann Pharmacother 2004;38(5):853–8.

19. Cox ZL, McCoy AB, Matheny ME, et al. Adverse drug events during AKI and its recovery. Clin J Am Soc Nephrol 2013;8(7):1070–8.

20. Barreto EF, Mueller BA, Kane-Gill SL, et al. Beta-lactams: The competing priorities of nephrotoxicity, neurotoxicity and stewardship. Ann Pharmacother 2018;52:1167–8.

21. Kashani K, Rosner MH, Haase M, et al. Quality improvement goals for acute kidney injury. Clin J Am Soc Nephrol 2019;14:941–53.

22. Kane-Gill SL, Dasta JF, Buckley MS, et al. Clinical practice guideline: safe medication use in the icu. Crit Care Med 2017;45(9):e877–915.

23. Rivosecchi RM, Kellum JA, Dasta JF, et al. Drug class combination-associated acute kidney injury. Ann Pharmacother 2016;50(11):953–72.

24. Kovacevic M, Vezmar Kovacevic S, Miljkovic B, et al. The prevalence and preventability of potentially relevant drug-drug interactions in patients admitted for cardiovascular diseases: a cross-sectional study. Int J Clin Pract 2017;71(10). https://doi.org/10.1111/ijcp.13005.

25. Zwart-van Rijkom JE, Uijtendaal EV, ten Berg MJ, et al. Frequency and nature of drug-drug interactions in a Dutch university hospital. Br J Clin Pharmacol 2009; 68(2):187–93. https://doi.org/10.1111/j.1365-2125.2009.03443.x.

26. Cabre M, Elias L, Garcia M, et al. Avoidable hospitalizations due to adverse drug reactions in an acute geriatric unit. Analysis of 3,292 patients. Med Clin (Barc) 2018;150(6):209–14. https://doi.org/10.1016/j.medcli.2017.06.075.

27. Patel TK, Patel PB. Mortality among patients due to adverse drug reactions that lead to hospitalization: a meta-analysis. Eur J Clin Pharmacol 2018;74(6):819–32. https://doi.org/10.1007/s00228-018-2441-5.

28. O'Shaughnessy M, Allen N, O'Regan J, et al. Agreement between renal prescribing references and determination of prescribing appropriateness in hospitalized patients with chronic kidney disease. QJM 2017;110(10):623–8.

29. By the American Geriatrics Society Beers Criteria Update Expert Panel. American Geriatrics Society 2015 updated Beers criteria for potentially inappropriate medication use in older adults. J Am Geriatr Soc 2015;63(11):2227–46.

30. Hanlon JT, Aspinall SL, Semla TP, et al. Consensus guidelines for oral dosing of primarily renally cleared medications in older adults. J Am Geriatr Soc 2009; 57(2):335–40.

31. Taji L, Battistella M, Grill AK, et al. Medications used routinely in primary care to be dose-adjusted or avoided in people with chronic kidney disease: results of a modified Delphi study. Ann Pharmacother 2020. https://doi.org/10.1177/1060028019897371. 1060028019897371.

32. Asberg A, Falck P, Undset LH, et al. Computer-assisted cyclosporine dosing performs better than traditional dosing in renal transplant recipients: results of a pilot study. Ther Drug Monit 2010;32(2):152–8.

33. Chawla LS, Bellomo R, Bihorac A, et al. Acute kidney disease and renal recovery: consensus report of the Acute Disease Quality Initiative (ADQI) 16 Workgroup. Nat Rev Nephrol 2017;13(4):241–57.

34. Coca SG, Singanamala S, Parikh CR. Chronic kidney disease after acute kidney injury: a systematic review and meta-analysis. Kidney Int 2012;81(5):442–8.

35. Davis-Ajami ML, Fink JC, Wu J. Nephrotoxic medication exposure in U.S. adults with predialysis chronic kidney disease: health services utilization and cost outcomes. J Manag Care Spec Pharm 2016;22(8):959–68.

36. Menon S, Kirkendall ES, Nguyen H, et al. Acute kidney injury associated with high nephrotoxic medication exposure leads to chronic kidney disease after 6 months. J Pediatr 2014;165(3):522–7.e2.

37. Kane-Gill SL, Dasta JF, Schneider PJ, et al. Monitoring abnormal laboratory values as antecedents to drug-induced injury. J Trauma 2005;59(6):1457–62.

38. Welch HK, Kellum JA, Kane-Gill SL. Drug-associated acute kidney injury identified in the United States Food and Drug Administration adverse event reporting system database. Pharmacotherapy 2018;38(8):785–93.

39. Kane-Gill S, Rea RS, Verrico MM, et al. Adverse-drug-event rates for high-cost and high-use drugs in the intensive care unit. Am J Health Syst Pharm 2006; 63(19):1876–81.

40. Kane-Gill SL, Goldstein SL. Drug-induced acute kidney injury: a focus on risk assessment for prevention. Crit Care Clin 2015;31(4):675–84.

41. Venkataramanan R, Shaw LM, Sarkozi L, et al. Clinical utility of monitoring tacrolimus blood concentrations in liver transplant patients. J Clin Pharmacol 2001; 41(5):542–51.

42. Hedayat S, Kershner RP, Su G. Relationship of whole-blood FK506 concentrations to rejection and toxicity in liver and kidney transplants. J Biopharm Stat 1996;6(4):411–24.

43. Ye ZK, Tang HL, Zhai SD. Benefits of therapeutic drug monitoring of vancomycin: a systematic review and meta-analysis. PLoS One 2013;8(10):e77169.

44. Zhang Y, Wang T, Zhang D, et al. Therapeutic drug monitoring coupled with bayesian forecasting could prevent vancomycin-associated nephrotoxicity in renal insufficiency patients: a prospective study and pharmacoeconomic analysis. Ther Drug Monit 2020. https://doi.org/10.1097/FTD.0000000000000750.

45. Frazee EN, Rule AD, Herrmann SM, et al. Serum cystatin C predicts vancomycin trough levels better than serum creatinine in hospitalized patients: a cohort study. Crit Care 2014;18(3):R110.

46. Barreto EF, Rule AD, Murad MH, et al. Prediction of the renal elimination of drugs with cystatin C vs creatinine: a systematic review. Mayo Clin Proc 2019;94(3): 500–14.

47. Kwong YD, Chen S, Bouajram R, et al. The value of kinetic glomerular filtration rate estimation on medication dosing in acute kidney injury. PLoS One 2019; 14(11):e0225601.

48. Bairy M. Using kinetic eGFR for drug dosing in AKI: concordance between kinetic eGFR, Cockroft-Gault estimated creatinine clearance, and MDRD eGFR for drug dosing categories in a pilot study cohort. Nephron 2020;144(6):299–303.

49. Sunder S, Jayaraman R, Mahapatra HS, et al. Estimation of renal function in the intensive care unit: the covert concepts brought to light. J Intensive Care 2014; 2(1):31.

50. Jones TE, Peter JV, Field J. Aminoglycoside clearance is a good estimate of creatinine clearance in intensive care unit patients. Anaesth Intensive Care 2009;37(6):944–52.

51. Zamoner W, Goncalves Pierri I, Zanchetta Cardoso Eid K, et al. Serum concentration of vancomycin is a diagnostic predictor of nephrotoxic acute kidney injury in septic patients in clinical and surgical wards. Infect Drug Resist 2020;13: 403–11.

52. Fitzmaurice MG, Wong A, Akerberg H, et al. Evaluation of potential drug-drug interactions in adults in the intensive care unit: a systematic review and meta-analysis. Drug Saf 2019;42(9):1035–44.

53. Gandhi S, Fleet JL, Bailey DG, et al. Calcium-channel blocker-clarithromycin drug interactions and acute kidney injury. JAMA 2013;310(23):2544–53.

54. Bentata Y. Tacrolimus: 20 years of use in adult kidney transplantation. What we should know about its nephrotoxicity. Artif Organs 2020;44(2):140–52.

55. Liu GJ, Wang YF, Zeng YJ, et al. The combined use of edaravone, diuretics, and nonsteroidal anti-inflammatory drugs caused acute kidney injury in an elderly patient with chronic kidney disease. CEN Case Rep 2012;1(2):96–103.

56. Thomas MC. Diuretics, ACE inhibitors and NSAIDs–the triple whammy. Med J Aust 2000;172(4):184–5.

57. Lapi F, Azoulay L, Yin H, et al. Concurrent use of diuretics, angiotensin converting enzyme inhibitors, and angiotensin receptor blockers with non-steroidal anti-

inflammatory drugs and risk of acute kidney injury: nested case-control study. BMJ 2013;346:e8525.

58. Ehrmann S, Helms J, Joret A, et al. Nephrotoxic drug burden among 1001 critically ill patients: impact on acute kidney injury. Ann Intensive Care 2019;9(1):106.

59. Cotner SE, Rutter WC, Burgess DR, et al. Influence of beta-Lactam infusion strategy on acute kidney injury. Antimicrob Agents Chemother 2017;61(10). https://doi.org/10.1128/AAC.00871-17.

60. Cartin-Ceba R, Kashiouris M, Plataki M, et al. Risk factors for development of acute kidney injury in critically ill patients: a systematic review and meta-analysis of observational studies. Crit Care Res Pract 2012;2012:691013.

61. Goldstein SL, Kirkendall E, Nguyen H, et al. Electronic health record identification of nephrotoxin exposure and associated acute kidney injury. Pediatrics 2013;132(3):e756–67.

62. Kirkendall ES, Spires WL, Mottes TA, et al. Development and performance of electronic acute kidney injury triggers to identify pediatric patients at risk for nephrotoxic medication-associated harm. Appl Clin Inform 2014;5(2):313–33.

63. Goldstein SL, Mottes T, Simpson K, et al. A sustained quality improvement program reduces nephrotoxic medication-associated acute kidney injury. Kidney Int 2016;90(1):212–21.

64. Goldstein SL, Dahale D, Kirkendall ES, et al. A prospective multi-center quality improvement initiative (NINJA) indicates a reduction in nephrotoxic acute kidney injury in hospitalized children. Kidney Int 2020;97(3):580–8.

65. Kane-Gill SL, Smithburger PL, Kashani K, et al. Clinical relevance and predictive value of damage biomarkers of drug-induced kidney injury. Drug Saf 2017;40(11):1049–74.

66. Rocha PN, Macedo MN, Kobayashi CD, et al. Role of urine neutrophil gelatinase-associated lipocalin in the early diagnosis of amphotericin B-induced acute kidney injury. Antimicrob Agents Chemother 2015;59(11):6913–21.

67. Pang HM, Qin XL, Liu TT, et al. Urinary kidney injury molecule-1 and neutrophil gelatinase-associated lipocalin as early biomarkers for predicting vancomycin-associated acute kidney injury: a prospective study. Eur Rev Med Pharmacol Sci 2017;21(18):4203–13.

68. Ostermann M, McCullough PA, Forni LG, et al. Kinetics of urinary cell cycle arrest markers for acute kidney injury following exposure to potential renal insults. Crit Care Med 2018;46(3):375–83.

69. Kane-Gill SL, Peerapornratana S, Wong A, et al. Use of tissue inhibitor of metalloproteinase 2 and insulin-like growth factor binding protein 7 [TIMP2]*[IGFBP7] as an AKI risk screening tool to manage patients in the real-world setting. J Crit Care 2020;57:97–101.

70. Meersch M, Schmidt C, Hoffmeier A, et al. Prevention of cardiac surgery-associated AKI by implementing the KDIGO guidelines in high risk patients identified by biomarkers: the PrevAKI randomized controlled trial. Intensive Care Med 2017;43(11):1551–61.

71. Gocze I, Jauch D, Gotz M, et al. Biomarker-guided intervention to prevent acute kidney injury after major surgery: the prospective randomized BigpAK Study. Ann Surg 2018;267(6):1013–20.

72. Barreto EF, Rule AD, Voils SA, et al. Innovative use of novel biomarkers to improve the safety of renally eliminated and nephrotoxic medications. Pharmacotherapy 2018;38(8):794–803.

73. Kellum JA, Lameire N, Group KAGW. Diagnosis, evaluation, and management of acute kidney injury: a KDIGO summary (Part 1). Crit Care 2013;17(1):204.

74. Malhotra R, Kashani KB, Macedo E, et al. A risk prediction score for acute kidney injury in the intensive care unit. Nephrol Dial Transplant 2017;32(5):814–22.

75. Basu RK, Wang Y, Wong HR, et al. Incorporation of biomarkers with the renal angina index for prediction of severe AKI in critically ill children. Clin J Am Soc Nephrol 2014;9(4):654–62.

76. Sutherland SM, Chawla LS, Kane-Gill SL, et al. Utilizing electronic health records to predict acute kidney injury risk and outcomes: workgroup statements from the 15(th) ADQI Consensus Conference. Can J Kidney Health Dis 2016;3:11.

77. Cai Q, Jing R, Zhang W, et al. Hydration strategies for preventing contrast-induced acute kidney injury: a systematic review and bayesian network meta-analysis. J Interv Cardiol 2020;2020:7292675.

78. Garcia S, Bhatt DL, Gallagher M, et al. Strategies to reduce acute kidney injury and improve clinical outcomes following percutaneous coronary intervention: a subgroup analysis of the PRESERVE Trial. JACC Cardiovasc Interv 2018; 11(22):2254–61.

79. Izzedine H, Launay-Vacher V, Deray G. Antiviral drug-induced nephrotoxicity. Am J Kidney Dis 2005;45(5):804–17.

80. Ostermann M, Chawla LS, Forni LG, et al. Drug management in acute kidney disease - report of the acute disease quality initiative XVI meeting. Br J Clin Pharmacol 2018;84(2):396–403.

81. Kane-Gill SL, Bauer SR. AKD-the time between AKI and CKD: what is the role of the pharmacist? Hosp Pharm 2017;52(10):663–5.

82. Kane-Gill SL, O'Connor MF, Rothschild JM, et al. Technologic distractions (Part 1): summary of approaches to manage alert quantity with intent to reduce alert fatigue and suggestions for alert fatigue metrics. Crit Care Med 2017;45(9): 1481–8.

83. Cassel CK, Guest JA. Choosing wisely: helping physicians and patients make smart decisions about their care. JAMA 2012;307(17):1801–2.

84. Rybak MJ, Le J, Lodise TP, et al. Therapeutic monitoring of vancomycin for serious methicillin-resistant *Staphylococcus aureus* infections: a revised consensus guideline and review by the American Society of Health-System Pharmacists, the Infectious Diseases Society of America, the Pediatric Infectious Diseases Society, and the Society of Infectious Diseases Pharmacists. Am J Health Syst Pharm 2020. https://doi.org/10.1093/ajhp/zxaa036.

85. Morrison AP, Melanson SE, Carty MG, et al. What proportion of vancomycin trough levels are drawn too early? Frequency and impact on clinical actions. Am J Clin Pathol 2012;137(3):472–8.

86. Collister D, Pannu N, Ye F, et al. Health care costs associated with AKI. Clin J Am Soc Nephrol 2017;12(11):1733–43.

87. Dasta JF, Kane-Gill S. Review of the literature on the costs associated with acute kidney injury. J Pharm Pract 2019;32(3):292–302.

Hepatorenal Syndrome

Saro Khemichian, MD[a], Claire Francoz, MD, PhD[b],
Francois Durand, MD[c], Constantine J. Karvellas, MD, SM, FRCPC[d],
Mitra K. Nadim, MD[e],*

KEYWORDS

- Acute on chronic liver failure • Acute kidney injury • Cirrhosis
- Hepatorenal syndrome • Biomarkers • Liver transplantation
- Simultaneous liver kidney transplantation • Model end-stage liver disease

KEY POINTS

- Assessment and evaluation of renal function and identifying cause of acute kidney injury (AKI) remain difficult in patients with liver cirrhosis.
- Various novel biomarkers have been developed that may be helpful in the diagnosis of AKI in patients with chronic liver disease and liver cirrhosis.
- Vasoconstrictor therapies, such as noradrenalin and terlipressin, along with albumin remain the main treatment for hepatorenal syndrome-AKI.
- Most recent Organ Procurement and Transplantation Network/United Network for Organ Sharing criteria for consideration of simultaneous liver and kidney transplantation have streamlined the decision-making process.
- Development of post–liver transplant AKI is multifactorial, relating to the recipient's pre-transplant course, the donor, surgical events, and the use of immunosuppression.

INTRODUCTION

Acute kidney injury (AKI) is a frequent complication of end-stage liver disease and occurs in as high as 50% of shospitalized patients.[1] The development of AKI impacts short- and long-term mortality and reduces kidney function following liver transplantation (LT).[2,3] Circulatory changes observed in end-stage cirrhosis, namely, hyperkinetic state, with renal vasoconstriction leading to decreased kidney blood flow are central in

[a] Division of Gastroenterology/Liver, Keck School of Medicine, University of Southern California, 1510 San Pablo Street, Los Angeles, CA 90033, USA; [b] Hepatology and Liver Intensive Care, Hospital Beaujon, 100 Boulevard Du General Leclerc, Clichy 92110, France; [c] Hepatology and Liver Intensive Care, Hospital Beaujon, University of Paris, 100 Boulevard Du General Leclerc, Clichy 92110, France; [d] Division of Gastroenterology (Liver Unit), Department of Critical Care Medicine, University of Alberta, 1-40 Zeidler Ledcor Building, Edmonton, Alberta T6G 2X8, Canada; [e] Division of Nephrology and Hypertension, Keck School of Medicine, University of Southern California, 1520 San Pablo Street, Suite 4300, Los Angeles, CA 90033, USA
* Corresponding author.
E-mail address: mitra.nadim@med.usc.edu

Crit Care Clin 37 (2021) 321–334
https://doi.org/10.1016/j.ccc.2020.11.011
0749-0704/21/© 2020 Elsevier Inc. All rights reserved.

the development of AKI.[4] Traditional diagnostic criteria focused on these changes, along with an increase in serum creatinine (sCr) >50% over baseline with value greater than 1.5 mg/dL as diagnostic for hepatorenal syndrome (HRS). Other studies, however, have shown that these criteria may be too narrow[5] and certainly may not encompass the spectrum of kidney injury in patients with end-stage liver disease. There are also no specific urine biomarkers that can reliably identify the cause of AKI in these patients.

ASSESSMENT OF KIDNEY FUNCTION IN CIRRHOSIS

Assessment of kidney function in patients with cirrhosis remains a challenging issue. Although sCr is the most commonly used clinical index of kidney function, it overestimates glomerular filtration rate (GFR) in patients with advanced cirrhosis because of the combination of decreased creatine production by the liver, muscle wasting, and large volume of distribution in the setting of fluid overload. In patients with AKI, sCr can lag by days despite a significant decrease in GFR especially in patients with fluid overload.[6,7] In addition, in patients with high serum bilirubin, sCr can be inaccurate if colorimetric-based Jaffe assays are used, as bilirubin interferes with the color reaction. There is no evidence that other serum markers of kidney function, such as cystatin C, are superior to sCr in patients with cirrhosis even though cystatin C is less influenced by confounding factors, such as age and muscle mass.[8]

The clearance of exogenous markers, such as radiocontrast media, inulin, or radioisotopes, is considered the gold standard for GFR assessment; however, they are not routinely used in clinical practice, because of cost, convenience, and availability, and have not been rigorously studied in patients with advanced cirrhosis and ascites. When properly performed, timed urinary collection of creatinine and urea overcomes some of these limitations. These limitations are, however, subject to errors because of inaccurate or incomplete collection and because of increased tubular secretion of creatinine as GFR declines.[9,10]

Estimation of GFR using mathematical equations based on sCr and/or cystatin-C is a simple method in the general population with stable sCr; however, in patients with cirrhosis, the precision of all estimated GFR (eGFR) equations is poor and tends to overestimate true GFR, especially in patients with GFR <40 mL/min and should be used with caution. The Modified Diet in Renal Disease-6 (MDRD-6) equation has been shown to be the most accurate creatinine-based equation in cirrhosis.[11] Equations based on cystatin C, with or without sCr (ie, Chronic Kidney Disease Epidemiology Collaboration creatinine-cystatin C equation), may be superior to creatinine-based equations.[12,13] More recently, in a single-center study of more than 10,000 iothalamate samples, GRAIL equation (Glomerular filtration rate in liver disease; http://www.bswh.md/grail) demonstrated more precision and less bias compared with MDRD-6 equation in patients with low GFR and correctly classified 75% of the cohort as having a measured GFR <30 mL/min/1.73 m^2 versus 52.8% in MDRD-6 (P<.01).[14,15]

DEFINITIONS

Historically, AKI in cirrhosis was defined by a fixed value of sCr >1.5 mg/dL (133 μmol/L).[16] However, this definition had limitations because patients with advanced cirrhosis and sCr values within the normal range may have a significant decrease in GFR because of reduced muscle mass and decreased creatine production.[11] In 2010, the Acute Disease Quality Initiative (ADQI) proposed a novel classification system of AKI in cirrhosis based on sCr changes and qualifying type 1 HRS as only one of the possible causes of AKI in end-stage liver disease.[17] In 2015, the International Club of Ascites (ICA) proposed revised definitions of AKI in cirrhosis based on the Kidney Disease Improving Global Outcomes Guidelines (KDIGO) (**Table 1**).[18] In line with the KDIGO criteria, AKI is defined by a change in sCr only and categorized into 3 stages of increasing severity. Baseline sCr is defined by a value of sCr obtained in the previous 3 months when available. Type 1 HRS is now considered one of the different phenotypes of AKI in cirrhosis termed AKI-HRS (see **Table 1**).[18] The prognostic relevance of these new definitions has been validated in several studies.[1,19]

Although oliguria was not included in the current definition of AKI in patients with liver disease, urine output (UO) has been found to be a sensitive and early marker for AKI and to be associated with adverse outcomes with more than 50% increase (14.6% vs 9%; $P<.001$) in mortality among critically ill patients with chronic liver disease and stage 1 AKI when defined by oliguria instead of sCr alone.[20] Furthermore, 61% of stage 2 to 3 AKI patients classified by oliguria were misclassified as non-AKI or stage 1 AKI based on sCr criteria. An international consensus meeting on management of critically ill cirrhotic patients has recommended that regardless of any increase in sCr, worsening oliguria or development of anuria should be considered AKI in patients with cirrhosis until proven otherwise.[21]

Recently, a group of experts proposed further changes in the definitions of HRS and other phenotypes of AKI in cirrhosis.[22] According to these changes, UO was reintroduced as one of the criteria defining HRS-AKI (UO $\leq$0.5 mL/kg for $\geq$6 hours). Type 2 HRS, which is a more chronic presentation of HRS, is termed HRS-NAKI (for non-AKI) and defined by eGFR $\leq$60 mL/min/1.73 m^2 for more than 3 months with initial fulfillment of ICA criteria for the diagnosis of HRS-AKI.[18,22,23] Whether these changes help better categorize cirrhotic patients with AKI or chronic kidney disease (CKD) needs further validation.

A major limitation of the HRS criteria is that they do not allow for the coexistence of other forms of acute or CKD, such as underlying diabetic nephropathy or other

Table 1
International club of ascites definition of acute kidney injury and hepatorenal syndrome in cirrhosis

Purpose	Definition
Definition of AKI	• Increase in sCr $\geq$0.3 mg/dL (26 μmol/L) within 48 h, or • A percentage increase in sCr $\geq$50% from baseline, which is known or presumed to have occurred within the previous 7 d
Staging of AKI	• Stage 1: increase in sCr $\geq$0.3 mg/dL (26 μmol/L) or increase in sCr $\geq$1.5 to 2-fold from baseline • Stage 2: increase in sCr >2- to 3-fold from baseline • Stage 3: increase in sCr >3-fold from baseline or sCr >4 mg/dL (353 μmol/L) with an acute increase $\geq$0.3 mg/dL (26 μmol/L) or initiation of renal replacement therapy
AKI-HRS	• AKI $\geq$ stage 2 • No improvement in sCr after $\geq$48 h of diuretic withdrawal and volume expansion with albumin at a dose of 1 g/kg up to a maximum of 100 g daily • Absence of hypovolemic shock or infection requiring vasoactive drugs to support blood pressure • No current or recent use of nephrotoxic drugs • Proteinuria <500 mg/d and hematuria <50 red blood cells per high-power field

glomerular diseases often associated with patients with liver disease (eg, immuno-globulin A, membranous or membranoproliferative disease). However, patients with underlying kidney disease can still develop "hepatorenal physiology." As a result, ADQI proposed that the term "hepatorenal disorders" be used to describe all patients with advanced cirrhosis and concurrent kidney dysfunction.[17] Such a definition would allow patients with cirrhosis and renal dysfunction to be properly classified and treated while maintaining the term HRS.

PATHOPHYSIOLOGY
Splanchnic and Systemic Circulatory Changes

Portal hypertension and splanchnic vasodilatation are characteristic features of cirrhosis that play a central role in HRS-AKI (**Fig. 1**).[4,24,25] In early stages of cirrhosis (compensated cirrhosis), mild reduction in arterial blood pressure is compensated for by an increase in cardiac output (CO) that preserves kidney perfusion. As portal hypertension increases and liver function deteriorates, systemic circulatory changes are more pronounced with a further decrease in systemic vascular resistance (SVR) and increase in CO. Splanchnic arterial vasodilatation increases as a result of increased synthesis of nitric oxide and other vasodilatory mediators. The state of central hypovolemia results in activation of systemic vasoconstrictors, including the renin angiotensin aldosterone system, the sympathetic system, and release of arginine vasopressin (AVP), which all contribute to maintain arterial pressure and kidney perfusion.[24] Although activation of RASS with elevated plasma renin activity and increased circulating levels of norepinephrine has a positive impact on arterial pressure, this response has a negative impact with retention of sodium and water, resulting in ascites, edema, and impaired free water excretion. Intense renal vasoconstriction also results in decreased kidney perfusion and decreased GFR, a central mechanism of HRS-AKI.[26] In recent years, it has been suggested that impaired cardiac function could also be one of the mechanisms leading to HRS-AKI.[27] Evidence suggests that cardiac work decreases in the most advanced stages of cirrhosis and that impaired cardiac work is more pronounced in patients receiving β-blockers.[28]

Kidney Factors

The main renal prostaglandins (prostaglandin I2 and prostaglandin E2) have vasodilator effects in the kidney and are increased in patients with cirrhosis and ascites.[29]

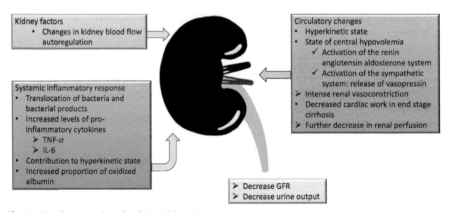

Fig. 1. Mechanisms involved in HRS-AKI.

Changes in renal blood flow autoregulation also exist in cirrhosis with a shift in the autoregulation curve, at least in part related to the activation of the sympathetic nervous system. As a result, for a given level of kidney perfusion pressure, kidney perfusion is lower in patients with cirrhosis as compared with patients without cirrhosis.

Systemic Inflammatory Response

There is now general agreement that cirrhosis is characterized by systemic inflammatory state and that inflammation contributes to complications, such as HRS-AKI. Even in the absence of documented infection, patients with cirrhosis have increased circulating levels of C-reactive proteins and proinflammatory cytokines, and this increase is correlated with disease severity, portal pressure, and hyperkinetic syndrome.[30] Bacterial translocation is one of the mechanisms involved in chronic systemic inflammatory response. Patients with bacterial translocation from gut lumen to mesenteric lymph nodes were shown to have increased levels of proinflammatory cytokines (tumor necrosis factor-α [TNF-α] and interleukin-6 [IL-6]), and vasoactive factors, including NO, in the splanchnic area.[31] In patients with spontaneous bacterial peritonitis (SBP) and HRS-AKI, TNF-α and IL-6 levels in ascitic fluid and blood are significantly higher than in patients with SBP and no HRS-AKI. This increased cytokine level is associated with increased NO levels also.[32] These findings suggest that systemic inflammatory response may trigger HRS-AKI by worsening circulatory dysfunction and further decreasing kidney perfusion.

CAUSE OF KIDNEY DYSFUNCTION

The most common causes of AKI in hospitalized patients are prerenal azotemia (most due to hypovolemia-induced AKI and only one-third due to HRS), followed by ATN. The cause of AKI should be determined promptly in order to prevent further worsening of AKI as progression to advanced stage AKI has been associated with a higher mortality. The cause of AKI is generally distinguished by the preceding history as well as urinalysis and response to diuretic withdrawal and volume challenge. However, these criteria may be misleading in certain circumstances, such as presence of CKD or recent diuretic use. Prompt diagnosis and identification of AKI phenotype in patients with cirrhosis allow for appropriate and timely intervention, whereby progression of AKI stage confers increasing mortality, particularly with HRS.[33] Given that sCr often lags in highlighting the timing and severity of renal injury, several urine biomarkers in addition to urine microalbuminuria or fractional excretion of sodium have been evaluated to allow earlier diagnosis and identification of the cause of AKI (ie, HRS vs ATN). This can potentially help identify patients who are less likely to benefit from volume resuscitation and vasopressor therapy.[34-36]

Urinary NGAL has emerged as the most sensitive marker to detect ATN or persistent AKI.[36] However, even though urinary NGAL level is higher in ATN when compared with HRS and other causes of AKI, there is a significant overlap between the groups.[34,36-38] Accurate biomarkers of underlying CKD are still lacking, and kidney biopsy is often contraindicated in this population. In most studies, the diagnosis of ATN was based on nonspecific criteria without a gold standard (biopsy) and therefore should be interpreted with caution.

PREVENTION AND TREATMENT OF HEPATORENAL SYNDROME

It is important to identify and remove potential precipitating agents in the development of AKI/HRS and to prevent factors that further impair circulatory status and reduce renal perfusion. It is also important to monitor the volume status closely in cirrhotic patients and to avoid hypovolemia. Early administration of broad-spectrum antibiotics should be prompt upon diagnosis of any infection. The patient's medication lists need to be carefully monitored daily. Long-term administration of albumin in patients with decompensated cirrhosis has been shown in a large randomized control trial to be associated with reduced rates of SBP, bacterial infections other than SBP, HRS, and improved survival.[39]

Volume expansion is not only important in the treatment of AKI but also in the differential diagnosis of cause of AKI. The type of fluid needed for resuscitation should be tailored based on the cause of AKI and volume status of the patient. It is imperative to exercise caution when administrating fluids in patients with AKI to avoid development of fluid overload and pulmonary edema. Diuretics should be discontinued, and any potentially nephrotoxic drug should also be stopped, whenever possible. Several treatments and therapies have been demonstrated to be beneficial for HRS, whereas LT remains the only definitive treatment. Other treatments have evolved to try to reverse some of the pathophysiological conditions that were described earlier. These are described in later discussion.

Albumin

Infusion of volume expanders, such as albumin, has been noted to be beneficial, and its use has become very common in the diagnosis and treatment of patients with HRS-AKI. Proposed mechanisms for this improvement include increased cardiac preload and peripheral vascular resistance, which may be due to the ability of albumin to bind vasodilators, such as nitric oxide, IL-6, and TNF-α.[40] Reduced levels of inflammatory markers have been noted in plasma and ascitic fluid of patients with SBP after albumin infusion.[41] In addition, albumin infusion has been shown in randomized trials to prevent HRS and improve survival in patients diagnosed with SBP.[42]

Pharmacologic Therapy

Once a diagnosis of HRS is made, the goal of medical therapy is to improve systemic hemodynamics with vasoconstrictors and restoring effective circulatory volume with albumin (**Table 2**). It is recommend to use concentrated albumin 1 g/kg with a maximum of 100 g initially followed by daily doses of 20 to 40 g/d. Choice of vasoconstrictors is guided by location of hospitalized patients (intensive care unit [ICU] vs general ward) and availability, as terlipressin is currently not available in several countries, including North America. Several randomized controlled trials have shown the efficacy of vasoconstrictors, particularly terlipressin and albumin, in treating HRS with a response rate ranging from 45% to 75% in more recent studies (**Table 3**). Recently, a large randomized controlled trial (n = 300) in North America demonstrated a higher rate of HRS reversal in patients who received terlipressin plus albumin versus albumin alone (29.1% vs 15.8%) for treatment of patients with HRS type 1.[43]

Noradrenaline or norepinephrine is an α-adrenergic agonist that has shown efficacy in treatment of HRS. A systematic review comparing terlipressin and noradrenaline demonstrated equivalent efficacy in regard to HRS reversal, 30-day mortality, and recurrence of HRS.[44] Adverse events were less frequent in patients who received noradrenaline.

Midodrine, which is an orally administered α-adrenergic agonist, in combination with octreotide, a somatostatin analogue, along with albumin infusion has also been used widely in management of type 1 HRS. Recently, a small randomized controlled trial of 49 patients comparing midodrine/octreotide to terlipressin, both with albumin, showed that the latter was more effective in reversing HRS (28.6% vs 70.4%; $P = .01$).[45]

Table 2
Vasoconstrictors for the treatment of hepatorenal syndrome

Drug	Mechanism of Action	Dose	Comments
Terlipressin	Vasopressin analogue	1.0 mg every 4–6 h either as IV bolus or through continuous IV infusion. Dose can be increased to 2 mg IV every 4–6 h after 48 h if sCr has not decreased by >25% from baseline up to a maximum of 12 mg/d as long as there are no side effects. Maximal treatment 14 d	Not available in the United States In countries where terlipressin is not available, the combination of octreotide/midodrine can be initiated, and if there is no decline in sCr within a maximum of 3 d, then the patient should be transferred to the ICU for a trial of noradrenaline Contraindicated in patients with preexisting ischemic heart disease, cerebrovascular disease, peripheral arterial, disease, hypertension, or asthma
Noradrenaline	α-Adrenergic agonist	0.5–3.0 mg/h (continuous infusion). Titrate to achieve a 15 mm Hg increase in MAP	Requires ICU
Midodrine + Octreotide	α-Adrenergic agonist (midodrine) Somatostatin analogue (octreotide)	7.5 mg orally tid with an increase to 12.5–15 mg tid as needed to increase MAP by 15 mm Hg Octreotide SQ 100 μg tid, titrated 200 μg tid on day 2, if renal function has not improved	

Abbreviations: IV, intravenous; MAP, mean arterial pressure; SQ, subcutaneous; tid, 3 times a day.
Note: All vasoconstrictors should be given in combination with 25% IV albumin, initially 1 g of albumin/kg for 2 d, up to a maximum of 100 g/d, followed by 20 to 40 g/d.

Table 3
Randomized controlled trials of terlipressin for the treatment of hepatorenal syndrome

Author, y (Country)	No. of Subjects	Patient Population	Definition of Complete HRS Reversal	Intervention and Comparator (Both with Albumin)	HRS Reversal, %	Mortality Without Transplant, %
Alessandria et al,[60] 2007 (Italy)	22	Type 1 HRS Type 2 HRS	≥30% decrease in sCr from baseline to a final value ≤1.5 mg/dL	Terlipressin Noradrenaline	83 70	90 100
Sharma et al,[61] 2008 (India)	40	Type 1 HRS	sCr ≤1.5 mg/dL	Terlipressin Noradrenaline	50 50	45 45
Sanyal et al,[62] 2008 (USA, Germany, Russia)	112 (double-blind, multicenter)	Type 1 HRS	sCr ≤1.5 mg/dL on 2 occasions at least 48 h apart	Terlipressin Placebo	34 13	87 91
Martin-Llahi et al,[63] 2008 (Spain)	46 (multicenter)	Type 1 HRS Type 2 HRS	sCr ≤1.5 mg/dL	Terlipressin Albumin	44 9	73 81
Singh,[64] 2012 (India)	46	Type 1 HRS	sCr ≤1.5 mg/dL	Terlipressin Noradrenaline	39 43	61 52
Cavallin et al,[45] 2015 (Italy)	49 (multicenter)	Type 1 HRS Type 2 HRS	sCr ≤1.5 mg/dL	Terlipressin Midodrine/ Octreotide	70 29	41 57
Boyer et al,[65] 2016 (USA, Canada)	196 (double-blind, multicenter)	Type 1 HRS	sCr ≤1.5 mg/dL on 2 occasions at least 48 h apart	Terlipressin Albumin	24 15	70 86
Arora,[66] 2020 (India)	120	Type 1 HRS (defined by new AKI-HRS criteria)	Return of sCr to a value within 0.3 mg/dL of baseline	Terlipressin Noradrenaline	40 17	52 80
Wong et al,[43] 2019 (North America)	300	Type 1 HRS	sCr ≤1.5 mg/dL on 2 occasions at least 2 h apart with subjects alive without RRT at least 10 d after second sCr	Terlipressin Placebo	29 16	63 61

Treatment with vasoconstrictors should be discontinued if there is no improvement in sCr after 5 to 7 days, if the patient is initiated on renal replacement therapy (RRT), or for those who exhibit side effects.

Renal Replacement Therapy

Initiation of RRT in patients who are not transplant candidates, especially those with HRS, has been controversial. However, the severity of illness and number of organ failure in patients with acute on chronic liver failure have been shown to be more predictive of mortality than cause of AKI.[46,47] Initiation of RRT should be considered in the broader clinical context, for therapeutic and/or supportive treatment of "nonkidney" indications, before overt complications from AKI have developed and the threshold for initiation should be lowered when AKI occurs as part of multiorgan failure. RRT should also be considered in patients if the daily fluid balance cannot be maintained as even or negative regardless of their UO in order to prevent fluid accumulation.[48] Continuous RRT should be preferred over other modalities, as it provides better cardiovascular stability. In patients undergoing LT, intraoperative RRT has the potential benefit of mitigating metabolic complications associated with LT; however, larger prospective studies are required to confirm benefit.[49,50]

Liver transplantation versus simultaneous liver-kidney transplantation

Prediction of recovery of kidney function following LT remains a challenge, as the relative contribution of preexisting comorbidities, such as diabetes and age, unrecognized intrinsic renal disease, perioperative events, and posttransplant immunosuppression on kidney dysfunction, following LT is difficult to delineate. Simultaneous liver-kidney (SLK) transplantation is a potential therapeutic option for patients with sustained kidney impairment before LT in whom renal recovery is less likely after LT. Which patients should receive an SLK transplant versus liver alone had been a difficult decision for LT programs with considerable regional variability in listing practices for SLK transplant.[51,52] In 2017, the US Organ Procurement and Transplantation Network and United Network for Organ Sharing (UNOS) approved a new allocation policy for these patients (**Box 1**).[53] The new policies also included a safety-net criteria such that patients that continued to have evidence of renal dysfunction in the form of either dialysis dependency or creatinine clearance or GFR of ≤20 mL/min would be prioritized for kidney transplant if they were placed on the kidney transplant waiting list

---

Box 1
Medical eligibility criteria for simultaneous liver and kidney transplantation[53]

- Patients with CKD with a measured GFR ≤60 mL/min for more than 90 consecutive days and at least one of the following:
  - ESRD on dialysis
  - Measured/calculated creatinine clearance or GFR ≤30 mL/min, at the time of placement of the patient on the LT waiting list

- Diagnosis of sustained AKI for 6 weeks including either:
  - Dialysis at least once every 7 days, or
  - Measured/calculated creatinine clearance or GFR of ≤25 mL/min documented at least once every 7 days

- Diagnosis of metabolic disease with either:
  - Hyperoxaluria
  - Atypical hemolytic uremic syndrome from mutations in factor H or factor I
  - Familial nonneuropathic systemic amyloidosis
  - Methylmalonic aciduria

between 60 and 365 days after LT. Currently, there is not a substantial number of studies analyzing the outcomes associated with changes implemented by UNOS with regards to SLK versus Liver-alone transplant. Emergence of these data will help with future policy changes to allow the best possible outcome for patients and utilization of scarce organs.

POST–LIVER TRANSPLANT ACUTE KIDNEY INJURY

AKI after LT is a common occurrence that can be seen in more than 50% of cases in some recent series.[54–57] Many patients undergoing LT have had some evidence of AKI and may have been on RRT, both of which are predisposing factors for development of CKD in the posttransplant setting.[58,59] Typically, posttransplant AKI is multifactorial, relating to the recipient's pretransplant course, the donor, surgical events, and the use of immunosuppression.

SUMMARY

Cirrhosis is a condition that predisposes to several phenotypes of AKI, and HRS-AKI is a specific complication of end-stage cirrhosis. AKI is especially common in critically ill cirrhotic patients, and it is associated with a worse outcome. Different phenotypes of AKI are associated with different outcomes. Early diagnosis of AKI is an important step in critically ill cirrhotic patients, and mild changes in sCr may a major decrease in GFR. Use of biomarkers may be able to differentiate ATN from other phenotypes, Prediction of reversibility after LT is an unresolved issue, and innovative biomarkers are needed. In critically ill cirrhotic patients who are not candidates for transplantation, a trial of RRT can be started for 48 to 72 hours with limitation in patients with multiple organ failures who do not improve rapidly.

CLINIC CARE POINTS

- Development of HRS portends a poor prognosis in patients with chronic liver disease.
- Determining the cause of AKI in patients with chronic liver disease can be challenging.
- HRS remains a diagnosis of exclusion and may coexist with patients with underlying CKD.
- It is imperative to identify and remove any potential precipitating agents that may predispose to development of HRS.
- Once a diagnosis of HRS is made, the goal of medical therapy is to improve systemic hemodynamics with vasoconstrictors and to restore effective circulatory volume with albumin with the goal to increase the mean arterial pressure by approximately 15 mm Hg.
- Patients with sustained kidney impairment who are eligible should be considered for SLK transplantation.

DISCLOSURE

All authors: none.

REFERENCES

1. Tandon P, James MT, Abraldes JG, et al. Relevance of new definitions to incidence and prognosis of acute kidney injury in hospitalized patients with cirrhosis: a retrospective population-based cohort study. PLoS One 2016;11(8):e0160394.

2. Nadim MK, Genyk YS, Tokin C, et al. Impact of the etiology of acute kidney injury on outcomes following liver transplantation: acute tubular necrosis versus hepatorenal syndrome. Liver Transpl 2012;18(5):539–48.

3. Hilmi IA, Damian D, Al-Khafaji A, et al. Acute kidney injury following orthotopic liver transplantation: incidence, risk factors, and effects on patient and graft outcomes. Br J Anaesth 2015;114(6):919–26.

4. Francoz C, Durand F, Kahn JA, et al. Hepatorenal syndrome. Clin J Am Soc Nephrol 2019;14(5):774–81.

5. Wong F, O'Leary JG, Reddy KR, et al. New consensus definition of acute kidney injury accurately predicts 30-day mortality in patients with cirrhosis and infection. Gastroenterology 2013;145(6):1280–1288 e1281.

6. Macedo E, Bouchard J, Soroko SH, et al. Fluid accumulation, recognition and staging of acute kidney injury in critically-ill patients. Crit Care 2010;14(3):R82.

7. Liu KD, Thompson BT, Ancukiewicz M, et al. Acute kidney injury in patients with acute lung injury: impact of fluid accumulation on classification of acute kidney injury and associated outcomes. Crit Care Med 2011;39(12):2665–71.

8. Xirouchakis E, Marelli L, Cholongitas E, et al. Comparison of cystatin C and creatinine-based glomerular filtration rate formulas with 51Cr-EDTA clearance in patients with cirrhosis. Clin J Am Soc Nephrol 2011;6(1):84–92.

9. Proulx NL, Akbari A, Garg AX, et al. Measured creatinine clearance from timed urine collections substantially overestimates glomerular filtration rate in patients with liver cirrhosis: a systematic review and individual patient meta-analysis. Nephrol Dial Transplant 2005;20(8):1617–22.

10. Francoz C, Glotz D, Moreau R, et al. The evaluation of renal function and disease in patients with cirrhosis. J Hepatol 2010;52(4):605–13.

11. Francoz C, Nadim MK, Baron A, et al. Glomerular filtration rate equations for liver-kidney transplantation in patients with cirrhosis: validation of current recommendations. Hepatology 2014;59(4):1514–21.

12. Mindikoglu AL, Dowling TC, Weir MR, et al. Performance of chronic kidney disease epidemiology collaboration creatinine-cystatin C equation for estimating kidney function in cirrhosis. Hepatology 2014;59(4):1532–42.

13. De Souza V, Hadj-Aissa A, Dolomanova O, et al. Creatinine- versus cystatine C-based equations in assessing the renal function of candidates for liver transplantation with cirrhosis. Hepatology 2014;59(4):1522–31.

14. Asrani SK, Jennings LW, Trotter JF, et al. A model for glomerular filtration rate assessment in liver disease (GRAIL) in the presence of renal dysfunction. Hepatology 2019;69(3):1219–30.

15. Asrani SK, Jennings LW, Kim WR, et al. MELD-GRAIL-Na: glomerular filtration rate and mortality on liver-transplant waiting list. Hepatology 2020;71(5):1766–74.

16. Salerno F, Gerbes A, Gines P, et al. Diagnosis, prevention and treatment of hepatorenal syndrome in cirrhosis. Gut 2007;56(9):1310–8.

17. Nadim MK, Kellum JA, Davenport A, et al. Hepatorenal syndrome: the 8th International Consensus Conference of the Acute Dialysis Quality Initiative (ADQI) group. Crit Care 2012;16(1):R23.

18. Angeli P, Gines P, Wong F, et al. Diagnosis and management of acute kidney injury in patients with cirrhosis: revised consensus recommendations of the International Club of Ascites. J Hepatol 2015;62(4):968–74.

19. Belcher JM, Garcia-Tsao G, Sanyal AJ, et al. Association of AKI with mortality and complications in hospitalized patients with cirrhosis. Hepatology 2013;57(2):753–62.

20. Amathieu R, Al-Khafaji A, Sileanu FE, et al. Significance of oliguria in critically ill patients with chronic liver disease. Hepatology 2017;66(5):1592–600.

21. Nadim MK, Durand F, Kellum JA, et al. Management of the critically ill patient with cirrhosis: a multidisciplinary perspective. J Hepatol 2016;64(3):717–35.

22. Angeli P, Garcia-Tsao G, Nadim MK, et al. News in pathophysiology, definition and classification of hepatorenal syndrome: a step beyond the International Club of Ascites (ICA) consensus document. J Hepatol 2019;71(4):811–22.

23. European Association for the Study of the Liver. Electronic address EEE, European Association for the Study of the L. EASL Clinical Practice Guidelines for the management of patients with decompensated cirrhosis. J Hepatol 2018; 69(2):406–60.

24. Durand F, Graupera I, Gines P, et al. Pathogenesis of hepatorenal syndrome: implications for therapy. Am J Kidney Dis 2016;67(2):318–28.

25. Ginès P, Solà E, Angeli P, et al. Hepatorenal syndrome. Nat Rev Dis Primers 2018; 4(1):23.

26. Salerno F, Gerbes A, Ginès P, et al. Diagnosis, prevention and treatment of hepatorenal syndrome in cirrhosis. Postgrad Med J 2008;84(998):662–70.

27. Wiese S, Hove JD, Bendtsen F, et al. Cirrhotic cardiomyopathy: pathogenesis and clinical relevance. Nat Rev Gastroenterol Hepatol 2014;11(3):177–86.

28. Giannelli V, Roux O, Laouenan C, et al. Impact of cardiac function, refractory ascites and beta blockers on the outcome of patients with cirrhosis listed for liver transplantation. J Hepatol 2020;72(3):463–71.

29. Elia C, Graupera I, Barreto R, et al. Severe acute kidney injury associated with non-steroidal anti-inflammatory drugs in cirrhosis: a case-control study. J Hepatol 2015;63(3):593–600.

30. Mehta G, Gustot T, Mookerjee RP, et al. Inflammation and portal hypertension - the undiscovered country. J Hepatol 2014;61(1):155–63.

31. Wiest R, Lawson M, Geuking M. Pathological bacterial translocation in liver cirrhosis. J Hepatol 2014;60(1):197–209.

32. Navasa M, Follo A, Filella X, et al. Tumor necrosis factor and interleukin-6 in spontaneous bacterial peritonitis in cirrhosis: relationship with the development of renal impairment and mortality. Hepatology 1998;27(5):1227–32.

33. Gluud LL, Christensen K, Christensen E, et al. Systematic review of randomized trials on vasoconstrictor drugs for hepatorenal syndrome. Hepatology 2010; 51(2):576–84.

34. Belcher JM, Sanyal AJ, Peixoto AJ, et al. Kidney biomarkers and differential diagnosis of patients with cirrhosis and acute kidney injury. Hepatology 2014;60(2): 622–32.

35. Francoz C, Nadim MK, Durand F. Kidney biomarkers in cirrhosis. J Hepatol 2016; 65(4):809–24.

36. Huelin P, Solà E, Elia C, et al. Neutrophil gelatinase-associated lipocalin for assessment of acute kidney injury in cirrhosis: a prospective study. Hepatology 2019;70(1):319–33.

37. Fagundes C, Pepin MN, Guevara M, et al. Urinary neutrophil gelatinase-associated lipocalin as biomarker in the differential diagnosis of impairment of kidney function in cirrhosis. J Hepatol 2012;57(2):267–73.

38. Verna EC, Brown RS, Farrand E, et al. Urinary neutrophil gelatinase-associated lipocalin predicts mortality and identifies acute kidney injury in cirrhosis. Dig Dis Sci 2012;57(9):2362–70.

39. Caraceni P, Riggio O, Angeli P, et al. Long-term albumin administration in decompensated cirrhosis (ANSWER): an open-label randomised trial. Lancet 2018; 391(10138):2417–29.

40. Fernández J, Navasa M, Garcia-Pagan JC, et al. Effect of intravenous albumin on systemic and hepatic hemodynamics and vasoactive neurohormonal systems in patients with cirrhosis and spontaneous bacterial peritonitis. J Hepatol 2004; 41(3):384–90.

41. Chen TA, Tsao YC, Chen A, et al. Effect of intravenous albumin on endotoxin removal, cytokines, and nitric oxide production in patients with cirrhosis and spontaneous bacterial peritonitis. Scand J Gastroenterol 2009;44(5):619–25.

42. Sort P, Navasa M, Arroyo V, et al. Effect of intravenous albumin on renal impairment and mortality in patients with cirrhosis and spontaneous bacterial peritonitis. N Engl J Med 1999;341(6):403–9.

43. Wong F, CM, Reddy R, et al. The confirm study: a North American randomized controlled trial (RCT) of terlipressin plus albumin for the treatment of hepatorenal syndrome type-1 (HRS-1). Boston (MA): AASLD; 2019.

44. Nassar Junior AP, Farias AQ, D' Albuquerque LA, et al. Terlipressin versus norepinephrine in the treatment of hepatorenal syndrome: a systematic review and meta-analysis. PLoS One 2014;9(9):e107466.

45. Cavallin M, Kamath PS, Merli M, et al. Terlipressin plus albumin versus midodrine and octreotide plus albumin in the treatment of hepatorenal syndrome: a randomized trial. Hepatology 2015;62(2):567–74.

46. Allegretti AS, Parada XV, Eneanya ND, et al. Prognosis of patients with cirrhosis and AKI who initiate RRT. Clin J Am Soc Nephrol 2018;13(1):16–25.

47. Angeli P, Rodríguez E, Piano S, et al. Acute kidney injury and acute-on-chronic liver failure classifications in prognosis assessment of patients with acute decompensation of cirrhosis. Gut 2015;64(10):1616–22.

48. Rosner MH, Ostermann M, Murugan R, et al. Indications and management of mechanical fluid removal in critical illness. Br J Anaesth 2014;113(5):764–71.

49. Nadim MK, Annanthapanyasut W, Matsuoka L, et al. Intraoperative hemodialysis during liver transplantation: a decade of experience. Liver Transpl 2014;20(7): 756–64.

50. Karvellas CJ, Taylor S, Bigam D, et al. Intraoperative continuous renal replacement therapy during liver transplantation: a pilot randomized-controlled trial (INCEPTION). Can J Anaesth 2019;66(10):1151–61.

51. Nadim MK, Davis CL, Sung R, et al. Simultaneous liver-kidney transplantation: a survey of US transplant centers. Am J Transplant 2012;12(11):3119–27.

52. Luo X, Massie AB, Haugen CE, et al. Baseline and center-level variation in simultaneous liver-kidney listing in the United States. Transplantation 2018;102(4): 609–15.

53. Formica RN, Aeder M, Boyle G, et al. Simultaneous liver-kidney allocation policy: a proposal to optimize appropriate utilization of scarce resources. Am J Transplant 2016;16(3):758–66.

54. Angeli P, Bezinover D, Biancofiore G, et al. Acute kidney injury in liver transplant candidates: a position paper on behalf of the liver intensive care group of Europe. Minerva Anestesiol 2017;83(1):88–101.

55. Leithead JA, Rajoriya N, Gunson BK, et al. The evolving use of higher risk grafts is associated with an increased incidence of acute kidney injury after liver transplantation. J Hepatol 2014;60(6):1180–6.

56. Nadim MK, Sung RS, Davis CL, et al. Simultaneous liver-kidney transplantation summit: current state and future directions. Am J Transplant 2012;12(11):2901–8.

57. Durand F, Francoz C, Asrani SK, et al. Acute kidney injury after liver transplantation. Transplantation 2018;102(10):1636–49.

58. Ojo AO, Held PJ, Port FK, et al. Chronic renal failure after transplantation of a non-renal organ. N Engl J Med 2003;349(10):931–40.

59. Levitsky J, O'Leary JG, Asrani S, et al. Protecting the kidney in liver transplant recipients: practice-based recommendations from the American Society of Transplantation Liver and Intestine Community of Practice. Am J Transplant 2016; 16(9):2532–44.

60. Alessandria C, Ottobrelli A, Debernardi-Venon W, et al. Noradrenalin vs terlipressin in patients with hepatorenal syndrome: a prospective, randomized, unblinded, pilot study. J Hepatol 2007;47(4):499–505.

61. Sharma P, Kumar A, Shrama BC, et al. An open label, pilot, randomized controlled trial of noradrenaline versus terlipressin in the treatment of type 1 hepatorenal syndrome and predictors of response. Am J Gastroenterol 2008;103(7): 1689–97.

62. Sanyal AJ, Boyer T, Garcia-Tsao G, et al. A randomized, prospective, double-blind, placebo-controlled trial of terlipressin for type 1 hepatorenal syndrome. Gastroenterology 2008;134(5):1360–8.

63. Martín-Llahí M, Pépin MN, Guevara M, et al. Terlipressin and albumin vs albumin in patients with cirrhosis and hepatorenal syndrome: a randomized study. Gastroenterology 2008;134(5):1352–9.

64. Singh V, Ghosh S, Singh B, et al. Noradrenaline vs. terlipressin in the treatment of hepatorenal syndrome: a randomized study. J Hepatol 2012;56(6):1293–8.

65. Boyer TD, Sanyal AJ, Wong F, et al. Terlipressin plus albumin is more effective than albumin alone in improving renal function in patients with cirrhosis and hepatorenal syndrome Type 1. Gastroenterology 2016;150(7):1579–89.e1572.

66. Arora V, Maiwall R, Rajan V, et al. Terlipressin is superior to noradrenaline in the management of acute kidney injury in acute on chronic liver failure. Hepatology 2020;71(2):600–10.

Cardiorenal Syndrome

Zaccaria Ricci, MD[a,b,]*, Stefano Romagnoli, MD, PhD[b,c],
Claudio Ronco, MD[d,e]

KEYWORDS

- Cardiorenal syndrome • Renocardiac syndrome • Heart failure • Acute kidney injury
- Heart transplantation • Ventricular-assist device • Pediatric cardiorenal syndrome

KEY POINTS

- Cardiorenal syndrome is common in patients suffering with initial severe forms of heart or kidney failure.
- A tight bidirectional link exists between these two organs and their reciprocal involvement is typical and progressive.
- Critically ill patients may have cardiorenal syndrome in the context of multiple organ failure.
- Prolonged (and artificial) organ support in end-stage heart and kidney failure has led to a novel form of cardiorenal syndrome where the organ is injured also by artificial support (chronic dialysis or ventricular-assist device).
- Pediatric cardiorenal syndrome is typical after cardiac surgery but the novel classification is revealing a frequent occurrence in this setting of frail patients.

INTRODUCTION: THE DEFINITION OF CARDIORENAL SYNDROME

The first time the term cardiorenal syndrome (CRS) was officially utilized was in 2004 during the National Heart, Lung, and Blood Institute Working Group conference, which defined CRS as the consequence of interactions between the kidneys and other circulatory compartments that increase blood volume, which worsens the symptoms of heart failure (HF) and disease progression.[1] A few years later, the Acute Dialysis Quality Initiative group proposed a practical classification of CRS dividing the syndrome into two main groups, "cardio → renal" and "reno → cardiac," focusing on the

[a] Department of Cardiology and Cardiac Surgery, Pediatric Cardiac Intensive Care Unit, Bambino Gesù Children's Hospital, IRCCS, P.zza S.Onofrio 4, Rome 00165, Italy; [b] Department of Health Science, University of Florence, Florence, Italy; [c] Department of Anesthesiology and Intensive Care, Azienda Ospedaliero-Universitaria Careggi, Largo Brambilla, 3, Florence 50139, Italy; [d] International Renal Research Institute of Vicenza (IRRIV), Vicenza, Italy; [e] Department of Nephrology, Dialysis and Transplantation, San Bortolo Hospital, Via Rodolfi 37, Vicenza 36100, Italy
* Corresponding author. Department of Cardiology and Cardiac Surgery, Pediatric Cardiac Intensive Care Unit, Bambino Gesù Children's Hospital, IRCCS, P.zza S.Onofrio 4, Rome 00165, Italy.
E-mail address: Zaccaria.ricci@opbg.net
Twitter: @RicciZaccaria (Z.R.); @StefanoRomagno9 (S.R.); @croncoIRRIV (C.R.)

Crit Care Clin 37 (2021) 335–347
https://doi.org/10.1016/j.ccc.2020.11.003
0749-0704/21/© 2020 Elsevier Inc. All rights reserved.
criticalcare.theclinics.com

primum movens of the disease process.[2,3] These two main groups were then split into acute (types 1 and 3 CRS) and chronic (types 2 and 4 CRS). A fifth group of diseases, including systemic illnesses affecting heart and kidneys, completed the classification (**Table 1**).

More precisely, the practical Acute Dialysis Quality Initiative classification clearly identified which is the primarily diseased organ and the secondary damaged one in acute and chronic conditions. In the first two groups cardiac (acute or chronic) diseases lead to kidney dysfunction, whereas in the third and fourth groups primary kidney (acute or chronic) diseases lead to cardiac dysfunction (**Fig. 1**). The last group includes all the systemic conditions (noncardiac [primary] and nonrenal [primary]) that cause a contemporary heart and kidney dysfunction (eg, sepsis).

This classification was meant to help the clinician to deliver a phenotype-based therapy for CRS once the patient suffers a renal or a cardiac disease even if a significant overlap between different subgroups and the evolution of one subtype to the other during disease progression may occur. In fact, the concept of CRS well matches with the more generalized principle of "organ crosstalk," which implies that the failure or dysfunction of one organ leads to the dysfunction of many other organs with a cascade of feedback mechanisms. As a consequence of the continuous and close interaction between organs and systems, even if the concept of CRS tends to focus on a two-organ interaction (first → second), the function of several organs and systems is usually disrupted simultaneously.[4] Consequently, even if CRS concept and classification may contribute to initially frame and analyze renal involvement in cardiac disease and vice versa, the clinical scenario may eventually complicate with a more

Table 1
Cardiorenal syndrome

Phenotype	Denomination	Description	Example
Type 1 CRS	Acute CRS (heart → kidney)	HF leading to AKI	Cardiogenic shock (eg, from ACS) leading to acute HF
Type 2 CRS	Chronic CRS (heart → kidney)	Chronic HF leading to CKD	Chronic HF
Type 3 CRS	Acute renocardiac syndrome (kidney → heart)	AKI leading to acute HF	AKI from various origins (eg, sepsis, nephrotoxic medications, cardiac surgery–associated) leading to HF with volume overload, systemic inflammation (CK clearance), and metabolic derangement in uremia
Type 4 CRS	Chronic renocardiac syndrome (kidney → heart)	CKD leading to chronic HF	Systolic-diastolic LV dysfunction (with LV hypertrophy) secondary to chronic HF
Type 5 CRS	Secondary CRS	Systemic disease leading to HF and kidney failure	Sepsis, vasculitis, diabetes mellitus, atherosclerosis, cirrhosis, thesaurismosis (eg, amyloidosis)

Classification proposed by the Acute Dialysis Quality Initiative in 2008 (modified).[48,49]
Abbreviations: ACS, acute coronary syndrome; AKI, acute kidney injury; CK, cytokines; CKD, chronic kidney disease; LV, left ventricle.

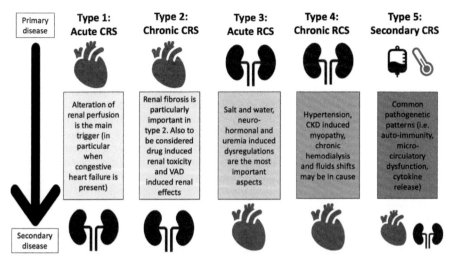

Fig. 1. Schematic representation of the five CRS types according to the organ direction (primary > secondary disease) and the time window (acute or chronic). According to this classification two CRS (acute and chronic), two renocardiac (acute and chronic) syndromes, and one secondary CRS are visualized. CKD, chronic kidney disease; RCS, renocardiac syndrome; VAD, ventricular-assist device.

complex multiple organ involvement (eg, lungs, liver, gut, brain), especially in critically ill cases.

CARDIORENAL SYNDROME IN ADULTS

Type 1 CRS (cardio → renal [acute]) includes all those conditions in which an acute cardiac dysfunction leads to acute kidney injury (AKI). Acute HF, commonly caused by ischemic disease, occurs in about 25% of patients hospitalized with acute HF. Less frequent causes are pulmonary embolism, pericardia effusion, myocarditis, papillary muscle rupture, post–cardiac surgery periods, or arrhythmias.[5,6] Noteworthy, in these patients, chronic kidney disease (CKD) is a common finding and AKI may easily occur in case of acute cardiac dysfunction and, on the other side, renal dysfunction may complicate chronic HF. All these forms of heart decompensation are characterized by renal retaining of sodium and extracellular fluid volume expansion.[7] Hemodynamic issues (eg, renal hypoperfusion) play a major role in type 1 CRS in the presence of acute HF. The decrease in renal artery flow and glomerular filtration rate (GFR), because of the inability of the failing heart to generate an adequate cardiac output (CO) and blood pressure (BP), are the mainly involved pathophysiologic mechanisms. HF and the consequent insufficient renal blood flow and BP activates the renin-angiotensin-aldosterone system (RAAS) axis, the sympathetic nervous system, and arginine vasopressin secretion, thus leading to further fluid retention and increased right ventricle and left ventricle (LV) preload, which in a failing heart leads to a worsening in pump function.[8] The activation of the sympathetic nervous system, persistent inflammation, and persistent RAAS activation may worsen heart and kidney function.[9] However, low CO/low BP cannot completely explain the pathophysiology of all type 1 CRS. HF is classified into three classes: (1) patients with normal LV ejection fraction (EF) who have values greater than or equal to 50% (HF with preserved EF), (2) those with reduced LVEF who have values less than 40% (HF with reduced EF), and (3) patients with an LVEF in the range of 40% to 49% (HF with midrange EF).[10] Patients with acute type 1 CRS may belong to any of the LV functional classes of HF and in many cases these patients are hospitalized with preserved or even elevated BP, LVEF, and CO.[11] The kidneys, which are characterized by a low-resistance vascular circuit, receive about 25% of CO and, to maintain a so elevated perfusion, the A (renal artery)-V (renal vein) delta pressure must be kept sufficiently large. Several clinical (cardiac and noncardiac) conditions are associated with acute or chronic increase in right atrial pressure (R_{ap}) that, physically in continuum with caval pressures (central venous pressure [CVP]), eventually leads to an increase in all the venous compartments of the abdominal organs (eg, suprahepatic veins, portal and mesenteric veins) including the renal veins. Therefore, an increase in CVP, as in LV diastolic dysfunction (potentially all the HF categories including HF with preserved EF, primary or secondary pulmonary hypertension, right ventricular systolic dysfunction, pericardial tamponade) may decrease the renal A-V pressure gradient, hence increasing the renal resistance, impairing intrarenal blood flow and reducing the GFR.[12,13] A post hoc analysis of the Evaluation Study of Congestive Heart Failure and Pulmonary Artery Catheterization Effectiveness (ESCAPE) trial showed that R_{ap} was the only hemodynamic parameter associated with baseline renal dysfunction.[14] A landmark study by Legrand and colleagues[15] showed a strong association between CVP and AKI in patients with sepsis thus suggesting the key role of venous congestion in the development of AKI. Specifically, a quasilinear association between CVP and new or persistent AKI was demonstrated even after adjustment for fluid balance and positive and expiratory pressure in mechanically ventilated patients (odds radio, 1.22 [1.08–1.39] for an increase of 1 mm Hg; $P = .002$).[15] Thus, low-flow, low BP, high CVP isolated or in combination, in the context of different states of HF (preserved, midrange, reduced EF) should always be considered in the evaluation of a patient who develops AKI.

Echocardiography can provide fundamental information for the diagnosis of CRS type 1: myocardial wall motion abnormalities, left ventricular hypertrophy, valvular diseases, endocarditis, aortic dissection.[16] Kidney ultrasound usually shows normal or large-sized kidneys with preserved corticomedullary ratio; color Doppler evaluation shows regular intraparenchymal blood flow, often associated with increased resistance index (>0.8 cm/s).

Early diagnosis of AKI in CRS type 1 (eg, in type 3) could be challenging because the classic AKI diagnostic criteria (creatinine, urine output) commonly fail at least in the early phases of the disease. New frontiers may be represented by more recent, more sensitive biomarkers (eg, serum and urinary neutrophil gelatinase–associated lipocalin, cystatin-C, kidney injury molecule 1, interleukin [IL]-18, and liver-type fatty acid–binding protein).[17–19] Definitive evidence that the application of such biomarkers may impact the course of cardiorenal disease is currently lacking.

Type 2 CRS (cardio → renal [chronic]) is characterized by chronic abnormalities in cardiac function leading to kidney injury or dysfunction (chronic HF). Chronic HF and CKD often coexist, and it is difficult to establish which of the two disease states is primary and which is secondary. CKD has been observed in 45% to 63% of patients with chronic HF and could be the evolution of a type 1 CRS.[20–22] Renal congestion caused by elevated R_{ap} and CVP and chronic hypoperfusion represent a cornerstone in renal dysfunction of these patients.[14]

Type 3 CRS (renal → cardiac [acute]) occurs when AKI contributes and/or precipitates to the development of acute HF. Volume overload, metabolic acidosis, and electrolyte disorders (eg, hyperkalemia and/or hypocalcemia) are the more common leading causes. A prospective, multicenter, community-based study in 748 patients with AKI reported heart disease as a cause of death in 15% of the cases.[23] Kidney and heart during AKI are closely interconnected (organ crosstalk) by means of macrophenomena (eg, volume overload, venous congestion, electrolyte abnormalities, acid-base disorders) and by the activation of immune (ie, release of proinflammatory and anti-inflammatory cytokines and chemokines) and sympathetic nervous system, activation of the RAAS, and coagulation cascades.

Ultrasound examination could be helpful in diagnosing and evaluating CRS type 3 patients. Kidney size and echogenicity provide primary features to discern between acute kidney disease and CKD: a hyperechogenic renal cortex with low corticomedullary ratio is suggestive of CKD.

However, cortical hyperechogenicity can also be present in acute tubular necrosis or acute glomerulonephritis.[24,25] Chest (cardiac and lung) ultrasound evaluation may show increased atrial volumes, pleural or pericardial effusion, and B lines on lung parenchyma.[16] Many potential biomarkers still under investigation have been proposed as tools for the CRS type 3 diagnosis (eg, neutrophil gelatinase–associated lipocalin, kidney injury molecule 1, IL-18, IL-6, cystatin C, N-acetyl-b-D-glucosamide, liver-type fatty acid–binding protein, Netrin-1, Klotho, and Midkine [neurite growth–promoting factor 2]).[26] Differently, cardiac biomarkers are routinely used in clinical practice to diagnose HF and to track the response to therapies (eg, troponins, B-type natriuretic peptide, and N-terminal pro–B-type natriuretic peptide).

Type 4 CRS (renal → cardiac [chronic]) defines cardiovascular involvement in patients with CKD. The relationships between CKD and cardiovascular risk have been acknowledged many years ago: acute cardiac events (eg, myocardial infarction) currently represent almost 50% of the causes of death in patients with CKD.[5] A large epidemiologic study, on 1,120,295 adults who have not undergone dialysis or kidney transplantation, estimated the longitudinal GFR with serum creatinine between 1996 and 2000. On a median follow-up of 2.8 years, the adjusted hazard ratio for cardiovascular events increased inversely with the estimated GFR (eGFR). The adjusted risk of hospitalization with a reduced eGFR followed a similar pattern.[27]

GFR is a strong independent factor of cardiovascular morbidity and mortality.[28] CKD leads to hyperphosphatemia (and secondary hyperparathyroidism), which, in turn, may cause coronary and valve calcifications. In addition, hypertension contributes to vascular calcification and consequent pressure overload, chronic inflammation, insulin-resistance, hyperhomocysteinemia, and lipid dysmetabolism all contribute to cardiovascular disease in patients with CKD.[29]

Many biomarkers, such as troponins, asymmetric dimethylarginine, plasminogen-activator inhibitor type I, homocysteine, natriuretic peptides, C-reactive protein, serum amyloid A protein, and ischemia-modified albumin, increase as GFR declines, although the therapeutic influence of these is not clearly understood.[30,31] In hyperechogenic kidney cortex with a reduced corticomedullary ratio, parapelvic and subcortical cysts are found during ultrasound investigation.[16] Swings of volume overload, left and right ventricular dysfunction, increased atrial volumes, pleural or pericardial effusion, valvular calcifications, and B lines are common findings in heart and lung echography.[16]

Type 5 CRS (systemic CRS) is characterized by simultaneous involvement of the heart and kidneys in several severe systemic clinical settings, such as sepsis; hepatorenal syndrome; and Fabry disease, a rare genetic lysosomal storage disease. Sepsis is the most common cause of renal-replacement therapy in intensive care units. Macrohemodynamic instability and microvascular alterations (distributive shock requiring high-dose vasopressors), and inflammation represent the basis of the pathophysiology involving the kidneys and heart (septic cardiomyopathy).[32,33] Although some aspects are still under investigation, many mediators and pathways have been implicated in pathogenesis of myocardial depression in sepsis.[34] The sepsis-induced, dysregulated inflammatory response has been directly linked to cardiomyocyte dysfunction. Cytokines (including IL-1β, tumor necrosis factor-α, IL-6, and the p38 mitogen activated protein kinases pathway), the complement system, nitric oxide dysregulation, high-mobility group box-1 (a damage and signaling molecule implicated in the pathogenesis of sepsis), and lipopolysaccharide together with oxidative stress have been identified as potential causative agents.[35] AKI is common during sepsis and septic shock occurring in 51% of patients with septic shock and positive blood cultures.[36]

Diagnosis of CRS type 5 is based on the global multiorgan evaluation of a systemic disease where clinical findings, ultrasound, and laboratory investigation are tiles of a big mosaic.

Finally, an increase in renal venous pressure, renal congestion, and AKI may occur in cases of elevated intra-abdominal pressures (IAPs; sustained or repeated elevation of IAP of >12 mm Hg), which, in turn, may happen in the setting of acute HF,[37] or independently, at least in part, from heart function (eg, sepsis complicated by severe capillary spillover, fluid overload, and tissue edema). The detrimental effects of increased IAPs on kidneys (and other intra-abdominal organs) have been known for a long time[38] and whether IAP is sustained greater than 20 mm Hg and associated with organ dysfunction (eg, AKI), it constitutes the abdominal compartment syndrome.[39]

CARDIORENAL SYNDROME IN PATIENTS SUPPORTED BY ARTIFICIAL HEART SUPPORT AND AFTER HEART TRANSPLANTATION

Patients with end-stage HF (ESHF) and with marked limitation in ordinary activity are scheduled for conventional left ventricular assist device (LVAD) implantation and heart transplantation.[40] LVAD is generally indicated as a bridge to heart transplant or as a destination therapy. The assessment of renal dysfunction in patients with ESHF is underestimated because of reduced creatinine production and sarcopenia. LVAD is an intracorporeal device that drains blood from the LV and pushes it to the systemic circulation through a mechanical pump. The technology of mechanical assist devices has significantly improved from the 1990s to the current third-generation machines and the number of implantations has increased accordingly.[41] Nowadays, a significant survival improvement, compared with standard medical therapy, has been attributed to the application of LVAD, especially with second- and third-generation devices.[42] The mechanical assistance of ESHF has opened a novel chapter of CRS type 2: as a matter of fact, patients with chronic heart dysfunction who suffer chronic renal failure undergo a sudden improvement of CO that ultimately impacts on kidney function and may have beneficial and harmful consequences.

Before deciding to implant an LVAD, risk stratification according to other organs functions is required. Kidney function before LVAD implantation has been shown to impact mortality[43] and a prediction model for the risk assessment of mortality in patients with LVAD demonstrated that every 1 mg/dL in creatinine increase doubles the chance of dying after implantation.[44] One of five patients with eGFR less than 30 mL/min/1.73 m² or those with dialysis dependence die in the first 3 months after LVAD surgery.[45] Current discussion is ongoing regarding the possibility to implant heart mechanical assistance to patients who are candidates for heart-kidney transplant or who are dialysis-dependent.[46] It is possible that with further improvements in LVAD technology this kind of ethical issue will be solved, and this approach will be extended to high-risk patients.

Kidney dysfunction after LVAD implantation can frequently occur (up to 12%).[47] This is AKI or acute-on-chronic kidney failure. Surgical "stress," infections, cardiopulmonary bypass (CPB), subclinical renal dysfunction, and reduced renal reserve all play a role for postsurgical AKI. The modifications of pulsatile blood flow and the flow adjustments required in the initial postimplantation days, added to increased hemolysis occurring in some cases, may impact renal perfusion in the midterm.[48] Also important is the effect of LVAD implantation on right ventricular function: although interventricular septum improves its shape because of the left chamber drainage of the pump, the increased left CO can exceed the dysfunctioning right ventricle capacity with a secondary increase in venous pressures and renal congestion.[48]

However, kidney function can also be positively affected by LVAD. Several studies have shown a sort of bidirectional trajectory depending on estimated function previous to device implantation. Essentially, it seems that patients with normal GFR tend to slightly decrease their renal function after 1-year follow-up, whereas those with impaired renal function had the most benefit.[43,49] With the increase of implantation indications and the inclusion of frailer patients added to the longer duration in transplant lists it is possible that progressive decrease in renal function will be observed in the next future. The INTERMACS database seemed to show that patients with significant improvement in eGFR ultimately had similar mortality to the patients with postimplantation CRS and the best outcomes where in the patients with slight improvement in kidney function (20%–50%).[43] Possibly, severe kidney dysfunction occurring either before or after LVAD implantation negatively affects patients' outcomes. A further reason to consider regarding the appearance of kidney dysfunction after LVAD is related to the inappropriate assessment of baseline GFR before implantation. CKD can be missed because of the absence of a recent (presurgical) creatinine measurement or it could be miscalculated because of patients' cardiac cachexia and muscles wasting with decreased creatinine production.[50] It is possible that improvement in physical activity and overall feeding could simply unmask a previously decreased GFR in these patients. Further improvement in assessment of actual renal function before LVAD implantation including the application of renal biomarkers is warranted and eagerly needed in this novel field of medicine.

Heart transplantation is the long-term treatment of ESHF and for most patients with LVAD. However, the impact of heart transplant on renal function is variable and depends on preoperative kidney status. Similarly to the data regarding LVAD, conflicting results are reported in the literature, with pediatric heart transplants being those with the longest renal follow-up.[51] In 46 children following heart-lung transplant, the percentage of recipients with normal renal function declined from 80% to 30% in the first 2 years, even after adjustment for nutritional conditions. A cause for post-transplantation renal function decrease is the frequent occurrence of right ventricular dysfunction and, above all, the nephrotoxicity of calcineurin inhibitors that are administered as immunosuppressants.[51] In a recent report, Kolsrud and co-workers[52] found that even if renal function declines after heart transplantation (around 10% decrease in the first year and a steady decline thereafter), preoperative renal function was not correlated with post–heart transplant outcomes and renal function. Clearly, those who had an early decrease greater than 25% in the first year had the worst outcomes. However, among the patients who survived the first year, only 12% developed end-stage renal disease requiring long-term dialysis. For this reason, candidates to heart transplantation with CRS and advanced CKD (pre–heart transplant GFR <45 mL/min) are generally scheduled for combined double heart and kidney transplantation, to optimize their cardiorenal interaction in the post-transplant period. It is currently suggested to perform a combined heart-kidney transplant procedure if preoperative eGFR is less than 30 mL/min or in dialysis, whereas a sequential heart-kidney procedure (in case a single donor is not available at the time of heart harvesting) is performed in patients with an eGFR between 30 and 45 mL/min.[53]

CARDIORENAL SYNDROME IN CHILDREN

Although pediatric AKI is a serious complication after CPB with an incidence ranging between 10% and 80%,[54] with the increased attention to CRS, all episodes of hemodynamic instability in the pediatric setting ultimately causing a decrease of renal function can be included as a form of CRS. The incidence of AKI requiring renal replacement following pediatric cardiac surgery ranges from 5% to 10% and is known to have an independent association with mortality.[55] Hence, all AKI episodes that can be considered a CRS type 1 manifestation, based on data collected in cardiac surgery children, should be considered a serious marker of multiorgan damage and a predictor of worse outcomes,[56] including long-term issues, such as CKD and hypertension.[57] The message is not to overlook any renal manifestation consequent to hemodynamic disorders, which in the past were erroneously tagged as "prerenal AKI" with an implicit and dangerous meaning of "less severe" condition. Another condition that is currently gaining importance from an epidemiology standpoint is pediatric ESHF. Established pediatric ESHF in children suffering from heart dysfunction after surgery for congenital heart diseases or a patient treated for dilative cardiomyopathy is classified as CRS type 2 if a secondary renal dysfunction (eg, acute and chronic) is present.[3] Pediatric CRS type 2 prevalence and long-term outcomes is currently poorly studied.

The risk factors of pediatric CRS include demographic (younger and neonatal age), preoperative, and perioperative variables[58]; hypotension and low CO[59]; nephrotoxic cardiac drugs use; humoral factors, such as renin-angiotensin system activation; immune-mediated mechanisms; metabolic products release[60]; and renal injury after cardiac catheterization.[61]

Fluid overload control is another important CRS pathogenetic mechanism in children with hemodynamic instability who require large amounts of fluid replacement.[62] Fluid overload is considered a cause and an effect of renal dysfunction[63] because it implies a reduced renal capacity of managing administered fluids and body water, and because of venous congestion and backward failure, it may eventually end up with AKI. Fluid accumulation is dose-dependent and affects ventilation time, length of stay in the intensive care unit, and postoperative infections.[64]

The therapy for pediatric CRS is based on awareness, early diagnosis, and prevention.[65] Diuretics and decongestion are the first-line treatment in adults and in this population. Short-term high-dose ethacrynic acid is effective in infants after cardiac surgery[66]: optimized fluid balance in the first postoperative period improved CO. Renal-replacement therapy is the most effective way of managing severe AKI.[67] Peritoneal dialysis[68] and extracorporeal renal-replacement therapy are frequently used in the pediatric setting with novel machines for pediatric continuous renal replacement therapy (CRRT) being available today.[69] Some studies on inodilators (eg, milrinone) have examined if postoperative AKI could be reduced by improving CO and peripheral vasodilation.[54] A recent randomized controlled trial showed that levosimendan is not able to prevent AKI in the postcardiosurgical phase, even if adult literature in this field showed different results.[70] There are not clearly identified hemodynamic goals in pediatric CRS studies.[71] A retrospective study on nesiritide infusion in children with resistance to diuretic therapy and pulmonary congestion[72] showed the ability to decrease CVP, serum creatinine levels, and the stage of AKI. Fenoldopam at high doses (1 µg/kg/min), administered continuously during CPB, was able to significantly reduce urine neutrophil gelatinase-associated lipocalin (uNGAL) levels and to increase urine output in a randomized trial in pediatric CPB patients.[73] With a similar hypothesis, dexmedetomidine has shown to attenuate the renal dysfunction after pediatric open heart surgery and its application in different settings of pediatric critical care as a pharmacologic approach for CRS is awaited.[74]

SUMMARY

CRS represents one of the most commonly identified organs crosstalk in severely ill patients. Early diagnosis and timely identification of the ongoing process has been simplified in recent years by the introduction of the CRS classification system. In CRS types 1 and 3, low CO and congestion are the cause of bidirectional interactions between the heart and the kidney. CRS types 2 and 4 are essentially the consequence of an interrupted pathophysiologic process ongoing chronically with these two organs. Support of heart function, control of fluid balance, and heart transplantation are the mainstay of therapy for CRS types 1 and 2 with important caveats regarding pharmacologic and artificial/mechanical support, which can become "nephrotoxic" and be involved in the CRS process. Prevention of AKI and optimal management of acute and chronic renal-replacement therapy play a crucial role in the avoidance of the development of CRS types 2 and 4, again by controlling efficiently the patient's fluid balance and renin-angiotensin axis activation. This is challenging in critically ill patients, especially when end-stage conditions are present and accelerated dialysis in these cases may be indicated.

DISCLOSURE

The authors have nothing to disclose.

REFERENCES

1. Cardio-renal connections in heart failure and cardiovascular disease. National Heart, Lung, and Blood Institute (NHLBI). Available at: https://www.nhlbi.nih.gov/events/2004/cardio-renal-connections-heartfailure-and-cardiovascular-disease. Accessed May 06, 2020.

2. House AA, Anand I, Bellomo R, et al. Acute dialysis quality initiative consensus group. definition and classification of cardio-renal syndromes: workgroup statements from the 7th ADQI consensus conference. Nephrol Dial Transplant 2010; 25:1416–20.

3. Ronco C, Haapio M, House AA, et al. Cardiorenal syndrome. J Am Coll Cardiol 2008;25:1527–39.

4. Vincent JL, Sakr Y, Sprung CL, et al. Sepsis Occurrence in Acutely Ill Patients investigators. Sepsis in European intensive care units: results of the SOAP study. Crit Care Med 2006;52:344–53.

5. Bagshaw SM, Cruz DN, Aspromonte N, et al. Acute Dialysis Quality Initiative Consensus Group. Epidemiology of cardio-renal syndromes: workgroup statements from the 7th ADQI consensus conference. Nephrol Dial Transplant 2010; 43:1406–16.

6. Damman K, Navis G, Voors AA, et al. Worsening renal function and prognosis in heart failure: systematic review and meta-analysis. J Card Fail 2007;13:599–608.

7. Ronco C, Cicoira M, McCullough PA. Cardiorenal syndrome type 1: pathophysiological crosstalk leading to combined heart and kidney dysfunction in the

setting of acutely decompensated heart failure. J Am Coll Cardiol 2012;60: 1031–42.

8. Schrier RW, Abraham WT. Hormones and hemodynamics in heart failure. N Engl J Med 1999;341:577–85.

9. Haase M, Muller C, Damman K, et al. Pathogenesis of cardiorenal syndrome type 1 in acute decompensated heart failure: workgroup statements from the Eleventh Consensus Conference of the Acute Dialysis Quality Initiative (ADQI). Contrib Nephrol 2013;182:99–116.

10. Ponikowski P, Voors AA, Anker SD, et al, Authors/Task Force Members. Document reviewers. 2016 ESC guidelines for the diagnosis and treatment of acute and chronic heart failure: the Task Force for the diagnosis and treatment of acute and chronic heart failure of the European Society of Cardiology (ESC). Developed with the special contribution of the Heart Failure Association (HFA) of the ESC. Eur J Heart Fail 2016;18:891–975.

11. Sweitzer NK, Lopatin M, Yancy CW, et al. Comparison of clinical features and outcomes of patients hospitalized with heart failure and normal ejection fraction (> or=55%) versus those with mildly reduced (40% to 55%) and moderately to severely reduced (<40%) fractions. Am J Cardiol 2008;101:1151–6.

12. Mullens W, Abrahams Z, Francis GS, et al. Importance of venous congestion for worsening of renal function in advanced decompensated heart failure. J Am Coll Cardiol 2009;53:589–96.

13. Damman K, Navis G, Smilde TD, et al. Decreased cardiac output, venous congestion and the association with renal impairment in patients with cardiac dysfunction. Eur J Heart Fail 2007;9:872–8.

14. Nohria A, Hasselblad V, Stebbins A, et al. Cardiorenal interactions: insights from the ESCAPE trial. J Am Coll Cardiol 2008;51:1268–74.

15. Legrand M, Dupuis C, Simon C, et al. Association between systemic hemodynamics and septic acute kidney injury in critically ill patients: a retrospective observational study. Crit Care 2013;17:R278.

16. Di Lullo L, Floccari F, Granata A, et al. Ultrasonography: Ariadne's thread in the diagnosis of the cardiorenal syndrome. Cardiorenal Med 2012;2:11–7.

17. Han WK, Bonventre JV. Biologic markers for the early detection of acute kidney injury. Curr Opin Crit Care 2004;10:476–82.

18. Hekmat R, Mohebi M. Comparison of serum creatinine, cystatin C, and neutrophil gelatinase-associated lipocalin for acute kidney injury occurrence according to risk, injury, failure, loss, and endstage criteria classification system in early after living kidney donation. Saudi J Kidney Dis Transpl 2016;27:659–64.

19. Vaidya VS, Ramirez V, Ichimura T, et al. Urinary kidney injury molecule-1: a sensitive quantitative biomarker for early detection of kidney tubular injury. Am J Physiol Renal Physiol 2006;290:F517–29.

20. Hebert K, Dias A, Delgado MC, et al. Epidemiology and survival of the five stages of chronic kidney disease in a systolic heart failure population. Eur J Heart Fail 2010;12:861–5.

21. Heywood JT, Fonarow GC, Costanzo MR, et al. High prevalence of renal dysfunction and its impact on outcome in 118,465 patients hospitalized with acute decompensated heart failure: a report from the ADHERE database. J Card Fail 2007;13:422–30.

22. Cruz DN, Bagshaw SM. Heart-kidney interaction: epidemiology of cardiorenal syndromes. Int J Nephrol 2010;2016:351291.

23. Liano F, Pascual J. Epidemiology of acute renal failure: a prospective, multicenter, community-based study. Madrid Acute Renal Failure Study Group. Kidney Int 1996;50:811–8.

24. Ozmen CA, Akin D, Bilek SU, et al. Ultrasound as a diagnostic tool to differentiate acute from chronic renal failure. Clin Nephrol 2010;74:46–52.

25. Licurse A, Kim MC, Dziura J, et al. Renal ultrasonography in the evaluation of acute kidney injury. Arch Intern Med 2010;2016:1900–7.

26. Chuasuwan A, Kellum JA. Cardio-renal syndrome type 3: epidemiology, pathophysiology, and treatment. Semin Nephrol 2012;32:31–9.

27. Go AS, Chertow GM, Fan D, et al. Chronic kidney disease and the risks of death, cardiovascular events, and hospitalization. N Engl J Med 2004;352:1296–305.

28. United States Renal Data System. USRDS 2009 annual data report: atlas of end-stage renal disease in the United States. Bethesda (MD): National Institute of Diabetes and Digestive and Kidney Diseases; 2009.

29. Olgaard K, Lewin E, Silver J. Calcimimetics, vitamin D and ADVANCE in the management of CKD-MBD. Nephrol Dial Transplant 2011;26:1117–9.

30. Austin WJ, Bhalla V, Hernandez-Arce I, et al. Correlation and prognostic utility of B-type natriuretic peptide and its amino-terminal fragment in patients with chronic kidney disease. Am J Clin Pathol 2006;126:506–12.

31. Ronco C, Di Lullo L. Cardiorenal syndrome. Heart Failure Clin 2014;10:251–80.

32. Ricci Z, Ronco C. Pathogenesis of acute kidney injury during sepsis. Curr Drug Targets 2009;10:1179–83.

33. Li X, Hassoun HT, Santora R, et al. Organ crosstalk: the role of the kidney. Curr Opin Crit Care 2009;15:481–7.

34. Virzì GM, Clementi A, Brocca A, et al. Molecular and genetic mechanisms involved in the pathogenesis of cardiorenal cross talk. Pathobiology 2016;83:201–10.

35. Beesley SJ, Weber G, Sarge T, et al. Septic cardiomyopathy. Crit Care Med 2018;46:625–34.

36. Rangel-Frausto MS, Pittet D, Costigan M, et al. The natural history of the systemic inflammatory response syndrome (SIRS). A prospective study. JAMA 1995;273:117–23.

37. Mullens W, Abrahams Z, Skouri HN, et al. Elevated intra-abdominal pressure in acute decompensated heart failure: a potential contributor to worsening renal function? J Am Coll Cardiol 2008;51:300–6.

38. Sugrue M, Buist MD, Hourihan F, et al. Prospective study of intra-abdominal hypertension and renal function after laparotomy. Br J Surg 1995;82:235–8.

39. Kirkpatrick AW, Roberts DJ, De Waele J, et al. Pediatric guidelines subcommittee for the World Society of the Abdominal Compartment Syndrome. Intra-abdominal hypertension and the abdominal compartment syndrome: updated consensus definitions and clinical practice guidelines from the World Society of the Abdominal Compartment Syndrome. Intensive Care Med 2013;39:1190–206.

40. Yancy CW, Jessup M, Bozkurt B, et al. American College of Cardiology Foundation; American Heart Association Task Force on Practice Guidelines. 2013 ACCF/AHA guideline for the management of heart failure: a report of the American College of Cardiology Foundation/American Heart Association Task Force on Practice Guidelines. J Am Coll Cardiol 2013;62:e147–239.

41. Benjamin EJ, Virani SS, Callaway CW, et al. American Heart Association Council on Epidemiology and Prevention Statistics Committee and Stroke Statistics

Subcommittee. Heart disease and stroke statistics-2018 update: a report from the American Heart Association. Circulation 2018;137:e67–492.

42. Rose EA, Gelijns AC, Moskowitz AJ, et al. Randomized evaluation of mechanical assistance for the treatment of congestive heart failure (REMATCH) Study Group. Long-term use of a left ventricular assist device for end-stage heart failure. N Engl J Med 2001;345:1435–43.

43. Brisco MA, Kimmel SE, Coca SG, et al. Prevalence and prognostic importance of changes in renal function after mechanical circulatory support. Circ Heart Fail 2014;7:68–75.

44. Cowger J, Sundareswaran K, Rogers JG, et al. Predicting survival in patients receiving continuous flow left ventricular assist devices: the HeartMate II risk score. J Am Coll Cardiol 2013;6:313–21.

45. Kirklin JK, Naftel DC, Kormos RL, et al. Quantifying the effect of cardiorenal syndrome on mortality after left ventricular assist device implant. J Heart Lung Transplant 2013;32:1205–13.

46. Cook JL, Colvin M, Francis GS, et al. American Heart Association Heart Failure and Transplantation Committee of the Council on Clinical Cardiology; Council on Cardiopulmonary, Critical Care, Perioperative and Resuscitation; Council on Cardiovascular Disease in the Young; Council on Cardiovascular and Stroke Nursing; Council on Cardiovascular Radiology and Intervention; and Council on Cardiovascular Surgery and Anesthesia. Recommendations for the use of mechanical circulatory support: ambulatory and community patient care: a scientific statement from the American Heart Association. Circulation 2017;135:e1145–58.

47. Kirklin JK, Naftel DC, Pagani FD, et al. Seventh INTERMACS annual report: 15,000 patients and counting. J Heart Lung Transplant 2015;34:1495–504.

48. Kamboj M, Kazory A. Left ventricular assist device and the kidney: getting to the heart of the matter. Blood Purif 2019;48:289–98.

49. Raichlin E, Baibhav B, Lowes BD, et al. Outcomes in patients with severe preexisting renal dysfunction after continuous-flow left ventricular assist device implantation. ASAIO J 2016;62:261–7.

50. Brisco MA, Hale A, Zile MR, et al. Patients undergoing LVAD placement demonstrate marked sarcopenia leading to overestimation of pre-implant glomerular filtration rate. J Heart Lung Transplant 2015;34:S165.

51. Pradhan M, Leonard MB, Bridges ND, et al. Decline in renal function following thoracic organ transplantation in children. Am J Transplant 2002;2:652–7.

52. Kolsrud O, Karason K, Holmberg E, et al. Renal function and outcome after heart transplantation. J Thorac Cardiovasc Surg 2018;155:1593–604.

53. Gallo M, Trivedi JR, Schumer EM, et al. Combined heart-kidney transplant versus sequential kidney transplant in heart transplant recipients. J Card Fail 2020; S1071-9164(19):30603–7.

54. Kumar TK, Allen CCP J, Spentzas Md T, et al. Acute kidney injury following cardiac surgery in neonates and young infants: experience of a single center using novel perioperative strategies. World J Pediatr Congenit Heart Surg 2016;7: 460–6.

55. Zappitelli M, Bernier PL, Saczkowski RS, et al. A small post-operative rise in serum creatinine predicts acute kidney injury in children undergoing cardiac surgery. Kidney Int 2009;76:885–92.

56. Blinder JJ, Goldstein SL, Lee VV, et al. Congenital heart surgery in infants: effects of acute kidney injury on outcomes. J Thorac Cardiovasc Surg 2012;143:368–74.

57. Madsen NL, Goldstein SL, Frøslev T, et al. Cardiac surgery in patients with congenital heart disease is associated with acute kidney injury and the risk of chronic kidney disease. Kidney Int 2017;92:751–6.
58. Blinder JJ, Asaro LA, Wypij D, et al. Acute kidney injury after pediatric cardiac surgery: a secondary analysis of the safe pediatric euglycemia after cardiac surgery trial. Pediatr Crit Care Med 2017;18:638–46.
59. Patterson T, Hehir DA, Buelow M, et al. Hemodynamic profile of acute kidney injury following the Fontan procedure: impact of renal perfusion pressure. World J Pediatr Congenit Heart Surg 2017;8:367–75.
60. Webb TN, Goldstein SL. Congenital heart surgery and acute kidney injury. Curr Opin Anaesthesiol 2017;30:105–12.
61. Bianchi P, Carboni G, Pesce G, et al. Cardiac catheterization and postoperative acute kidney failure in congenital heart pediatric patients. Anesth Analg 2013; 117:455–61.
62. Alobaidi R, Basu RK, DeCaen A, et al. Fluid accumulation in critically ill children. Crit Care Med 2020. https://doi.org/10.1097/CCM.0000000000004376.
63. Hassinger AB, Wald EL, Goodman DM. Early postoperative fluid overload precedes acute kidney injury and is associated with higher morbidity in pediatric cardiac surgery patients. Pediatr Crit Care Med 2014;15:131–8.
64. Ricci Z. Fluid overload after neonatal cardiac surgery is bad: keep the bottles on the shelf, squeeze the patients or both? Pediatr Crit Care Med 2016;17:463–5.
65. Park SK, Hur M, Kim E, et al. Risk factors for acute kidney injury after congenital cardiac surgery in infants and children: a retrospective observational study. PLoS One 2016;11:e0166328.
66. Ricci Z, Haiberger R, Pezzella C, et al. Furosemide versus ethacrynic acid in pediatric patients undergoing cardiac surgery: a randomized controlled trial. Crit Care 2015;19:2.
67. Ricci Z, Romagnoli S. Prescription of dialysis in pediatric acute kidney injury. Minerva Pediatr 2015;67:159–67.
68. Kwiatkowski DM, Goldstein SL, Cooper DS, et al. Peritoneal dialysis vs furosemide for prevention of fluid overload in infants after cardiac surgery: a randomized clinical trial. JAMA Pediatr 2017;171:357–64.
69. Ricci Z, Goldstein SL. Pediatric continuous renal replacement therapy. Contrib Nephrol 2016;187:121–30.
70. Thorlacius EM, Suominen PK, Wåhlander H, et al. The effect of levosimendan versus milrinone on the occurrence rate of acute kidney injury following congenital heart surgery in infants: a randomized clinical trial. Pediatr Crit Care Med 2019;20:947–56.
71. Pappachan VJ, Brown KL, Tibby SM. Paediatric cardiopulmonary bypass surgery: the challenges of heterogeneity and identifying a meaningful endpoint for clinical trials. Intensive Care Med 2017;43:113–5.
72. Bronicki RA, Domico M, Checchia PA, et al. The use of nesiritide in children with congenital heart disease. Pediatr Crit Care Med 2017;18:151–8.
73. Ricci Z, Luciano R, Favia I, et al. High-dose fenoldopam reduces postoperative neutrophil gelatinase-associated lipocaline and cystatin C levels in pediatric cardiac surgery. Crit Care 2011;15:R160.
74. Kwiatkowski DM, Axelrod DM, Sutherland SM, et al. Dexmedetomidine is associated with lower incidence of acute kidney injury after congenital heart surgery. Pediatr Crit Care Med 2016;17:128–34.

Neonatal Acute Kidney Injury

Understanding of the Impact on the Smallest Patients

Keegan J. Kavanaugh, MD[a], Jennifer G. Jetton, MD[b],*,
Alison L. Kent, BMBS, FRACP, MD[c,d]

KEYWORDS

- Neonate • Acute kidney injury • Prematurity • Biomarkers • Outcomes

KEY POINTS

- Neonatal acute kidney injury (AKI) is common and associated with adverse short and long-term outcomes.
- The field of neonatal kidney injury research is expanding rapidly, supported by collaboration between neonatologists and nephrologists.
- Advances in the care of critically ill newborns will depend on ongoing improvement in AKI biomarkers and development of evidence-based clinical practice guidelines for AKI surveillance and fluid balance monitoring.

INTRODUCTION

There has been significant progress in the study of neonatal acute kidney injury (AKI), particularly in the past 5 years.[1,2] Much of this new work corroborates what already is known about AKI in general and efforts are being made for advancement in understanding of how this complex syndrome has an impact on neonates. As in older patient groups, AKI is common in neonates, occurring in 40% to 70% of babies cared for in the neonatal intensive care unit (NICU), and neonates with AKI have significantly

[a] Stead Family Department of Pediatrics, University of Iowa, 200 Hawkins Drive, 2015-26 BT, Iowa City, IA 52241, USA; [b] Division of Pediatric Nephrology, Dialysis, and Transplantation, Stead Family Department of Pediatrics, University of Iowa, 200 Hawkins Drive, 2029 BT, Iowa City, IA 52241, USA; [c] Division of Neonatology, Golisano Children's Hospital, University of Rochester School of Medicine, 601 Elmwood Avenue, Box 651, Rochester, NY 14642, USA; [d] College of Health and Medicine, Australian National University, Canberra, Australian Capital Territory 2601, Australia
* Corresponding author.
E-mail address: Jennifer-jetton@uiowa.edu
Twitter: @atomic_kidney (J.G.J.); @Aussiekidney (A.L.K.)

Crit Care Clin 37 (2021) 349–363
https://doi.org/10.1016/j.ccc.2020.11.007
0749-0704/21/© 2020 Elsevier Inc. All rights reserved.

higher mortality rates than those without AKI.[2] With these points in mind, progress is imperative; however, knowledge gaps remain, and more data are needed to support evidence-based clinical practice guidelines. As illustrated in a recent survey examining the perceptions of neonatologists and pediatric nephrologists, there remain significant differences between the fields regarding aspects of assessment and management, such as the utilization of standardized AKI definitions, recognition of early stage AKI, and use of renal support therapy in this setting.[1] In addition, both specialties lack evidence-based guidelines for kidney function monitoring and long-term follow-up after NICU discharge.[1,2]

This article highlights some of the recent advances in the field of neonatal nephrology to aid in understanding of the incidence of AKI and its impact on the smallest patients.[3,4] Using 2 case scenarios, those aspects of neonatal physiology and medical comorbidities are addressed that make the diagnosis and management of neonatal AKI different from those in older populations. Current research in this area is highlighted, much of which is occurring through collaboration between neonatologists and nephrologists. In so doing, the authors hope to tighten the gaps in the collective understanding of neonatal AKI to realize a brighter future for babies with or at risk for kidney disease.

CASE SCENARIO 1

A woman with preexisting hypertension has been reviewed regularly in the high-risk pregnancy clinic. Her baby was noted at 20 weeks' gestation to be in the tenth percentile for estimated fetal weight, with symmetric growth measurements for head circumference and abdominal circumference. By 26 weeks, she has severe preeclampsia, requiring treatment with 3 antihypertensives (methyldopa, labetalol, and intermittent nifedipine). Fetal ultrasound indicates an estimated fetal weight now on the third percentile (560 g), and there is reverse umbilical arterial Doppler flow. She is administered antenatal steroids 48 hours prior to delivery as well as magnesium sulfate infusion for 24 hours for management of hypertension and fetal neuroprotection. Maternal creatinine prior to delivery is 1.2 mg/dL (106 μmol/L). The male baby is delivered by cesarean section at 26 3/7 weeks' gestation, weighing 530 g, managed with intubation and early surfactant, and requires ongoing respiratory support with mechanical ventilation (MV). An echocardiogram at 36 hours detects a 2.4-mm patent ductus arteriosus (PDA) with evidence of hemodynamic significance, and the baby is treated at 48 hours of age with indomethacin. The baby's creatinine at 24 hours of age is 1.4 mg/dL (124 μmol/L), remains 1.4 on day 2 and 1.5 on day 3, but by day of life (DOL) 4 is 2.2 mg/dL (195 μmol/L). The baby has an episode of necrotizing enterocolitis (NEC) treated with piperacillin/tazobactam for 7 days at day 15 and has poor growth, continuing to grow along the first percentile. Creatinine at 5 weeks of life has leveled out at 0.85 mg/dL (75 μmol/L).

Case scenario 1 illustrates the spectrum of issues related to kidney injury in the neonatal period, some unique to this patient group and some common to all critically ill patients. This is not an uncommon scenario—critically ill babies may face multiple exposures and renal insults in the first weeks of life, both prenatal and postnatal. These include growth restriction related to maternal factors, preterm birth associated with chorioamnionitis, postnatal nephrotoxic medication use, and critical events, such as PDA and NEC. This scenario also highlights challenges with interpreting serum creatinine (SCr) changes using standard AKI definitions in the first week of life, especially in preterm infants.

PREMATURITY, LOW BIRTHWEIGHT, AND ACUTE KIDNEY INJURY

Nephron mass plays an important role in susceptibility to AKI as well as long-term kidney health. Nephrogenesis occurs from 5-8 weeks to 34-36 weeks of gestation, with a majority of nephrons formed during the third trimester.[5–8] Nephron counts also show correlation with birthweight. Bertram and colleagues[9] found an increase of 185,000 to 300,000 nephrons per kidney for every kilogram increase in birthweight. Autopsy studies of premature kidneys show that nephrogenesis continues briefly in the newborn period, although in altered and diminished capacity.[6,7,9–11] Thus, babies born extremely premature or with very low birthweight (VLBW) are born with less nephron endowment and nephrons that are abnormal in appearance and likely in function.

Single-center data have shown that VLBW babies are at risk for AKI, with incidence ranging from 4% to 40% across studies.[12] In addition, AKI is associated with increased mortality, with 1 study finding 3.5-fold (adjusted odds ratio [aOR] 3.44; 95% CI, 1.23–9.61) and 2-fold (aOR 1.90; 95% CI, 1.10–3.27) increases in adjusted odds of death, using 1-mg/dL increase and 100% increase in SCr as AKI surrogates, respectively.[13] These data also were confirmed in the recent multicenter Assessment of Worldwide Acute Kidney Injury Epidemiology in Neonates (AWAKEN) study, in which babies in the 22-week to 29-week gestational age (GA) group had a 47.9% incidence of AKI compared with 36.7% in term babies and 18.3% in the 29-week to 36-week GA group.[3]

HIGH-RISK EXPOSURES FOR PRETERM BABIES

In addition to the risks for kidney injury associated with preterm birth, these infants also are at risk for morbidities unique to prematurity that are associated with increased mortality and AKI. Two of these, PDA and NEC, are illustrated in the case scenario 1. The relationship between PDA and AKI is bivariate, depending on both PDA size and treatment. Hemodynamically significant PDA can produce the phenomenon called ductal steal, shunting blood left to right away from systemic circulation, thus compromising perfusion to vital organs, including the kidneys.[14] Management includes either surgical ligation or medical treatment with nonsteroidal anti-inflammatory drugs (NSAIDs), which are known to reduce renal blood flow and alter intrarenal circulation via both cyclooxygenase and prostaglandin inhibition.[15] In 1 recent study of 206 premature neonates in their first month of life, PDA was independently associated with a 5-fold increase in the development of any-stage AKI (OR 5.31; 95% CI, 3.75–7.53), even after adjusting for PDA intervention, including NSAID exposure.[16] This is consistent with findings from previous studies: one showing increased incidence of PDA in infants with AKI compared with those without AKI (41% vs 22.5, respectively; P<.05)[17] and another demonstrating increased incidence of AKI in neonates with PDA versus without PDA (45% vs 11%, respectively; P<.05).[18]

Similarly, NEC is a life-threatening occurrence in premature infants that increases the risk for AKI for several reasons, including its association with a severe systemic inflammatory response, sepsis, hypotension, and treatment, often with several nephrotoxic antimicrobials.[19] Criss and colleagues[20] found an overall incidence of AKI of 54% in neonates with NEC as well as significantly increased mortality in neonates with NEC and AKI (44.1%) compared with neonates without AKI (25.6%; P = .008). This association also was seen in Weintraub and colleagues'[18] (53.3% NEC + AKI vs 26.9% AKI without NEC; P = .000) and Stojanović and colleagues[17] (35.8% vs 9.9%, respectively; P<.001) studies.

NEPHROTOXIC MEDICATION EXPOSURE

Both the conditions, described previously, involve nephrotoxic medications as part of their treatment. The burden of nephrotoxic medication exposure, particularly in VLBW infants, is high. In a study of 107 VLBW neonates, 87% were exposed to at least 1 nephrotoxin during the NICU course.[21] Furthermore, 26% of the exposed group developed AKI, with AKI episodes occurring after nephrotoxin exposure in 47% of cases.[21] Antimicrobials represented a majority of nephrotoxin exposures (5 of the top 6) as expected, given that premature neonates have many sepsis risk factors, including potential infection instigating preterm birth, immature skin, and need for central line access.

Whether or not the AKI risk for these patients is related to the underlying condition, the nephrotoxic therapy, or a combination not always is clear, and balancing the risks and benefits of various treatment strategies is challenging. In the absence of alternatives for these therapies, nephrotoxin stewardship programs, such as Baby Nephrotoxic Injury Negated by Just-in-Time Action (NINJA), are critical for mitigating AKI risk. In an extension of the larger multicenter quality improvement project NINJA in noncritically ill hospitalized children, Stoops and colleagues[22,23] assessed AKI surveillance and incidence rates in the NICU after implementation of an electronic medical record alert system. The investigators compared data over 3 time frames—pre-NINJA, NINJA initiation, and sustainability—in a cohort of 476 newborns over a 30-month period. From the initiation to sustainability phases, they found (1) the prevalence of high nephrotoxin exposure decreased from 16.4 per 1000 patient days to 9.6 per 1000 patient days ($P = .03$); (2) the prevalence of AKI dropped from 5.1 to 1.1 ($P<.001$); (3) the rate of AKI in patients with high nephrotoxin exposure decreased from 30.9% to 11.0% ($P<.001$); and (4) AKI intensity was reduced from 9.1 per 100 susceptible patient-days to 2.9 per 100 susceptible patient-days ($P<.001$).[23] These findings suggest that systematic surveillance of nephrotoxin use is possible and can significantly reduce neonatal AKI events.

ACUTE KIDNEY INJURY DIAGNOSIS AND BIOMARKERS

Case scenario 1 illustrates recognizable AKI risk factors (eg, VLBW, PDA, nephrotoxin exposure, and NEC). Identifying at-risk neonates is critical because traditional AKI biomarkers—SCr and urine output—are limited in their ability to identify AKI early. Although these limitations are common in all patient groups, there are several that are unique to neonates. SCr levels in newborns during the first week of life are not in steady state due to changes in renal blood flow in the transition from intrauterine to extrauterine life, with variability in normal neonatal SCr levels depending on GA and pre/term status.[24,25] Term neonatal glomerular filtration rate (GFR) rises rapidly after birth from 10 mL/min/1.73 m^2 to 40 mL/min/1.73 m^2 through week 1 to week 2 of life, reaching adult function of 100 mL/min/1.73 m^2 to 120 mL/min/1.73 m^2 by age 1.5 years to 2 years.[6,8,11] Preterm neonatal GFR is lower and takes longer to rise. Because the usual AKI definitions rely on a steady-state baseline, SCr, application in these cohorts is difficult. The same is true for urine output. Following birth, babies have an obligate diuresis. Premature neonates have limited ability to concentrate urine, and, although they may have an AKI event, their urine output may not reduce below 0.5 mL/kg/h. As with SCr changes, these physiologic changes in urine production are not captured adequately in AKI definitions used in pediatric and adult patients and likely account, at least in part, for why the widespread use of a standardized definition has not occurred in neonatal AKI research until recently. In addition, both the Baby NINJA and AWAKEN studies showed that frequency of SCr monitoring is highly variable across centers. In the AWAKEN study, the median frequency of SCr checks over the 3-month period ranged from 1 to 11, with some trend toward higher rates of AKI in the centers that check more frequently.[3] In the Baby NINJA study, SCr compliance (obtaining daily SCr until the end of AKI or 2 days after end of nephrotoxin exposure) was 56.5% in the pre-NINJA era, compared with 90.7% and 86.1% in initiation and sustainability eras, respectively.[23]

In an effort to advance neonatal AKI research efforts, a modification of the Kidney Disease: Improving Global Outcomes (mKDIGO) AKI definition (neonatal mKDIGO) was endorsed at a multidisciplinary, National Institutes of Health–sponsored conference for use and further validation (**Table 1**).[26–28] Although empiric, the adaptation of this definition has allowed for testing in a range of NICU subpopulations and GAs. Moreover, the use of a common definition has enabled cross-study comparisons, an important development because many studies have small sample sizes.

Although the development of a standardized definition for neonatal AKI represents a critical step, additional validation and optimization are needed. This definition has been tested mostly in small, single-center samples.[4,27,29] More recently, the mKIDGO definition was used in AWAKEN, the largest study of neonatal AKI to date.[3,4,29] This international study of more than 2000 newborns showed that neonates who met AKI criteria using this definition had higher risk of mortality (aOR 4.6; 95% CI, 2.5–8.3; $P<.0001$) and longer hospital stay (8.8 days; 95% CI, 6.1–11.5; $P<.0001$), even after controlling for multiple confounders.[3,26,29,30]

In an effort to optimize the definition, Askenazi and colleagues[4] sought to clarify the variability in SCr thresholds by GA.[4,30] The results showed that absolute SCr rise outperformed percent change rise in SCr in the ability to predict mortality. In addition, the absolute SCr rise cutoffs are higher in < 29 week GA neonates than in >29 weeks GA babies (> 0.6 in <29 weeks vs. > 0.3 mg/dL in > 29 weeks GA).[30] This analysis looked only at the first week of life, and the biomarker cutpoints took into account only changes in SCr and not urine output. More work is needed to optimize the standardized neonatal AKI definition, recognizing that different definitions may be required for premature and term infants as well as those in and past the first week of life.

NOVEL ACUTE KIDNEY INJURY BIOMARKERS

As discussed previously, it is well known that SCr is a suboptimal biomarker for AKI because it is a marker of kidney function, not damage.[26,27,30] SCr changes are delayed, up to 72 hours after insult, and may not be apparent until there is greater than 50% loss of GFR.[20,26,27,30] Thus, more accurate biomarkers are needed, with some now showing promise.[31,32]

Table 1
Modified Kidney Disease: Improving Global Outcomes classification

Stage	Serum Creatinine	Urine Output
0	No change in SCr or rise <0.3 mg/dL	>1 mL/kg/h
I	SCr rise $\geq$ 0.3 mg/dL within 48 h OR SCr rise $\geq$ 1.5–1.9 × reference SCr within 7 d	>0.5 and $\leq$ 1 mL/kg/h
II	SCr rise $\geq$ 2.0–2.9 × reference SCr	>0.3 and $\leq$ 0.5 mL/kg/h
III	SCr rise $\geq$ 3 × reference SCr OR SCr $\geq$ 2.5 mg/dL OR dialysis	$\leq$ 0.3 mL/kg/h

Although many urinary biomarkers have been identified, neutrophil gelatinase–associated lipocalin (NGAL), cystatin C (CysC), and tissue inhibitor of metalloproteinases-2 (TIMP2)/insulinlike growth factor binding protein 7 (IGFBP7) show the most potential to be incorporated into routine clinical practice (**Table 2**).[31] NGAL, a protein bound to neutrophil granules present in multiple tissue types, is thought to have numerous functional roles, including innate immune response and the promotion of epithelial proliferation in times of injury.[31,33] Serum NGAL normally is filtered by the glomerulus and reabsorbed in the proximal tubule, with increased urine NGAL suggestive of AKI, especially when AKI is associated with tubular damage.[31,33] CysC is a cysteine protease inhibitor produced by all nucleated cells; it is freely filtered by the glomerulus and completely reabsorbed and catabolized by the proximal tubule.[31,33] Both serum and urine levels have been considered in AKI diagnostics, with increases in serum and urine levels indicative of changes in GFR and tubular injury, respectively.[31,34,35]

In VLBW neonates with SCr-diagnosed AKI on DOL4 (as in case scenario 1), Askenazi and colleagues[36] found urinary NGAL and urinary CysC levels already peaking on DOL0 and DOL1, respectively.[31] Similarly, in another study, urinary NGAL and urinary CysC levels both were significantly elevated in preterm neonates with AKI versus non-AKI controls (NGAL: 0.598 µg/mL vs 4.24 µg/mL, respectively; $P<.0001$; CysC control: 0.98 µg/mL vs AKI 6.09 µg/mL, respectively; $P<.001$) on the day of and day before AKI diagnosis by KDIGO criteria.[37] In sepsis, urine NGAL and serum NGAL have been shown to be elevated in neonates without AKI, whereas CysC remained stable, suggestive of diminished utility of NGAL in this subpopulation.[31,38,39] Finally, there are robust data investigating these biomarkers in neonates with hypoxic ischemic insults. Sweetman and colleagues[34] found urinary NGAL and urinary CysC levels were significantly elevated on DOL1, DOL3, and DOL10 in newborns with AKI and hypoxic ischemic encephalopathy (HIE).[31,40] Furthermore, Sarafidis and colleagues[41] found similar results in asphyxiated newborns, with elevated levels of urinary NGAL and urinary CysC strongly predictive of AKI on DOL1[31,34,42] (**Fig. 1**).

Urinary TIMP2/IGFBP7 has shown promise in detecting AKI in critically ill adults, pediatric and adult patients undergoing cardiac surgery,[2,43,44] and children and neonates in other settings.[31,43] In a retrospective study of 237 neonates, urinary TIMP2/IGFBP7 levels measured 0 to 5 days prior to AKI diagnosis were significantly higher in the severe AKI group compared with the non-AKI group.[43]

Table 2
Potential clinical urinary biomarkers to diagnose acute kidney injury

Urinary Biomarker	Renal Area of Injury	Increase or Decrease	Normal Values	Area Under the Curve
CysC	Proximal tubule	Increases	1.64–2.59 mg/L 0–3 DOL 1.52–2.40 mg/L 3–30 DOL	Term neonates—0.89–0.93 Preterm neonates—0.68
NGAL	Ascending limb and proximal tubule	Increases	2–150 ng/mL	Term neonates —0.86–0.91 Preterm neonates—0.73 Following bypass—0.85
TIMP2/ IGFBP7	Proximal and distal tubule	Increases	>0.03 (ng/mL)^2	Neonates—0.71 Following bypass—0.85

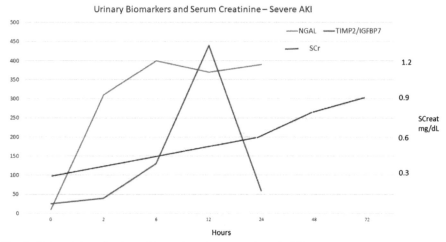

Fig. 1. Rate of rise of urinary biomarkers in comparison to SCr.

Although novel AKI biomarkers have potential, reference ranges for these may vary by GA, sex, and birthweight.[31] The studies of these urinary biomarkers in neonates has been confined to specific subpopulations, and more extensive normative data for neonates is required.[31] As in adult and pediatric populations, urinary biomarkers are being compared with the gold standard of SCr, which requires a reduction in function of up to 50% before a change is detected. AKI diagnosis may require a different approach in the future, utilizing biomarkers in place of SCr.

CASE SCENARIO 2

A term infant is delivered at an outlying hospital with HIE. Apgar scores were 1, 1, and 3 at 1 minute, 5 minutes, and 10 minutes of life, respectively. Cord pH was 6.95, base excess 17, and lactate 15. The baby was intubated and ventilated, and cooling was commenced at the outlying center. Following transfer to a tertiary referral center, the neonate had evidence of multiorgan injury, requiring several antiepileptic medications to control seizures, hypotension requiring dobutamine and epinephrine infusions, disseminated intravascular coagulopathy requiring fresh frozen plasma infusions, and thrombocytopenia requiring platelet transfusions. In total, the baby received 6 bolus infusions and gained 20% over birthweight. SCr at 6 hours of life was 1.4 mg/dL (124 μmol/L) (maternal creatinine 0.5 mg/dL [44 μmol/L]) and increased to 2.8 mg/dL (248 μmol/L) at 48 hours of life, with urine output 0.3 mL/kg/h.

This common scenario demonstrates an AKI event in a term infants, occurring intrapartum and then continuing with postnatal insult from poor perfusion and subsequent fluid overload (FO). Although preterm infants have unique factors that make them vulnerable to AKI, term babies also are at risk. As discussed previously, the rate of AKI in term babies (≥36 weeks' GA) in AWAKEN was 38% compared with the 18.1% incidence in the 29-week to 36-week GA group.[3] Even after discharge, term infants who become ill are at risk, as shown in a study of 80 term neonates less than 28 days admitted to a pediatric ICU. In this cohort, the overall incidence of AKI was high, 35% and 46% by KDIGO and pRIFLE criteria, respectively.[45] Mortality also was significantly higher than in subjects without AKI (28.6 vs 9.6%, respectively; $P = .03$).[45]

ACUTE KIDNEY INJURY AND THE INTERPLAY WITH OTHER ORGAN SYSTEMS

Case scenario 2 highlights AKI as part of a complex syndrome involving multiple organs. Several recent studies have examined the relationship between AKI and the brain in neonatal cohorts. Stoops and colleagues[46] studied 825 premature neonates from the AWAKEN cohort, finding increased likelihood of intraventricular hemorrhage in the AKI group compared with the non-AKI group (27% vs 11%, respectively; P<.0001). After adjustment for potential confounders, babies with AKI had a 1.6-times higher odds of developing any stage intraventricular hemorrhage (95% CI, 1.04–2.56; P = .0347) than those without AKI.[46] Similarly, Kirkley and colleagues[47] examined 113 near-term/term infants with HIE and found that AKI was common (41.6%) and associated with an 8.5-day longer hospital stay (95% CI, 0.79–16.2 d; P = .03). These data are consistent with previous studies. Sarkar and colleagues[48] found AKI independently associated with hypoxic-ischemic lesions on brain magnetic resonance imaging at DOL7 to DOL10 in a population of asphyxiated neonates treated with therapeutic hypothermia (odds ratio [OR] 2.9; 95% CI, 1.1–7.6). In addition, Cavallin and colleagues[49] evaluated the prognostic role of AKI in neurodevelopmental outcomes in neonates with HIE treated with therapeutic hypothermia, finding increased likelihood of unfavorable outcome (death or disability) in neonates with AKI compared with those without AKI at both 12 months (78% AKI vs 39% no AKI; P = .03) and 24 months (100% with unfavorable outcome in AKI group vs 59% in the no AKI group).

The association between AKI and lung disease has been described in adult patients; several recent studies also have explored this relationship in neonates. Starr and colleagues[50] examined the association between bronchopulmonary dysplasia and AKI in 546 premature infants. Infants 29 weeks' GA to 32 weeks' GA with AKI had 4-times higher odds of developing moderate/severe bronchopulmonary dysplasia or death (aOR 3.82; CI, 1.84–7.96; P<.001), although this association was not seen in the GA less than or equal to 29 weeks group. In a companion study of 1348 near-term/term neonates, babies with AKI had a nearly 5-fold increased odds of chronic lung disease/death (aOR 4.57; CI, 2.92–7.17; P<.0001).[51] These infants also required longer duration of both invasive and noninvasive respiratory support as well as longer need for oxygen supplementation.

Other morbidity associated with neonatal AKI includes hypertension. Kraut and colleagues[52] showed that both diagnosed and undiagnosed neonatal hypertension were 2 times more likely in those with AKI (aOR 2.1; 95% CI, 1.4–3.1; P = .004). Mechanistically, AKI results in hypertension through complex intrarenal and extrarenal effects, including parenchymal renal damage and the formation of inflammatory mediators, that ultimately disrupt renal autoregulation via aberrant functionality of pathways like the renin-angiotensin-aldosterone system. Along with hypertension, this dysregulation can further result in electrolyte abnormalities, reduced urine output, and FO.[52]

All these disease processes involve systemic inflammation such that there may be potential inflammatory communication pathways through which to 1 organ may have an impact on and communicate to others. Further examination of AKI responses and relationships to other organs and disease processes is required.

FLUID BALANCE AND FLUID OVERLOAD

Fluid balance and its pathogenic extension, FO, has been shown in pediatric and adult populations to impact outcomes. Data supporting this relationship in neonates are not as robust.[53–55] Case scenario 2 demonstrates how quickly FO can occur in a baby with multiorgan failure and AKI. In a small study of AKI and FO in sick near-term/term neonates, Askenazi and colleagues[53] found a positive 8.2% weight change by DOL3 in neonates with AKI compared to negative 4% in the non-AKI group (P<.001).[26] The positive weight change in AKI is striking when accounting for the obligate diuresis of 5% to 10% of body weight expected following birth. Survival in the AKI group was lower than in the non-AKI group (77% vs 100%, respectively; P = .02).[26,53] Selewski and colleagues[54] demonstrated a similar association between FO and AKI in this GA group using AWAKEN data. Babies with AKI had consistently higher fluid balances throughout that week.[55] Furthermore, the need for MV on DOL7 was independently associated with peak fluid balance in week 1 of life and fluid balance on DOL7.[54] In a related analysis of preterm infants (<36 weeks), the relationship between AKI, ability to achieve a negative fluid balance by day 7, and need for MV on day 7 again was seen.[55] These studies together demonstrate important implications of fluid balance on clinical outcomes across GA: with every 1% rise in maximum fluid balance, there were 12% and 14% increased odds of receiving MV at postnatal day 7 (term: aOR 1.12; 95% CI, 1.08–1.17; P<.0001; premature: aOR 1.14; 95% CI, 1.10–1.19; P<.0001).[54,55] Fluid management in sick neonates thus requires careful consideration, and strategies to minimize FO, especially those with AKI, require an understanding of its influence on poor outcomes.

NEONATAL ACUTE KIDNEY INJURY AND LONG-TERM OUTCOMES

Follow-up of adult and pediatric patients who have sustained an AKI event have shown an increased risk of chronic kidney disease (CKD), challenging the notion that AKI is an isolated event after which the return to full kidney function is expected. The association between prematurity, low birthweight, and long-term CKD risk has been described for some time, although only limited data are available exploring the relationship of neonatal AKI to outcomes. In their review of long-term renal outcomes after neonatal AKI, Harer and colleagues[56] found that in 3 of 4 studies there was a significant increase in evidence of CKD as assessed by estimated GFR, renal volume, proteinuria, and hypertension. One study found no difference in rates of CKD between patients with a history of neonatal AKI and those without,[57] whereas 2 others found rates of renal dysfunction as high as 55% to 65%.[56,58,59] Although these data are compelling, large, multicenter longitudinal cohorts are needed to understand more fully the risks related to neonatal AKI and long-term CKD, controlling for confounders.

CURRENT DEVELOPMENTS IN NEONATAL ACUTE KIDNEY INJURY MANAGEMENT: CAFFEINE AND CONTINUOUS RENAL REPLACEMENT THERAPY

As in all patient groups, there are no proved treatment strategies for AKI once it has occurred. However, 2 pharmacologic interventions, theophylline and caffeine, both adenosine receptor antagonists thought to act on A_1 and A_{2A} receptors in the kidneys (thereby inhibiting vasoconstrictive effects of adenosine), have been examined in neonatal populations. Four small studies of the use of theophylline in babies with perinatal asphyxia demonstrated some modest effect in preventing or ameliorating AKI as evidenced by improved urine output.[60,61] All these studies, however, were conducted prior to the widespread use of cooling. Based on these limited but positive data, KDIGO AKI guidelines suggest consideration for a single dose of theophylline to be given within 6 hours of birth to babies with perinatal asphyxia, although this strategy needs to be confirmed in a randomized controlled trial.[62] Two more recent studies have examined the relationship between caffeine and AKI in preterm babies. In a small single-center study, Carmody and colleagues[63] found decreased incidence of (AKI in 17.8% patients treated with caffeine vs. 43.6% in patients not treated). More recently, Harer and colleagues[64] examined the association between early caffeine administration (within first 7 DOLs) in preterm infants less than 33 weeks and AKI utilizing AWAKEN data. Caffeine-exposed babies had a decreased incidence of AKI compared with non–caffeine-exposed group (50 of 447 [11.2%] vs 72 of 228 [31.6%], respectively; P<.01).[64] Furthermore, neonates treated with caffeine had significantly reduced odds of severe AKI (stage II–III) (aOR 0.20; 95% CI, 0.12–0.34), despite the fact they had increased risk factors, including lower average GA, lower birthweight, increased likelihood of intubation and requirement of further respiratory support, higher severity of illness scores, and increased nephrotoxin exposure.[64] These results suggest prophylactic use of caffeine in preterm neonates may be reasonable to mitigate AKI risk though additional investigation, specifically regarding dosage and timing of administration, is still warranted.

For management of severe AKI and FO, continuous renal replacement therapy (CRRT) frequently is used in pediatric and adult populations. Use in the neonatal population, however, has remained limited primarily due to lack of equipment designed and appropriately sized for small infants.[65–68] Peritoneal dialysis is well tolerated in infants, although for babies as small as the neonate in case scenario 1 (generally <1–1.5 kg), there are no commercially available catheters small enough for use in this patient group. A handful of case reports and case series are available in the literature describing novel uses of a variety of lines and catheters in extreme circumstances. There currently is only1 CRRT device with Food and Drug Administration (FDA) approval specifically designed for patients less than 20 kg. The Cardio-Renal Pediatric Dialysis Emergency Machine (CARPEDIEM) has been used in Europe in neonates as small as 2 kg and received FDA approval in April 2020 for use in patients 2.5-10 kg with AKI and fluid overload in the United States.[2,65,66] The Aquadex FlexFlow System (CHF Solutions, Eden Prairie, Minnesota) is another device, originally designed for adults with congenital heart failure, that has been adapted for use for CRRT in infants.[67] The benefits of this circuit are the small extracorporeal volume, as low as 33 mL; the ability to use a smaller vascular catheter; and the ability to avoid blood prime in babies as small as 4 kg. Experience from 3 centers using this device recently was published in a multicenter retrospective study by Menon and colleagues.[68] This study included 72 patients less than 10 kg with AKI, with the smallest patient being 1.4 kg. As documented in other studies, hospital survival rates for the patients less than 10 kg supported with CRRT were much lower than those seen in patients greater than 20 kg (32% vs 68%, respectively).[68] Treatment survival in patients less than 10 kg was 60% compared with 97% of those greater than 20 kg.[68] Whether the widespread use of machines specifically designed for neonates like CARPEDIEM allows for improved survival outcomes remains to be seen.

SUMMARY

This review highlights recent progress in the field of neonatal AKI. Through intensification of research in this area, there has been a better understanding of the impact of AKI on both short-term and long-term outcomes as well as the factors that put babies most at risk. More also is understood about how those risk factors and outcomes differ between premature and near-term/term infants. As in older patients, AKI in neonates appears to be part of a systemic inflammatory process with the potential for profound complications across organ systems. It thus is imperative to continue to accumulate high-quality data to support the development of guidelines that will allow progressing in the diagnosis and management of this complex syndrome. Research priorities include ongoing optimization of the neonatal AKI definition as well as more widespread acceptance and use of alternative AKI biomarkers independent of SCr. Additionally, it is paramount to make continued efforts at AKI prevention. The Baby NINJA study offers proof of concept that surveillance and mitigation strategies aimed specifically at nephrotoxin stewardship and kidney function monitoring and documentation can and should be implemented more widely across NICUs. Center-specific investigation and protocols could be developed further through quality improvement programs. The development of evidence-based, long-term follow-up guidelines also is a priority in order to understand improve the impact of neonatal AKI on long-term kidney health as the smallest patients enter childhood and adulthood.

CLINICS CARE POINTS[15,69,70]

Short-term AKI mitigation strategies
- Develop center-specific AKI surveillance guidelines to increase AKI monitoring (while minimizing laboratory burden) during high-risk clinical events (eg, NEC, PDA, and HIE), with input from interdisciplinary teams, including neonatologists, nephrologists, pharmacists, and nursing staff.
- Develop center-specific guidelines aimed at nephrotoxin stewardship (eg, SCr and drug level monitoring and limiting number of nephrotoxic medication exposures when clinically feasible).
- Document parameters related to kidney health and AKI in the daily progress note, including urine output, fluid balance, and blood pressure.
- Document AKI episodes in the daily progress note and discharge summary.
- Develop outpatient referral guidelines in collaboration with pediatric nephrology colleagues. High-risk babies could include those with AKI stage 2 or higher, history of multiple AKI events, and/or severe AKI requiring dialysis, especially in low-birthweight/preterm babies.

Strategies to support long-term renal health
- Document birth history and birthweight in the medical record.
- Support healthy kidney habits throughout childhood through primary and specialty nephrology care when appropriate (eg, maintain a healthy weight, monitor blood pressure, avoid NSAIDs, and avoid dehydration).
- Reduce other risk factors for CKD (obesity, diabetes, hypertension, and dyslipidemia), especially in patients with history of LBW/prematurity.

DISCLOSURE

The authors have nothing to disclose.

REFERENCES

1. Kent A, Charlton J, Guillet R, et al. Neonatal acute kidney injury: a survey of neonatologists' and nephrologists' perceptions and practice management. Am J Perinatol 2018;35(01):001–9.
2. Goldstein SL. Pediatric acute kidney injury—the time for nihilism is over. Front Pediatr 2020;8:16.
3. Jetton JG, Boohaker LJ, Sethi SK, et al. Incidence and outcomes of neonatal acute kidney injury (AWAKEN): a multicentre, multinational, observational cohort study. Lancet Child Adolesc Health 2017;1(3):184–94.
4. Askenazi DJ. AWAKEN-ing a new frontier in neonatal nephrology. Front Pediatr 2020;8:21.

5. Matsell DG, Hiatt MJ. Functional development of the kidney in Utero. In: Polin RA, Abman SH, Rowitch DH, et al, editors. Fetal and Neonatal Physiology. 5th Edition. Elsevier; 2017. p. 965–76.e3.

6. Jetton JG, Selewski DT, Charlton JR, et al. Pathophysiology of neonatal acute kidney injury. Fetal and Neonatal Physiology 2017;1668–76.e3. Elsevier.

7. Faa G, Gerosa C, Fanni D, et al. Marked interindividual variability in renal maturation of preterm infants: lessons from autopsy. J Matern Fetal Neonatal Med 2010;23(sup3):129–33.

8. Sulemanji M, Vakili K. Neonatal renal physiology. Semin Pediatr Surg 2013;22(4):195-8.

9. Bertram JF, Douglas-Denton RN, Diouf B, et al. Human nephron number: implications for health and disease. Pediatr Nephrol 2011;26(9):1529.

10. Rodríguez MM, Gómez AH, Abitbol CL, et al. Histomorphometric analysis of postnatal glomerulogenesis in extremely preterm infants. Pediatr Dev Pathol 2004; 7(1):17–25.

11. Nada A, Bonachea EM, Askenazi DJ. Acute kidney injury in the fetus and neonate. Paper presented at: Seminars in Fetal and Neonatal Medicine2017.

12. Perico N, Askenazi D, Cortinovis M, et al. Maternal and environmental risk factors for neonatal AKI and its long-term consequences. Nat Rev Nephrol 2018;14(11): 688–703.

13. Askenazi DJ, Griffin R, McGwin G, et al. Acute kidney injury is independently associated with mortality in very low birthweight infants: a matched case–control analysis. Pediatr Nephrol 2009;24(5):991–7.

14. Benitz WE. Patent ductus arteriosus in preterm infants. Pediatrics 2016;137(1): e20153730.

15. Murphy HJ, Thomas B, Van Wyk B, et al. Nephrotoxic medications and acute kidney injury risk factors in the neonatal intensive care unit: clinical challenges for neonatologists and nephrologists. Pediatr Nephrol 2019;35(11):1–12.

16. Majed B, Bateman DA, Uy N, et al. Patent ductus arteriosus is associated with acute kidney injury in the preterm infant. Pediatr Nephrol 2019;34(6):1129–39.

17. Stojanović V, Barišić N, Milanović B, et al. Acute kidney injury in preterm infants admitted to a neonatal intensive care unit. Pediatr Nephrol 2014;29(11):2213–20.

18. Weintraub A, Connors J, Carey A, et al. The spectrum of onset of acute kidney injury in premature infants less than 30 weeks gestation. J Perinatol 2016;36(6): 474–80.

19. Garg PM, Tatum R, Ravisankar S, et al. Necrotizing enterocolitis in a mouse model leads to widespread renal inflammation, acute kidney injury, and disruption of renal tight junction proteins. Pediatr Res 2015;78(5):527–32.

20. Criss CN, Selewski DT, Sunkara B, et al. Acute kidney injury in necrotizing enterocolitis predicts mortality. Pediatr Nephrol 2018;33(3):503–10.

21. Rhone ET, Carmody JB, Swanson JR, et al. Nephrotoxic medication exposure in very low birth weight infants. J Matern Fetal Neonatal Med 2014;27(14):1485–90.

22. Goldstein SL, Mottes T, Simpson K, et al. A sustained quality improvement program reduces nephrotoxic medication-associated acute kidney injury. Kidney Int 2016;90(1):212–21.

23. Stoops C, Stone S, Evans E, et al. Baby NINJA (Nephrotoxic injury negated by just-in-time action): reduction of nephrotoxic medication-associated acute kidney injury in the neonatal intensive care unit. J Pediatr 2019;215:223–8. e226.

24. Askenazi DJ, Ambalavanan N, Goldstein SL. Acute kidney injury in critically ill newborns: what do we know? What do we need to learn? Pediatr Nephrol 2009;24(2):265.

25. Zappitelli M, Ambalavanan N, Askenazi DJ, et al. Developing a neonatal acute kidney injury research definition: a report from the NIDDK neonatal AKI workshop. Pediatr Res 2017;82(4):569–73.
26. Selewski DT, Charlton JR, Jetton JG, et al. Neonatal acute kidney injury. Pediatrics 2015;136(2):e463–73.
27. Jetton JG, Askenazi DJ. Acute kidney injury in the neonate. Clin Perinatol 2014; 41(3):487–502.
28. Jetton JG, Askenazi DJ. Update on acute kidney injury in the neonate. Curr Opin Pediatr 2012;24(2):191.
29. Jetton JG, Guillet R, Askenazi DJ, et al. Assessment of worldwide acute kidney injury epidemiology in neonates: design of a retrospective cohort study. Front Pediatr 2016;4:68.
30. Askenazi D, Abitbol C, Boohaker L, et al. Optimizing the AKI definition during first postnatal week using assessment of worldwide acute kidney injury epidemiology in neonates (AWAKEN) cohort. Pediatr Res 2019;85(3):329–38.
31. Dyson A, Kent A. Diagnosis of acute kidney injury in neonates: can urinary biomarkers help? Curr Treat Options Pediatr 2018;4(4):425–37.
32. Basu RK. Dynamic biomarker assessment: a diagnostic paradigm to match the AKI syndrome. Front Pediatr 2020;7:535.
33. Mishra J, Mori K, Ma Q, et al. Amelioration of ischemic acute renal injury by neutrophil gelatinase-associated lipocalin. J Am Soc Nephrol 2004;15(12): 3073–82.
34. Sweetman DU. Neonatal acute kidney injury–Severity and recovery prediction and the role of serum and urinary biomarkers. Early Hum Dev 2017;105:57–61.
35. Kandasamy Y, Smith R, Wright IM. Measuring cystatin C to determine renal function in neonates. Pediatr Crit Care Med 2013;14(3):318–22.
36. Askenazi DJ, Koralkar R, Patil N, et al. Acute kidney injury urine biomarkers in very low-birth-weight infants. Clin J Am Soc Nephrol 2016;11(9):1527–35.
37. Hanna M, Brophy PD, Giannone PJ, et al. Early urinary biomarkers of acute kidney injury in preterm infants. Pediatr Res 2016;80(2):218–23.
38. Li Y, Li X, Zhou X, et al. Impact of sepsis on the urinary level of interleukin-18 and cystatin C in critically ill neonates. Pediatr Nephrol 2013;28(1):135–44.
39. Smertka M, Wroblewska J, Suchojad A, et al. Serum and urinary NGAL in septic newborns. Biomed Res Int 2014;2014:717318.
40. Sweetman DU, Onwuneme C, Watson WR, et al. Renal function and novel urinary biomarkers in infants with neonatal encephalopathy. Acta Paediatr 2016;105(11): e513–9.
41. Sarafidis K, Tsepkentzi E, Agakidou E, et al. Serum and urine acute kidney injury biomarkers in asphyxiated neonates. Pediatr Nephrol 2012;27(9):1575–82.
42. El Raggal N, Khafagy SM, Mahmoud N, et al. Serum neutrophil gelatinase-associated lipocalin as a marker of acute kidney injury in asphyxiated neonates. Indian Pediatr 2013;50(5):459–62.
43. Chen J, Sun Y, Wang S, et al. The effectiveness of urinary TIMP-2 and IGFBP-7 in predicting acute kidney injury in critically ill neonates. Pediatr Res 2019; 87(6):1–8.
44. Meersch M, Schmidt C, Hoffmeier A, et al. Prevention of cardiac surgery-associated AKI by implementing the KDIGO guidelines in high risk patients identified by biomarkers: the PrevAKI randomized controlled trial. Intensive Care Med 2017;43(11):1551–61.
45. Kriplani DS, Sethna CB, Leisman DE, et al. Acute kidney injury in neonates in the PICU. Pediatr Crit Care Med 2016;17(4):e159–64.

46. Stoops C, Boohaker L, Sims B, et al. The association of intraventricular hemorrhage and acute kidney injury in premature infants from the assessment of the worldwide acute kidney injury epidemiology in neonates (AWAKEN) study. Neonatology 2019;116(4):321–30.

47. Kirkley MJ, Boohaker L, Griffin R, et al. Acute kidney injury in neonatal encephalopathy: an evaluation of the AWAKEN database. Pediatr Nephrol 2019;34(1): 169–76.

48. Sarkar S, Askenazi DJ, Jordan BK, et al. Relationship between acute kidney injury and brain MRI findings in asphyxiated newborns after therapeutic hypothermia. Pediatr Res 2014;75(3):431–5.

49. Cavallin F, Rubin G, Vidal E, et al. Prognostic role of acute kidney injury on long-term outcome in infants with hypoxic-ischemic encephalopathy. Pediatr Nephrol 2020;35(3):477–83.

50. Starr MC, Boohaker L, Eldredge LC, et al. Acute kidney injury and bronchopulmonary dysplasia in premature neonates born less than 32 weeks' gestation. Am J Perinatol 2020;37(03):341–8.

51. Starr MC, Boohaker L, Eldredge LC, et al. Acute kidney injury is associated with poor lung outcomes in infants born≥ 32 weeks of gestational age. Am J Perinatol 2020;37(02):231–40.

52. Kraut EJ, Boohaker LJ, Askenazi DJ, et al. Incidence of neonatal hypertension from a large multicenter study [Assessment of worldwide acute kidney injury epidemiology in neonates—AWAKEN]. Pediatr Res 2018;84(2):279–89.

53. Askenazi DJ, Koralkar R, Hundley HE, et al. Fluid overload and mortality are associated with acute kidney injury in sick near-term/term neonate. Pediatr Nephrol 2013;28(4):661–6.

54. Selewski DT, Akcan-Arikan A, Bonachea EM, et al. The impact of fluid balance on outcomes in critically ill near-term/term neonates: a report from the AWAKEN study group. Pediatr Res 2019;85(1):79–85.

55. Selewski DT, Gist KM, Nathan AT, et al. The impact of fluid balance on outcomes in premature neonates: a report from the AWAKEN study group. Pediatr Res 2020;87(3):550–7.

56. Harer MW, Charlton JR, Tipple TE, et al. Preterm birth and neonatal acute kidney injury: implications on adolescent and adult outcomes. J Perinatol 2020; 40(9):1–10.

57. Maqsood S, Fung N, Chowdhary V, et al. Outcome of extremely low birth weight infants with a history of neonatal acute kidney injury. Pediatr Nephrol 2017;32(6): 1035–43.

58. Abitbol CL, Bauer CR, Montané B, et al. Long-term follow-up of extremely low birth weight infants with neonatal renal failure. Pediatr Nephrol 2003;18(9): 887–93.

59. Harer MW, Pope CF, Conaway MR, et al. Follow-up of acute kidney injury in neonates during childhood years (FANCY): a prospective cohort study. Pediatr Nephrol 2017;32(6):1067–76.

60. Bhatt GC, Gogia P, Bitzan M, et al. Theophylline and aminophylline for prevention of acute kidney injury in neonates and children: a systematic review. Arch Dis Child 2019;104(7):670–9.

61. Kellum JA, Lameire N, Group KAGW. Diagnosis, evaluation, and management of acute kidney injury: a KDIGO summary (Part 1). Crit Care 2013;17(1):204.

62. Kellum JA, Lameire N, Aspelin P, et al. Kidney disease: improving global outcomes (KDIGO) acute kidney injury work group. KDIGO clinical practice guideline for acute kidney injury. Kidney Int Suppl 2012;2(1):1–138.

63. Carmody JB, Harer MW, Denotti AR, et al. Caffeine exposure and risk of acute kidney injury in a retrospective cohort of very low birth weight neonates. J Pediatr 2016;172:63–8. e61.

64. Harer MW, Askenazi DJ, Boohaker LJ, et al. Association between early caffeine citrate administration and risk of acute kidney injury in preterm neonates: results from the AWAKEN Study. JAMA Pediatr 2018;172(6):e180322.

65. Ronco C, Garzotto F, Brendolan A, et al. Continuous renal replacement therapy in neonates and small infants: development and first-in-human use of a miniaturised machine (CARPEDIEM). Lancet 2014;383(9931):1807–13.

66. Lorenzin A, Garzotto F, Alghisi A, et al. CVVHD treatment with CARPEDIEM: small solute clearance at different blood and dialysate flows with three different surface area filter configurations. Pediatr Nephrol 2016;31(10):1659–65.

67. Askenazi D, Ingram D, White S, et al. Smaller circuits for smaller patients: improving renal support therapy with Aquadex™. Pediatr Nephrol 2016;31(5):853–60.

68. Menon S, Broderick J, Munshi R, et al. Kidney support in children using an ultra-filtration device: a multicenter, retrospective study. Clin J Am Soc Nephrol 2019;14(10):1432–40.

69. Dyson A, Kent AL. The effect of preterm birth on renal development and renal health outcome. Neoreviews 2019;20(12):e725–36.

70. Vincent K, Murphy HJ, Ross JR, et al. Acute kidney injury guidelines are associated with improved recognition and follow-up for neonatal patients. Adv Neonatal Care 2020;20(4):269–75.

Onconephrology

Jaya Kala, MD*, Kevin W. Finkel, MD, FCCM

KEYWORDS

- Acute kidney injury in cancer • Tumor lysis syndrome • Cast nephropathy
- CAR-T cell therapy • Chemotherapy induced kidney injury
- Cancer related thrombotic microangiopathy • Sinusoidal occlusion syndrome
- Hematopoietic stem cell transplantation induced kidney injury

KEY POINTS

- Acute kidney injury is common in patients with cancer.
- Patients with cancer who are critically ill have the highest risk of acute kidney injury.
- Acute kidney injury is associated with increased morbidity, mortality, length of stay, and costs in hospitalized patients with cancer.
- Patients with malignancy can develop kidney diseases similar to other acutely and chronically ill patients and are also at risk for unique kidney syndromes because of either the cancer itself or its treatment.
- It is important for nephrologists to have knowledge about newer chemotherapeutics and understand the pathophysiology of the renal injury caused by them, which will help guide treatment.

INTRODUCTION

Onconephrology is a rapidly growing field within nephrology. According to the American Cancer Society, Cancer Facts & Figures 2020 Annual report, more than 1.8 million new cancer cases are expected to be diagnosed in 2020. About 606,520 Americans are expected to die of cancer in 2020, which translates to about 1660 deaths per day. Cancer is the second most common cause of death in the United States, exceeded only by heart disease.

Acute kidney injury (AKI) is common in patient with cancer[1].[2] Nearly 80% of patients who were studied in the BIRMA study received nephrotoxic medications and were in need of dose adjustments.[1] The development of AKI can further limit cancer treatment options, increase toxicity to chemotherapeutics, reduce drug delivery, exclude patients from potential clinical trials, and exclude them from eligibility for hematopoietic

Division of Renal Diseases and Hypertension, Department of Internal Medicine, University of Texas Health Science Center at Houston-McGovern Medical School, 6431 Fannin Street, MSB 5. 134, Houston, TX 77030, USA
* Corresponding author.
E-mail address: jaya.kala@uth.tmc.edu

Crit Care Clin 37 (2021) 365–384
https://doi.org/10.1016/j.ccc.2020.11.004
0749-0704/21/© 2020 Elsevier Inc. All rights reserved.

stem cell transplantation (HSCT). The etiology of AKI in patients with cancer is quite varied and is often multifactorial. Causes vary from those common to all hospitalized patients to factors unique to the underlying malignancy or its treatment.

EPIDEMIOLOGY

AKI is associated with increased morbidity, mortality, length of stay, and costs.[3] In a northern Denmark study with a 1.2 million population in the catchment area, incident cancer was found in 44,116 patients. The 1-year and 5-year risks of AKI in this population were 17.5% and 27.5%, respectively. The incidence of AKI was greatest for kidney cancer (44%), multiple myeloma (33%), liver cancer (32%), and acute leukemia (28%). Renal replacement therapy was required in 5.1% of these patients within 1 year of AKI onset.[4]

Among critically ill patients, 20% have an underlying malignancy with an overall prognosis strongly dependent on the admitting diagnosis and the type of cancer.[5] Patients with solid tumors have a lower mortality rate (56%) than those with hematologic malignancies (67%). In the Sepsis Occurrence in Critically Ill Patients (SOAP) study, in the subset of patients with more than 3 failing organs, more than 75% of patients with cancer died; this finding compares with 50% of those without cancer. In a retrospective analysis of 1009 critically ill patients with hematologic malignancies, Darmon and colleagues[6] reported an AKI incidence of 66.5%. After adjustment, the factors associated with the development of AKI were older age, a history of hypertension, tumor lysis syndrome, multiple myeloma, exposure to nephrotoxins, and the Sequential Organ Failure Assessment score. In a study of 163,071 patients undergoing systemic therapy for cancer in Canada over a 7-year period, 1 in 10 patients experienced hospitalization or received dialysis for AKI.[7] The rate of AKI was 27 per 1000 person-years, with a cumulative incidence of 9.3%. The cancer-related AKI was commonly associated with advanced stage, chronic kidney disease, diabetes, and treatment with diuretics or angiotensin-converting enzyme inhibitor, or angiotensin receptor blockers. Patients with multiple myeloma, bladder cancer, cervical cancer, and leukemia were at highest risk. In yet another study on patients with hematologic malignancies, AKI was present in 36% patients with acute myelogenous leukemia and high-risk myelodysplastic syndrome undergoing induction therapy.[8] The predictors of AKI that were identified were age greater than 55 years; mechanical ventilation; vasopressors; low white cell counts; hypoalbuminemia; use of vancomycin, diuretics, and amphotericin B; and use of non–fludarabine-based chemotherapy. After a diagnosis of renal cell carcinoma, many patients undergo radical nephrectomy. This procedure itself is associated with a 33.7% risk of AKI and predicts future development of chronic kidney disease at 1 year.[9]

DISCUSSION

The etiologies of AKI in patients with cancer include those that occur in the general population as well as those that are specific to the cancer itself or its treatment. These etiologies can be categorized into prerenal, intrinsic, and postrenal causes. In a majority of cases, the cause of AKI is multifactorial.

PRERENAL

The most frequent causes of AKI in patients with cancer is prerenal disease (**Fig. 1**). Uses of diuretics, nonsteroidal anti-inflammatory drugs, angiotensin-converting

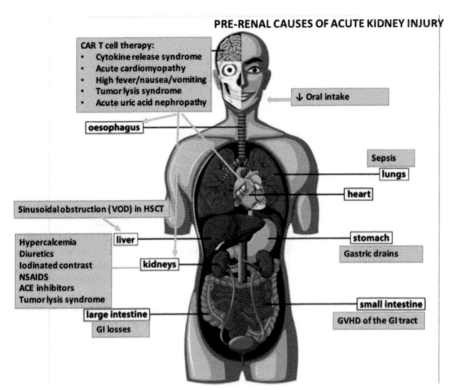

PRE-RENAL CAUSES OF ACUTE KIDNEY INJURY

CAR T cell therapy:
- Cytokine release syndrome
- Acute cardiomyopathy
- High fever/nausea/vomiting
- Tumor lysis syndrome
- Acute uric acid nephropathy

↓ Oral intake

oesophagus

Sepsis

lungs

heart

Sinusoidal obstruction (VOD) in HSCT

Hypercalcemia
Diuretics
Iodinated contrast
NSAIDS
ACE inhibitors
Tumor lysis syndrome

liver

kidneys

stomach

Gastric drains

small intestine

GVHD of the GI tract

large intestine

GI losses

Fig. 1. Prerenal causes of AKI (human anatomy image courtesy of VectorStock.com). HSCT, hematopoietic stem cell transplantation; NSAIDs, nonsteroidal anti-inflammatory drugs; VOD, veno-occlusive disease.

enzyme inhibitors or angiotensin receptor blockers have also been implicated in causing AKI.[8] We have reviewed a few of the prerenal causes herein.

Tumor Lysis Syndrome

Tumor lysis syndrome is often a dramatic presentation of AKI in patients with malignancy.[10] It is characterized by the development of hyperphosphatemia, hypocalcemia, hyperuricemia, and hyperkalemia. Tumor lysis syndrome can occur spontaneously during the rapid growth phase of malignancies, such as bulky lymphoblastomas and Burkitt and non-Burkitt lymphomas that have extremely rapid cell turnover rates, or when cytotoxic chemotherapy induces the lysis of malignant cells in patients with large tumor burdens.

The pathophysiology of AKI associated with tumor lysis syndrome is classically attributed to 2 main factors, namely, preexisting volume depletion before the onset of renal failure, and the precipitation of uric acid and calcium phosphate complexes in the renal tubules and tissue. Patients may be volume depleted from anorexia or nausea and vomiting associated with the malignancy, or from increased insensible losses from fever or tachypnea.

Hyperuricemia is either present before treatment with chemotherapy or develops after therapy despite prophylaxis with allopurinol. Uric acid is nearly completely ionized at a physiologic pH, but becomes progressively insoluble in the acidic environment of the renal tubules. Precipitation of uric acid causes intratubular obstruction leading to increased renal vascular resistance and a decreased glomerular filtration rate.

Hyperphosphatemia and hypocalcemia also occur in tumor lysis syndrome. In patients who do not develop hyperuricemia, AKI has been attributed to metastatic intrarenal calcification or acute nephrocalcinosis. Tumor lysis with the release of inorganic phosphate results in acute hypocalcemia and metastatic calcification, resulting in AKI.

The optimal management of the tumor lysis syndrome decreases the risk of AKI and prevents the development of symptomatic electrolyte abnormalities. Key components to its management include ensuring a high urine output (maintained at a rate of 200 mL/h), decreasing uric acid levels, and controlling serum phosphate levels. The use of loop diuretics should avoided because they acidify the urine and can lead to volume depletion. A consensus statement on the treatment of tumor lysis syndrome was published by the American Society of Clinical Oncology in 2008.[11]

In patients at low risk of tumor lysis syndrome, allopurinol is administered to inhibit uric acid formation. During massive tumor lysis, uric acid excretion can still increase despite the administration of allopurinol, so that intravenous hydration is still necessary to prevent AKI. Because allopurinol and its metabolites are excreted in the urine, the dose should be decreased in the face of impaired renal function.

Therapy with intravenous sodium bicarbonate is associated with several potential side effects, such as severe hypocalcemia-induced tetany and seizures, and its use is no longer recommended. An alkaline pH markedly decreases the urinary solubility of calcium phosphate and can precipitate phosphate nephropathy.

In medium-risk and high-risk patients, rasburicase (recombinant urate oxidase) should be started if evidence of tumor lysis syndrome is present. It converts uric acid to water-soluble allantoin, thereby decreasing the serum uric acid levels and urinary uric acid excretion.[12] The use of rasburicase obviates the need for urinary alkalinization, but a good urine flow with hydration should be maintained given the probability of preexisting volume depletion. Rasburicase treatment should be avoided in patients with glucose-6-phosphate dehydrogenase deficiency because hydrogen peroxide, a breakdown product of uric acid, can cause methemoglobinemia and, in severe cases, hemolytic anemia.

Sinusoidal Occlusion Syndrome

Sinusoidal occlusion syndrome (SOS) is a unique kidney disorder that occurs between 10 and 21 days after HSCT and is associated with the development of SOS, formerly referred to as veno-occlusive disease of the liver.[13] It is characterized by tender hepatomegaly, fluid retention with ascites formation, and jaundice. It is the result of fibrous narrowing of small hepatic venules and sinusoids triggered by the pretransplant cytoreductive regimen, and is more common after allogeneic than autologous HSCT. The development of SOS is most commonly associated with pretreatment with cyclophosphamide, busulfan, and/or total body irradiation.[14] The resultant AKI is similar in appearance to the hepatorenal syndrome.

Patients are usually resistant to diuretics and spontaneous recovery is rare. Risk factors for the development of AKI include weight gain; hyperbilirubinemia; the use of amphotericin B, vancomycin, or acyclovir; and a baseline serum creatinine level of greater than 0.7 mg/dL. The development of AKI adversely affects survival. In patients who require dialysis, the mortality rate approaches 80%. Small trials using infusions of prostaglandin E, pentoxifylline, or low-dose heparin to prevent the development of SOS have been promising.[15] Smaller trials with defibrotide, an antithrombotic and fibrinolytic agent, have shown a benefit in patients with SOS.[15] However, their use is not commonplace because of the associated risk of bleeding.

Hypercalcemia

Malignancy is the most common cause of hypercalcemia in hospitalized patients. Hypercalcemia is diagnosed in advanced disease and is associated with a poor prognosis. The major mechanisms involved in malignancy associated hypercalcemia are (1) secretion of parathyroid hormone-related protein; (2) direct osteolytic metastases with release of local cytokines; and (3) secretion of 1-25, dihydroxy vitamin D.[16]

Hypercalcemia induces prerenal azotemia by causing nephrogenic diabetes insipidus, renal vasoconstriction, and intratubular calcium deposition. When the serum calcium level is greater than 13 mg/dL, patients will have some degree of volume depletion. Volume repletion with isotonic saline should be infused intravenously in large volumes to increase calcium excretion. The effectiveness of loop diuretics in decreasing serum calcium levels has been questioned and its use can no longer be recommended.[17]

Bisphosphonates, pyrophosphate analogs with a high affinity for hydroxyapatite, may be necessary to control the serum calcium in severe cases.[18] Pamidronate and clodronate, 2 second-generation bisphosphonates, are commonly used preparations. Pamidronate can be given as a single intravenous dose of 30 to 90 mg and may normalize the calcium level for several weeks. However, its onset is somewhat delayed with a mean time to achieve normocalcemia of 4 days. Therefore, other means of lowering the calcium level must be implemented in the immediate period.

Calcitonin, derived from the thyroid C-cell, inhibits osteoclast activity. The onset of action of calcitonin is rapid, but with a short half-life, and is usually not given as a sole therapy, often being combined with pamidronate.[19] Tachyphylaxis to calcitonin is frequently seen at 48 hours as a result of downregulation of the calcitonin receptor. The concomitant administration of glucocorticoids can prolong calcitonin's effective duration of action.[20]

Glucocorticoids are also effective in the therapy for hypercalcemia in patients with hematologic malignancies or multiple myeloma. In these cases, glucocorticoids inhibit osteoclastic bone resorption by decreasing tumor production of locally active cytokines.

A more recent addition to agents used to treat hypercalcemia of malignancy is denosumab.[21] It is a humanized monoclonal antibody directed against receptor of nuclear factor κB ligand, thereby decreasing osteoclast differentiation and proliferation. Denosumab has been effective in decreasing calcium levels in patients with breast or prostate cancers, as well as those with multiple myeloma.

Hemodialysis with a low calcium bath is the preferred method of decreasing serum calcium levels in patients with severe symptomatic hypercalcemia.

Chimeric Antigen Receptor T Cell Therapy

Chimeric antigen receptor T (CAR-T) cell therapy was first approved by the US Food and Drug Administration in 2017 as an adaptive cell transfer treatment. The initial development of CAR-T cell therapy had been largely focused on acute lymphoblastic leukemia. Currently, this therapy has been used on hematologic malignancies and solid cancers, such as glioblastoma multiforme, ovarian cancer, pancreatic cancer, mesothelioma, and prostate cancer.[22]

The nephrotoxicities associated with CAR-T cell therapy are related to cytokine release syndrome and tumor lysis syndrome (**Fig. 2**). In published trials, cytokine release syndrome was observed in more than 40% of patients, regardless of the target

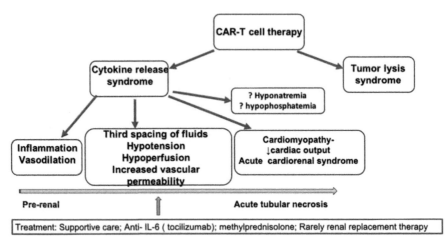

Fig. 2. CAR T-cell therapy and its nephrotoxicities.

of the CAR-T cell therapy. These patients present initially with fever for 6 to 7 days and often rising ferritin levels. Organ dysfunction is manifested in 14 to 15 days. This syndrome results from a high level of circulating inflammatory cytokines, predominantly IL-6.[22] Cytokines are produced either directly from the CAR-T cells or from the immune cells activated by the CAR-T cells.

In a recent retrospective review of 46 patients with non-Hodgkin lymphoma treated with CAR-T cell therapy between February 2018 and February 2019, serum creatinine values before treatment and until 100 days after treatment were used to assess AKI.[23] The overall incidence of cytokine release syndrome was found to be 78.3%, and the cumulative incidence of any grade of AKI was 30% by day 100. Grade 1 AKI was seen in 21.7% of patients, grades 2 to 3 in 8.7%, and no patient required renal replacement therapy. Most patients recovered their renal function within 30 days, which was attributed to early recognition of cytokine release syndrome and management of the complications of CAR-T cell therapy.[23]

INTRINSIC

There are multiple intrinsic causes of AKI among patients with cancer (**Fig. 3**). Etiologies that are specific to cancer are discussed with examples of a few cases from our clinical practice.

GLOMERULAR AND PARANEOPLASTIC CAUSES

Several solid and hematologic malignancies have been associated with glomerular diseases. It is thought to be a result of abnormal tumor cell products. Membranous nephropathy is most commonly associated with solid malignancies, such as lung and gastric tumors.[24] Minimal change disease is classically associated with Hodgkin's lymphoma. It usually occurs at the time the malignancy is diagnosed and is associated with high rate of steroid and cyclosporine resistance. The most common glomerular disease seen with thymoma is minimal change disease. Focal segmental glomerulosclerosis is associated with solid malignancies, kidney cancer and thymoma. Membranoproliferative glomerulonephritis is associated with lung, kidney, and stomach cancers. IgA nephropathy has been most frequently associated with kidney cell

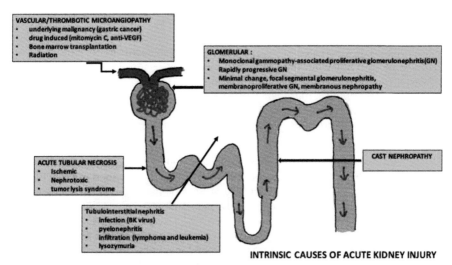

Fig. 3. Intrinsic causes of AKI. GN, glomerulonephritis; VEGF, vascular endothelial growth factor.

cancer. It is also associated with T-cell lymphoma. Glomerular diseases associated with hematologic cancers are minimal change disease, focal segmental glomerulosclerosis, membranoproliferative glomerulonephritis, membranous nephropathy, amyloidosis, immunotactoid glomerulonephritis, fibrillary glomerulonephritis, and crescentic glomerulonephritis.

Dysproteinemia-Related Acute Kidney Injury

AKI complicates multiple myeloma in 20% to 50% of patients.[25–27] Dysproteinemic kidney diseases occur when B-cells or plasma cell clones produce pathogenic monoclonal immunoglobulins or light chains that cause kidney damage. Their presentation ranges from subnephrotic range proteinuria or microscopic hematuria with preserved kidney function to severe nephrotic syndrome to severe AKI or rapidly progressive glomerulonephritis.[28] The overproduction of monoclonal immunoglobulins and free light chains often cause nephrotoxic effects. Cast nephropathy is the most common cause of AKI. Light chain–related proximal tubular injury, and various glomerulopathies such as light-chain deposition disease and amyloid light chain amyloidosis, hypercalcemia, hyperuricemia, sepsis, and nephrotoxin exposure are also implicated in paraprotein-related AKI.

Proliferative glomerulonephritis with monoclonal immunoglobulin deposits is characterized by mesangioproliferative, membranoproliferative, and/or endocapillary proliferative glomerulonephritis on light microscopy; monoclonal immunoglobulin deposition on immunofluorescence microscopy; and nonorganized electron dense deposits on electron microscopy.[28] The renal prognosis is poor during its initial description, with approximately one-half the patients progressing to kidney failure within 2 to 5 years of diagnosis. In a case series of 19 patients with proliferative glomerulonephritis with monoclonal immunoglobulin deposits, 13 without detectable clones, empirical therapy directed at the hypothesized underlying clone led to a 90% renal response rate, with 30% of patients achieving a complete renal response.[29] This approach often involved combination chemotherapeutic regimens. This finding needs to be validated in prospective studies. There is a high rate of recurrence of proliferative glomerulonephritis with monoclonal immunoglobulin deposits after renal transplantation.

Proliferative or Crescentic Glomerulonephritis

Membranoproliferative and rapidly progressive glomerulonephritis have been described in patients with lymphomas and solid tumors. There also seems to be some evidence that patients with antineutrophil cytoplasmic antibody–associated vasculitis have an increased risk of preceding or concurrent malignancy.[30] In a series of patients with crescentic glomerulonephritis, malignancy was seen in 20% of patients.[31] Renal biopsy in patients with cancer presenting with AKI is crucial in making an accurate diagnosis, which may turn out to be different from the presumptive diagnosis.

Case

A 54-year-old gentleman being treated with midostaurin for acute myeloid leukemia was admitted with AKI. He was in remission as proven by his bone marrow biopsy. Within a few days, he developed hemoptysis from diffuse alveolar hemorrhage. His AKI continued to worsen, requiring hemodialysis. Antibodies to proteinase-3, myeloperoxidase, and glomerular basement membrane were negative. Renal biopsy (Fig. 4) confirmed acute pauci-immune focal necrotizing glomerulonephritis with fibrin crescents, indicating rapidly progressing glomerulonephritis. He improved with pulse methylprednisolone, intravenous cyclophosphamide, and plasma exchange with resolution of hemoptysis. Because he was in remission, the glomerulonephritis was considered to be potentially due to the use of midostaurin and not due to the paraneoplastic syndrome from acute myeloid leukemia.[32]

TUBULOINTERSTITIAL CAUSES

Although a variety of cancers can metastasize to the kidneys and invade the parenchyma, the most common malignancies to do so are lymphomas and leukemia. The true incidence of renal involvement is unknown because it is usually a silent disease and only occasionally causes renal impairment. Rarely, renal infiltration from metastatic ovarian cancer may present as severe AKI requiring dialysis, such as in our patient (Fig. 5), who shows a high-grade serous carcinoma of the ovary primary infiltrating the entire renal biopsy specimen. The patient had no known history of cancer and AKI was her presenting diagnosis.

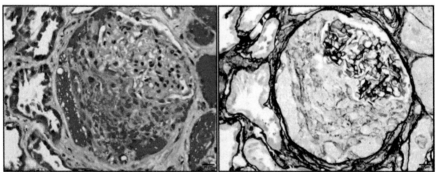

| Crescent composed primarily of fibrin with early epithelial proliferation indicating very acute necrotizing glomerulonephritis. | Jones Silver stain: very segmentally interrupted Glomerular Basement Membrane |

Fig. 4. Acute pauci-immune focal necrotizing glomerulonephritis (GN) with fibrin crescents indicating rapidly progressing GN (RPGN) considered to be potentially owing to the use of midostaurin (hematoxylin-eosin, original magnification ×40). The renal biopsy was done with a presumptive diagnosis of paraneoplastic syndrome from acute myeloid leukemia (AML) (Jones Silver, original magnification ×40).

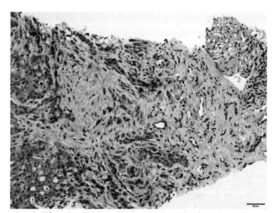

Poorly differentiated high-grade adenocarcinoma involving almost the entire sample, favoring high grade serous carcinoma of ovarian primary.

Fig. 5. Kidney biopsy of patient with AKI and no known history of ovarian cancer, hematoxylin and eosin staining (original magnification ×20) shows a high-grade serous carcinoma of the ovary primary infiltrating the entire renal biopsy specimen as the cause of AKI.

Lymphoma

Renal involvement in lymphoma is often clinically silent and requires a high index of suspicion to make a diagnosis. Patients may present with AKI, but this scenario is rare and is most commonly seen in highly malignant and disseminated disease.[33] Other presentations include proteinuria in both the nephrotic and non-nephrotic range, as well as a variety of glomerular lesions including pauci-immune crescentric glomerulonephritis.[34] Patients may also present with flank pain and hematuria.

The diagnosis may be suspected from clinical features and imaging studies. Renal ultrasound examination (**Fig. 6**) and computed tomography scanning may reveal diffusely enlarged kidneys, sometimes with multiple focal lesions.[35] The following criteria support the diagnosis of kidney disease owing to lymphomatous infiltration: (1) renal enlargement without obstruction; (2) the absence of other causes of kidney

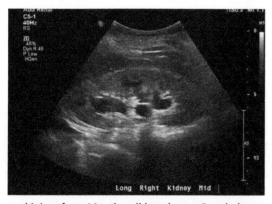

Fig. 6. Infiltrative renal injury from Mantle cell lymphoma. Renal ultrasound image of a patient with Mantle cell lymphoma (MCL), a rare subtype of non-Hodgkin's lymphoma. The patient's MCL had infiltrated the entire kidney causing AKI. The patient responded well to low dose radiation therapy with return of creatinine to baseline.

disease; and (3) rapid improvement of kidney function after radiotherapy or systemic chemotherapy.

Leukemia

Leukemia cells can infiltrate any organ, and the kidneys are the most frequent extramedullary site of infiltration. Autopsy studies reveal that 60% to 90% of patients have renal involvement.[36] Leukemic infiltration of the kidneys is often an indolent and clinically silent disease. Most often, it is incidentally noted on autopsy or by the detection of renal enlargement on ultrasound examination or a computed tomography scan. Although uncommon, many cases of AKI attributable to leukemic infiltration have been described.[37] Patients may also experience hematuria or proteinuria. Occasionally, renal enlargement is accompanied by flank pain or fullness. Patients with significantly elevated white cell counts can develop AKI from leukostasis. Treatment is directed by the type of leukemia. Although some patients do not recover, in the majority of cases renal function does improve as the leukemia responds to systemic treatment.

Chemotherapy-Induced Kidney Injury

Chemotherapeutic agents can result in a variety of kidney manifestations including AKI, tubulointerstitial nephritis with several acid–base and electrolyte disturbances, hypertension, proteinuria and nephrotic syndrome, and thrombotic microangiopathy.

The kidney effects of chemotherapy can be differentiated by the primary site of injury such as the endothelium (hypertension and thrombotic microangiopathy), visceral podocyte (proteinuria and nephrotic syndrome), renal tubules (AKI), and tubulointerstitium (renal tubular acidosis, Fanconi syndrome, and electrolyte wasting). A listing of agents and the associated kidney effects are found in **Table 1**.

Acute Interstitial Nephritis

Drug-induced acute interstitial nephritis is a common cause of AKI, affecting 20% of patients with unexplained AKI.[38] The most frequently implicated drugs are antibiotics, nonsteroidal anti-inflammatory drugs and proton pump inhibitors. It is important to exclude these drugs as being the offending agents before chemotherapeutics are implicated as the cause of the acute interstitial nephritis. In doing so, we can avoid unnecessary discontinuation of life-saving chemotherapeutics. The classic triad of rash, fever, and eosinophilia occurring within a few days of drug therapy is seen in as few as 10% of patients. The diagnosis often gets delayed and not all biopsy-proven acute interstitial nephritis presents with AKI.[39] This factor makes diagnosis challenging. A high index of suspicion and careful drug history taking is crucial in making this diagnosis (**Fig. 7**).

Check Point Inhibitors

Upon activation by an immunologic event (infection or injury), cytotoxic T cells undergo a damping of the response to maintain "immunohomeostasis" by expressing several receptors including cytotoxic T-lymphocyte-associated antigen 4, programmed death 1 protein, and programmed death ligand-1 that downregulate T-cell function.[40] By inhibiting T-lymphocyte-associated antigen-4 and programmed death 1 protein/programmed death ligand-1, check point inhibitors enhance tumor-directed immune responses and are new agents for the treatment of solid and hematologic malignancies. However, with this enhanced immune response several immune-related adverse events have been reported such as hepatitis, rash, colitis, and myocarditis. In a recent case report in 13 patients with AKI while receiving check

Table 1
Chemotherapy and kidney manifestations

Chemotherapeutic Agents	Kidney Effects
Cisplatin	AKI Proximal tubulopathy Fanconi syndrome Nephrogenic diabetes insipidus Salt-wasting nephropathy Magnesium wasting
Ifosfamide	AKI Proximal tubulopathy Fanconi syndrome Nephrogenic diabetes insipidus
Methotrexate	AKI (crystalline nephropathy)
Pamidronate	AKI Collapsing focal segmental glomerulosclerosis
Zoledronic acid	AKI
Calcineurin inhibitors	AKI Thrombotic microangiopathy Hypertension Hyperkalemia
Biologic agents	
Interferon-α	AKI Minimal change disease Focal segmental glomerulosclerosis
IL-2	AKI (prerenal) Capillary leak syndrome
Targeted therapies	
Anti-vascular endothelial growth factor and tyrosine kinase inhibitors	AKI Thrombotic microangiopathy Hypertension Proteinuria
BRAF inhibitors	AKI Electrolyte disorders
ALK inhibitors	AKI Electrolyte disorders Renal microcysts
Immunotherapeutic agents	

T-lymphocyte-associated antigen-4
    inhibitors (cytotoxic T-lymphocyte
    antigens)
	AKI
	Proteinuria

Programmed death 1 protein (programmed death)	AKI
Chimeric antigen receptor T cells	Capillary leak with prerenal AKI

point inhibitors, 12 of 13 had acute tubulointerstitial nephritis on kidney biopsy, which seemed to respond to steroid administration.[41] The estimated incidence of immune check point inhibitor-associated AKI ranges from 1.4% to 4.9%.[42]

A multicenter study of 138 patients with immune check point inhibitor AKI was conducted to identify clinical features and outcomes. A low baseline glomerular filtration rate, proton pump inhibitor use, and combination immune check point

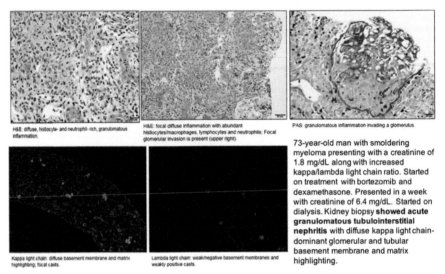

H&E: diffuse, histiocyte- and neutrophil- rich, granulomatous inflammation.

H&E: focal diffuse inflammation with abundant histiocytes/macrophages, lymphocytes and neutrophils; Focal glomerular invasion is present (upper right).

PAS: granulomatous inflammation invading a glomerulus.

73-year-old man with smoldering myeloma presenting with a creatinine of 1.8 mg/dL along with increased kappa/lambda light chain ratio. Started on treatment with bortezomib and dexamethasone. Presented in a week with creatinine of 6.4 mg/dL. Started on dialysis. Kidney biopsy **showed acute granulomatous tubulointerstitial nephritis** with diffuse kappa light chain-dominant glomerular and tubular basement membrane and matrix highlighting.

Kappa light chain: diffuse basement membrane and matrix highlighting; focal casts.

Lambda light chain: weak/negative basement membranes and weakly positive casts.

Fig. 7. Case of acute tubulointerstitial nephritis. H&E, hematoxylin and eosin; PAS, periodic acid-Schiff.

inhibitor therapy were independent risk factors for AKI. The concurrent use of potential tubulointerstitial nephritis–causing medication was seen in 69% of patients. Tubulointerstitial nephritis was the dominant lesion in 93% of the 60 patients biopsied. Immune check point inhibitor therapy was held at AKI diagnosis in 134 patients and 119 (86%) received corticosteroids. The treatment with steroids was associated with a greater odds of complete kidney recovery. With rechallenge, recurrent immune check point inhibitor AKI was found in 23% of patients. The latency period between rechallenge and recurrent immune check point inhibitor AKI was shorter than with initial AKI.[43]

Cast Nephropathy

Multiple myeloma is a plasma cell proliferative disorder that commonly involves the kidneys. Up to 40% of patients have a serum creatinine that is greater than the upper normal of limit at diagnosis, with 10% requiring.[44] The severity of renal injury has a negative correlation with the overall survival rate. Patients on dialysis owing to multiple myeloma have a 3-fold increased mortality risk within the first year of starting renal replacement therapy. The most common cause of AKI in patients with multiple myeloma is light chain cast nephropathy or myeloma kidney. Light chain cast nephropathy–induced renal failure is a myeloma-defining event.[45]

   The precipitating factors are hypercalcemia, dehydration, infection, contrast agents, and the use of nonsteroidal anti-inflammatory drugs and angiotensin-converting enzyme inhibitors. The precipitation of casts is triggered by the decreased glomerular filtration rate, decreased tubular flow, and increased interaction between filtered monoclonal light chains and Tamm-Horsfall protein. Patients with light chain cast nephropathy often present with severe AKI and require dialysis. The recovery of renal function depends on the early initiation of chemotherapeutic agents and other supportive measures to decrease the ongoing damage from light chains.[45] The algorithm for the diagnosis of cast nephropathy is presented in **Fig. 8**.[27,44,45]

Bortezomib-based chemotherapy is of considerable benefit in patients with myeloma cast nephropathy compared with conventional agents and the rate of kidney recovery is significantly higher than in the past.[46] In addition to chemotherapeutic agents, the removal of free light chains using therapeutic plasma exchange or hemodialysis with the use of high cutoff hemodialysis has been controversial. Studies in patients with Multiple Myeloma and Renal Failure Due to Myeloma Cast Nephropathy (MYRE) and the European Trial of Free Light Chain Removal by Extended Hemodialysis in Cast Nephropathy (EuLITE) trials both randomized patients with dialysis-dependent AKI owing to biopsy-confirmed myeloma cast nephropathy to bortezomib-based chemotherapy and either conventional hemofiltration and hemodialysis or high cutoff hemodialysis with a primary end point of discontinuation of Renal replacement therapy. Because both studies were small and had equivocal results, the routine use of high cutoff hemodialysis cannot be recommended.

VASCULAR OR THROMBOTIC MICROANGIOPATHY

Thrombotic microangiopathy manifests as nonimmune hemolytic anemia, thrombocytopenia, and organ dysfunction, including AKI. The characteristic renal lesion consists of vessel wall thickening in capillaries and arterioles, with swelling and detachment of endothelial cells from the basement membranes and accumulation of subendothelial fluffy material. Distinguishing between cancer induced thrombotic microangiopathy, thrombotic thrombocytopenic purpura (TTP)–induced thrombotic microangiopathy, and complement-mediated thrombotic microangiopathy is important. This practice will help avoid unnecessary plasma exchange or the use of complement-directed

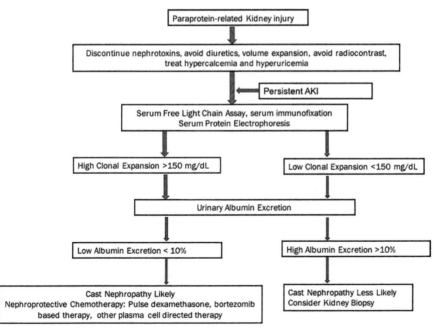

Fig. 8. Diagnostic algorithm for light chain cast nephropathy. (*Adapted from* Finkel KW, Cohen EP, Shirali A, Abudayyeh A, American Society of Nephrology Onco-Nephrology F. Paraprotein-Related Kidney Disease: Evaluation and Treatment of Myeloma Cast Nephropathy. Clin J Am Soc Nephrol. 2016;11(12):2273-9.)

therapy. The presence of thrombotic microangiopathy could be a presenting feature of an underlying cancer or seen in end-stage or advanced cancer. There is also extensive involvement of the bone marrow, causing bone pain at presentation. These patients do not respond well to plasma exchange.[47] In comparison with TTP, patients with cancer-induced thrombotic microangiopathy have more frequent respiratory symptoms (70% of patients), abnormal liver functions (transaminases, alkaline phosphatase, direct bilirubin), elevated creatinine, infiltrating carcinomas, or bone marrow necrosis.[48] Cancer-induced thrombotic microangiopathy occurs as a result of induction of coagulation cascade from the hypoxia and inflammation induced release of tissue factors, cancer procoagulants, tumor-derived cytokines, and plasminogen activator inhibitor-1. The endothelial injury can occur from direct invasion, venous catheter use, chemotherapeutics, radiation therapy, or substances produced from the tumor.[49] The majority of these injuries are seen with solid tumors, such as gastric and colon cancers, but hematologic cancers such as lymphomas are seen in approximately 8% of cases. Chemotherapy agents are likewise associated with the development of thrombotic microangiopathy (**Table 2**).[50]

The treatment of renal failure and thrombotic microangiopathy in patients with cancer from any etiology is mainly supportive, with the initiation of dialysis as necessary.

Table 2
Chemotherapy induced thrombotic microangiopathy

Drug	Characteristics
Mitomycin C (2%–15%)	Cumulative dose of 40–60 mg May occur in 4–6 mo after treatment Noncardiogenic pulmonary edema Renal failure Permanent and irreversible damage High probability of recurrent damage on rechallenge High incidence of acute mortality Treatment: needs dialysis, steroids, plasma exchange, rituximab, ecluzimab
Gemcitabine (0.25%–0.4%)	Cumulative dose of >22.5 mg/dL Hypertension Proteinuria Hematuria Acute renal failure Treatment: with drug discontinuation and complement inhibition
Anti-VEGF therapy (bevacizumab)	Any time after drug initiation (1 dose to 29 mo) Not dose related Reversible after discontinuing Hypertension Proteinuria Renal failure Safer with rechallenge Survival good after discontinuing drug Treatment: with drug discontinuation and complement inhibition
Tyrosine kinase inhibitor	Hypertension Proteinuria Renal failure Treatment: with drug discontinuation and complement inhibition

Adapted from reference Weitz IC. Thrombotic Microangiopathy in Cancer. Semin Thromb Hemost. 2019;45(4):348-53.

Table 3
HSCT-induced AKI

| Prerenal | Intrinsic | | | Postrenal |
	Tubular/Interstitial	Vascular/Thrombotic Microangiopathy		
Sepsis	Ischemic	Calcineurin inhibitors mTOR inhibitors		BK-induced bladder disease
Hypotension	Toxic (infections)	Acute graft-versus-host disease		Retroperitoneal fibrosis
Capillary leak syndrome	Drugs (aminoglycosides, vancomycin, amphotericin-B, methotrexate, fludarabine)	Viral mediated		Adenovirus cystitis
Engraftment syndrome		Complement dysregulation		
Calcineurin inhibitors Contrast nephropathy	Infections (pyelonephritis, BK, cytomegalovirus, parvovirus B19, adenovirus)	Total body irradiation		
Veno-occlusive disease	Tumor lysis syndrome			

Adapted from reference Wanchoo R, Stotter BR, Bayer RL, Jhaveri KD. Acute kidney injury in hematopoietic stem cell transplantation. Curr Opin Crit Care. 2019;25(6):531-8.

Any offending agent should be discontinued. The role of TPE is controversial because it has not been uniformly beneficial. If stopping or treating any underlying cause for thrombotic microangiopathy is unsuccessful and the patient continues to deteriorate. TPE should be initiated; however, it is mandatory that ADAMTS13 activity be measured. A low activity level (<5%) confirms the diagnosis of TTP and TPE should continue. If the activity level is normal, TTP is excluded as a diagnosis and TPE can be discontinued. At that point, the diagnosis of atypical hemolytic uremic syndrome is likely and strong consideration should be given to administering eculizumab, a humanized monoclonal antibody, which inhibits terminal complement activation by binding to complement C5 and preventing the formation of the terminal membrane attack complex.[51,52]

Stem Cell Transplantation

HSCT can result in both AKI and CKD. The incidence of AKI is found to be 10% in autologous transplants and 50% (with reduced-intensity conditioning) and 73% (high intensity) in those who receive allogeneic transplant. Causes of AKI include acute graft-versus-host disease, SOS, thrombotic microangiopathy, use of calcineurin inhibitors, and viral infections.[53] In addition, engraftment syndrome, cytokine storm, transplant associated thrombotic microangiopathy and infections such as BK virus and adenovirus nephritis, have been found to cause AKI (**Table 3**). AKI after HSCT confers a poor short-term and long-term prognosis. These patients have an increased risk of death in the first 6 months after HSCT.[54] Their 5-year survival is 20% lower than those without AKI. The treatment of AKI is mainly supportive. Treatment of a specific cause, holding nephrotoxins, and treating infections may lead to an improvement in kidney function. Decreased intensity conditioning, non–amphotericin-based antifungal therapy, and the prompt recognition of engraftment syndrome, graft-versus-host disease, VOD, and thrombotic microangiopathy is important. Most patient develop multiorgan

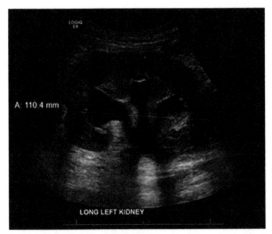

**Post Renal Acute Kidney Injury caused
by
obstruction secondary to
lymphadenopathy**

Fig. 9. Postrenal AKI caused by obstruction owing to lymphadenopathy. The hydronephrosis is caused by obstruction.

Table 4	
Postrenal causes of AKI	
Intrarenal	**Extrarenal**
Uric acid	Retroperitoneal fibrosis
Methotrexate acyclovir	Direct invasion
	Lymphadenopathy

failure. Adequate management by monitoring intake and output is preventing fluid overload.[54] Patient admitted to the intensive care unit have a poor prognosis. In a retrospective study of patients admitted in the intensive care unit after HSCT, 70.2% required mechanical ventilation and 66% required dialysis.[55] Studies to understand the management strategies in HSCT-associated AKI are needed.

POSTRENAL

Urinary tract obstruction (as seen in **Fig. 9**) is the most common cause of postrenal AKI in cancers associated with rectal, bladder, prostate, or gynecologic tumors. The causes of postrenal AKI are listed in **Table 4**.

SUMMARY

The field of onconephrology has recently developed for a variety of reasons. Although patients with malignancy can develop kidney diseases, similar to other acutely and chronically ill patients, they are also at risk for unique kidney syndromes because of either the cancer itself or its treatment. Understanding these unique disorders is a prerequisite to providing outstanding clinical care. Providing expert advice on drug response, toxicity, and clearance, as well as clinical study eligibility are important considerations in onconephrology. Patients with advanced malignancies can develop severe AKI with multiple organ dysfunction syndrome. In these cases, the nephrologist is an essential partner in discussions about end-of-life issues and the appropriateness of initiating kidney replacement therapies.

CLINICS CARE POINTS

- There are several kidney disorders that are unique to patients with cancer owing to either the underlying malignancy or its treatment.
- The most frequent causes of AKI in patients with cancer is prerenal disease.
- The nephrotoxicities associated with CAR-T cell therapy are related to cytokine release syndrome (>40% of patients) and tumor lysis syndrome.
- AKI complicates multiple myeloma in 20% to 50% of patients. Cast nephropathy is the most common cause of AKI.
- The estimated incidence of immune check point inhibitor-associated AKI ranges from 1.4% to 4.9%. Tubulointerstitial nephritis is the most common biopsy finding and best treated with steroids.
- Light chain cast nephropathy–induced renal failure is a myeloma-defining event.
- The presence of thrombotic microangiopathy could be a presenting feature of an underlying cancer or be seen in end-stage or advanced cancer.

- AKI after HSCT confers a poor short-term and long-term prognosis with a 5-year survival that is 20% lower than for those without AKI.

DISCLOSURE

The authors have nothing to disclose.

REFERENCES

1. Janus N, Launay-Vacher V, Byloos E, et al. Cancer and renal insufficiency results of the BIRMA study. Br J Cancer 2010;103(12):1815–21.
2. Canet E, Zafrani L, Lambert J, et al. Acute kidney injury in patients with newly diagnosed high-grade hematological malignancies: impact on remission and survival. PLoS One 2013;8(2):e55870.
3. Taccone FS, Artigas AA, Sprung CL, et al. Characteristics and outcomes of cancer patients in European ICUs. Crit Care 2009;13(1):R15.
4. Christiansen CF, Johansen MB, Langeberg WJ, et al. Incidence of acute kidney injury in cancer patients: a Danish population-based cohort study. Eur J Intern Med 2011;22(4):399–406.
5. Lameire N, Vanholder R, Van Biesen W, et al. Acute kidney injury in critically ill cancer patients: an update. Crit Care 2016;20(1):209.
6. Darmon M, Vincent F, Canet E, et al. Acute kidney injury in critically ill patients with haematological malignancies: results of a multicentre cohort study from the Groupe de Recherche en Reanimation Respiratoire en Onco-Hematologie. Nephrol Dial Transplant 2015;30(12):2006–13.
7. Kitchlu A, McArthur E, Amir E, et al. Acute kidney injury in patients receiving systemic treatment for cancer: a population-based cohort study. J Natl Cancer Inst 2019;111(7):727–36.
8. Lahoti A, Kantarjian H, Salahudeen AK, et al. Predictors and outcome of acute kidney injury in patients with acute myelogenous leukemia or high-risk myelodysplastic syndrome. Cancer 2010;116(17):4063–8.
9. Cho A, Lee JE, Kwon GY, et al. Post-operative acute kidney injury in patients with renal cell carcinoma is a potent risk factor for new-onset chronic kidney disease after radical nephrectomy. Nephrol Dial Transplant 2011;26(11):3496–501.
10. Howard SC, Jones DP, Pui CH. The tumor lysis syndrome. N Engl J Med 2011; 364(19):1844–54.
11. Coiffier B, Altman A, Pui CH, et al. Guidelines for the management of pediatric and adult tumor lysis syndrome: an evidence-based review. J Clin Oncol 2008; 26(16):2767–78.
12. Jeha S, Pui CH. Recombinant urate oxidase (rasburicase) in the prophylaxis and treatment of tumor lysis syndrome. Contrib Nephrol 2005;147:69–79.
13. Zager RA. Acute renal failure in the setting of bone marrow transplantation. Kidney Int 1994;46(5):1443–58.
14. McDonald GB, Hinds MS, Fisher LD, et al. Veno-occlusive disease of the liver and multiorgan failure after bone marrow transplantation: a cohort study of 355 patients. Ann Intern Med 1993;118(4):255–67.
15. Lam AQ, Humphreys BD. Onco-nephrology: AKI in the cancer patient. Clin J Am Soc Nephrol 2012;7(10):1692–700.
16. Grill V, Martin TJ. Hypercalcemia of malignancy. Rev Endocr Metab Disord 2000; 1(4):253–63.

17. LeGrand SB, Leskuski D, Zama I. Narrative review: furosemide for hypercalcemia: an unproven yet common practice. Ann Intern Med 2008;149(4):259–63.

18. Singer FR, Minoofar PN. Bisphosphonates in the treatment of disorders of mineral metabolism. Adv Endocrinol Metab 1995;6:259–88.

19. Hosking DJ, Gilson D. Comparison of the renal and skeletal actions of calcitonin in the treatment of severe hypercalcaemia of malignancy. Q J Med 1984;53(211): 359–68.

20. Binstock ML, Mundy GR. Effect of calcitonin and glutocorticoids in combination on the hypercalcemia of malignancy. Ann Intern Med 1980;93(2):269–72.

21. Castellano D, Sepulveda JM, Garcia-Escobar I, et al. The role of RANK-ligand inhibition in cancer: the story of denosumab. Oncologist 2011;16(2):136–45.

22. Jhaveri KD, Rosner MH. Chimeric antigen receptor T cell therapy and the kidney: what the nephrologist needs to know. Clin J Am Soc Nephrol 2018;13(5):796–8.

23. Gutgarts V, Jain T, Zheng J, et al. Acute Kidney Injury after CAR-T cell therapy: low incidence and rapid recovery. Biol Blood Marrow Transplant 2020;26(6): 1071–6.

24. Jhaveri KD, Shah HH, Patel C, et al. Glomerular diseases associated with cancer, chemotherapy, and hematopoietic stem cell transplantation. Adv Chronic Kidney Dis 2014;21(1):48–55.

25. Eleutherakis-Papaiakovou V, Bamias A, Gika D, et al. Renal failure in multiple myeloma: incidence, correlations, and prognostic significance. Leuk Lymphoma 2007;48(2):337–41.

26. Hutchison CA, Batuman V, Behrens J, et al. The pathogenesis and diagnosis of acute kidney injury in multiple myeloma. Nat Rev Nephrol 2011;8(1):43–51.

27. Finkel KW, Cohen EP, Shirali A, et al. Paraprotein-related kidney disease: evaluation and treatment of myeloma cast nephropathy. Clin J Am Soc Nephrol 2016;11(12):2273–9.

28. Hogan JJ, Alexander MP, Leung N. Dysproteinemia and the kidney: core curriculum 2019. Am J Kidney Dis 2019;74(6):822–36.

29. Gumber R, Cohen JB, Palmer MB, et al. A clone-directed approach may improve diagnosis and treatment of proliferative glomerulonephritis with monoclonal immunoglobulin deposits. Kidney Int 2018;94(1):199–205.

30. Pankhurst T, Savage CO, Gordon C, et al. Malignancy is increased in ANCA-associated vasculitis. Rheumatology (Oxford) 2004;43(12):1532–5.

31. Bacchetta J, Juillard L, Cochat P, et al. Paraneoplastic glomerular diseases and malignancies. Crit Rev Oncol Hematol 2009;70(1):39–58.

32. Pankow JD, Richard-Carpentier G, Daver NG, et al. Unique case of ANCA-negative pauci-immune necrotizing glomerulonephritis with diffuse alveolar hemorrhage, potentially associated with midostaurin. CEN Case Rep 2020;9(2): 147–51.

33. Malbrain ML, Lambrecht GL, Daelemans R, et al. Acute renal failure due to bilateral lymphomatous infiltrates. Primary extranodal non-Hodgkin's lymphoma (p-EN-NHL) of the kidneys: does it really exist? Clin Nephrol 1994;42(3):163–9.

34. Henriksen KJ, Hong RB, Sobrero MI, et al. Rare association of chronic lymphocytic leukemia/small lymphocytic lymphoma, ANCAs, and pauci-immune crescentic glomerulonephritis. Am J Kidney Dis 2011;57(1):170–4.

35. Bach AG, Behrmann C, Holzhausen HJ, et al. Prevalence and patterns of renal involvement in imaging of malignant lymphoproliferative diseases. Acta Radiol 2012;53(3):343–8.

36. Suh WM, Wainberg ZA, de Vos S, et al. Acute lymphoblastic leukemia presenting as acute renal failure. Nat Clin Pract Nephrol 2007;3(2):106–10.

37. Phillips JK, Bass PS, Majumdar G, et al. Renal failure caused by leukaemic infiltration in chronic lymphocytic leukaemia. J Clin Pathol 1993;46(12):1131–3.

38. Perazella MA, Markowitz GS. Drug-induced acute interstitial nephritis. Nat Rev Nephrol 2010;6(8):461–70.

39. Moledina DG, Perazella MA. Drug-induced acute interstitial nephritis. Clin J Am Soc Nephrol 2017;12(12):2046–9.

40. Postow MA, Callahan MK, Wolchok JD. Immune checkpoint blockade in cancer therapy. J Clin Oncol 2015;33(17):1974–82.

41. Cortazar FB, Marrone KA, Troxell ML, et al. Clinicopathological features of acute kidney injury associated with immune checkpoint inhibitors. Kidney Int 2016; 90(3):638–47.

42. Mamlouk O, Selamet U, Machado S, et al. Nephrotoxicity of immune checkpoint inhibitors beyond tubulointerstitial nephritis: single-center experience. J Immunother Cancer 2019;7(1):2.

43. Cortazar FB, Kibbelaar ZA, Glezerman IG, et al. Clinical features and outcomes of immune checkpoint inhibitor-associated AKI: a multicenter study. J Am Soc Nephrol 2020;31(2):435–46.

44. Sathick IJ, Drosou ME, Leung N. Myeloma light chain cast nephropathy, a review. J Nephrol 2019;32(2):189–98.

45. Rajkumar SV, Dimopoulos MA, Palumbo A, et al. International Myeloma Working Group updated criteria for the diagnosis of multiple myeloma. Lancet Oncol 2014;15(12):e538–48.

46. LeBlanc R, Song K, White D, et al. Updates from the 2019 American Society of Clinical Oncology and European Hematology Association annual meetings: a Canadian perspective on high-risk cytogenetics in multiple myeloma. Curr Oncol 2019;26(4):e581–94.

47. Thomas MR, Scully M. Microangiopathy in cancer: causes, consequences, and management. Cancer Treat Res 2019;179:151–8.

48. Morton JM, George JN. Microangiopathic hemolytic anemia and thrombocytopenia in patients with cancer. J Oncol Pract 2016;12(6):523–30.

49. Mukai M, Komori K, Oka T. Mechanism and management of cancer chemotherapy-induced atherosclerosis. J Atheroscler Thromb 2018;25(10): 994–1002.

50. Weitz IC. Thrombotic microangiopathy in cancer. Semin Thromb Hemost 2019; 45(4):348–53.

51. Vasu S, Wu H, Satoskar A, et al. Eculizumab therapy in adults with allogeneic hematopoietic cell transplant-associated thrombotic microangiopathy. Bone Marrow Transplant 2016;51(9):1241–4.

52. Al Ustwani O, Lohr J, Dy G, et al. Eculizumab therapy for gemcitabine induced hemolytic uremic syndrome: case series and concise review. J Gastrointest Oncol 2014;5(1):E30–3.

53. Hingorani S. Renal complications of hematopoietic-cell transplantation. N Engl J Med 2016;374(23):2256–67.

54. Wanchoo R, Stotter BR, Bayer RL, et al. Acute kidney injury in hematopoietic stem cell transplantation. Curr Opin Crit Care 2019;25(6):531–8.

55. Nakamura M, Fujii N, Shimizu K, et al. Long-term outcomes in patients treated in the intensive care unit after hematopoietic stem cell transplantation. Int J Hematol 2018;108(6):622–9.

Biomarkers in Acute Kidney Injury

Win Kulvichit, MD[a,b], John A. Kellum, MD, MCCM[c],
Nattachai Srisawat, MD, PhD[a,b,c,d,e,f,g,*]

KEYWORDS

- AKI • Biomarkers • NGAL • TIMP-2 • IGFBP7 • CCL14

KEY POINTS

- The continuum of acute kidney injury natural history has provided a clinically relevant framework to develop suitable biomarkers for a variety of clinical uses.
- Several novel biomarkers currently are being investigated through several phases of the development pipeline.
- The routine use of biomarkers should be evidence based because many implementation trials are now available.

INTRODUCTION
Evolution of Acute Kidney Injury

Historically, the definition of acute kidney injury (AKI) (previously termed, acute renal failure) was based on clinical observations, such as oliguria/anuria and signs and symptoms of uremia. Although the first discovery of creatinine, the most widely used AKI biomarker, dates back to 1847 when Liebig[1] named a substance, creatinine, obtained by heating creatine, the use of endogenous serum creatinine as a marker of renal function was not introduced until the 1940s. Subsequently, more than 35 different definitions have been proposed to define AKI. In the twenty-first century, AKI definitions were developed by international consensus: Risk, Injury, Failure,

[a] Division of Nephrology, Faculty of Medicine, Chulalongkorn University, 10th Floor, Bhumisiri mangkhalanusorn Building, Ratchadamri Road, Pathum Wan, Bangkok 10330, Thailand; [b] Excellence Center for Critical Care Nephrology, King Chulalongkorn Memorial Hospital, 1873 Rama IV Road, Pathum Wan, Bangkok 10330, Thailand; [c] Department of Critical Care Medicine, Center for Critical Care Nephrology, The CRISMA Center, University of Pittsburgh School of Medicine, 3347 Forbes Avenue, Suite 220, Pittsburgh, PA 15213, USA; [d] Critical Care Nephrology Research Unit, Chulalongkorn University, Bangkok, Thailand; [e] Academy of Science, Royal Society of Thailand, Bangkok, Thailand; [f] Tropical Medicine Cluster, Chulalongkorn University, Bangkok, Thailand; [g] Excellence Center for Critical Care Medicine, King Chulalongkorn Memorial Hospital, Bangkok, Thailand
* Corresponding author. Division of Nephrology, Faculty of Medicine, Chulalongkorn University, 10th Floor, Bhumisiri mangkhalanusorn Building, Ratchadamri Road, Pathum Wan, Bangkok 10330, Thailand.
E-mail address: drnattachai@yahoo.com

Crit Care Clin 37 (2021) 385–398
https://doi.org/10.1016/j.ccc.2020.11.012   criticalcare.theclinics.com

Loss, End-Stage (RIFLE) criteria, Acute Kidney Injury Network (AKIN) criteria, and Kidney Disease: Improving Global Outcomes (KDIGO) criteria.[2-4] These definitions were proposed in 2002, 2005, and 2012, consecutively, by consensus of nephrologists and intensivists, and all were based on serum creatinine and urine output. The use of serum creatinine and urine output as the current gold standard for AKI diagnosis, however, has several limitations.

LIMITATIONS OF CURRENT ACUTE KIDNEY INJURY DIAGNOSIS
Serum creatinine

Creatinine, derived from creatine, a waste product produced from muscle, typically is cleared from the blood primarily by glomerular filtration and also by proximal tubular secretion. Although it has been used extensively as a marker of renal function, serum creatinine is not an ideal biomarker for AKI for several reasons. First, the delay of creatinine elevation can range up to 24 hours to 48 hours from the onset of a renal dysfunction due to the creatinine accumulation time.[5] Second, changes of serum creatinine are not sensitive enough to detect acute injury involving less than 50% of the nephrons in a previously normal person because of the compensatory response of the remaining nephrons (renal reserve).[6-10] Moreover, the amount of tubular secretion becomes an increasingly important fraction of creatinine excretion inverse to the amount of creatinine excreted from glomerular filtration. Thus, accumulation of creatinine is not linear with reduced glomerular filtration. Third, serum creatinine is not specific for AKI because it can be affected by many confounding factors. In some conditions, serum creatinine might overestimate the acute reduction of glomerular filtration rate (GFR) (eg, chronic kidney disease [CKD]; rhabdomyolysis; and exposure to medications blocking tubular secretion of creatinine, such as cimetidine, trimethoprim, and so forth) In other conditions, serum creatinine can underestimate the reduction of GFR (eg, low muscle mass, poor nutritional status, dilutional effect in fluid overload, and hyperbilirubinemia).[11-15] Fourth, sepsis, an important cause of AKI, reduces energy production and lowers the muscle perfusion, which explained the late detection of serum creatinine change for AKI in sepsis.[16] Fifth, because serum creatinine can be confounded by CKD and muscle mass, baseline serum creatinine always is necessary to adjudicate AKI diagnosis. Many patients, however, do not have baseline serum creatinine data at the time of hospital admission.[17]

Urine output

Decreased urine output generally is perceived as a more sensitive marker for AKI diagnosis compared with serum creatinine because urine production is directly affected by the reduction of GFR. But, like creatinine, urine output is not specific for AKI. Oliguria can be caused by many physiologic factors, such as prolonged fasting, hypovolemia, stress, and pain, via the action of antidiuretic hormone. The other common extrarenal factor affecting urine output is urinary tract obstruction. On the other hand, urine output can persist until GFR almost ceases in nonoliguric AKI, such as nephrotoxin-induced AKI or leptospirosis.[18,19] Lastly, weight-adjusted urine output criteria can be misleading in obese patients. Using the ideal body weight rather than the true weight might be more appropriate to avoid overdiagnosing AKI in this population.[20]

BIOMARKERS AND THE CONTINUUM OF ACUTE KIDNEY INJURY

The continuum of AKI from initial kidney stress, to early injury, to dysfunction, and to long-term outcomes is the current conceptual model of the clinical course of AKI (**Fig. 1**). In each point of the continuum, biomarkers may help define the mechanisms and predict the evolution of AKI.

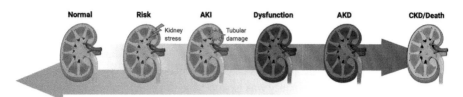

Fig. 1. Continuum of AKI.

In the recent past, the search for an ideal biomarker for AKI once was viewed to be similar to the discovery of cardiac troponin for myocardial infarction. Unlike myocardial infarction, however, in which ischemic injury was the dominant cause, AKI can be caused by multiple conditions with different mechanisms. Due to the limitations of serum creatinine and the complexity of AKI, a great effort has been made to develop biomarkers to augment the diagnosis and management of AKI. According to the continuum of AKI, biomarkers can be classified broadly into 2 main categories: markers of damage and markers of dysfunction (**Fig. 2**).

The development of novel biomarkers

The process of biomarker development can be divided into 4 main phases: discovery, quantification/verification, validation, and implementation.[21] Although hundreds of biomarker candidates had been screened through the biomarker development

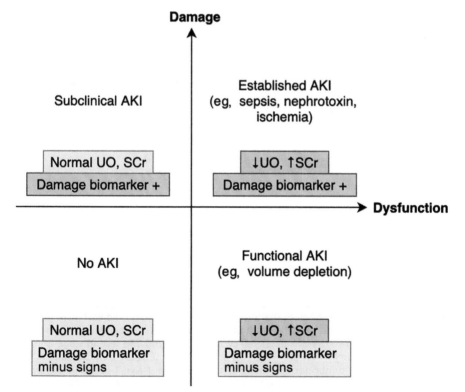

Fig. 2. Simplified paradigm of AKI biomarkers by damage and dysfunction. SCr, serum creatinine; UO, urine output.

pipeline, only a select few were launched onto the market and incorporated into the clinical practice.

Neutrophil gelatinase–associated lipocalin

Human neutrophil gelatinase–associated lipocalin (NGAL) is a 25-kDa glycoprotein of the lipocalin superfamily. It originally was isolated and identified from activated neutrophil granules in 1993.[22] NGAL later was found to be expressed at low constant rates by various tissues, including kidney, lung, liver, gastrointestinal tract, and adipose tissue.[23] The main production sites of NGAL in the kidneys are the intercalated cells of the collecting duct. An important function of NGAL under physiologic conditions is to act as a bacteriostatic agent by binding to the bacterial siderophore, enterochelin, thereby interrupting bacterial iron uptake.[24] NGAL also plays a role in the iron transport pathway, which regulates iron-dependent gene translation critical for cell growth and development (**Fig. 3**).[25] NGAL exists in 3 different molecular forms, a 25-kDa monomer, a 45-kDa homodimer, and also a 135-kDa heterodimer conjugated with matrix metalloproteinase (MMP)-9. Although neutrophils mainly secrete the homodimeric form, the injured kidney epithelial cells predominantly release monomeric and heterodimeric

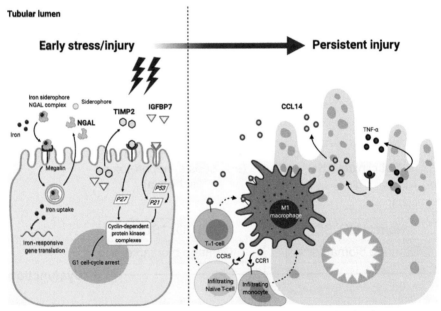

Fig. 3. Mechanisms of novel markers in AKI depicted in 2 stages. (*Left*) The first stage is an early stage of stress/injury with NGAL and TIMP2-IGFBP7. NGAL is produced and secreted from the tubular cells and binds iron and siderophore to form iron-siderophore complex and then enters the cells via megalin receptor. Iron-siderophore complex is stored in endosome, which releases iron to activate the function of iron-responsive genes. TIMP2-IGFBP7 also is produced and secreted from the tubular cells, which in turn bind each own receptor and stimulate p53, p21, and p27. The result of inhibition of cyclin-dependent protein kinase complexes by p21 and p27 results in G1 cell-cycle arrest. (*Right*) The second stage is a later stage of persistent injury with CCL14. CCL14 is produced and secreted from the tubular cells with a stimulation of tumor necrosis factor (TNF)-α receptor. Naïve T cells and monocytes then were recruited from blood circulation and were activated by the binding of CCL14 to CCR5 and CCR1, respectively. Naïve T cells differentiate to T_H1 cells, whereas monocytes differentiate to M1 macrophages. These 2 cell types are proinflammatory and involved in the phagocytosis of damaged tubular cells.

forms.[26] Under normal conditions, urinary NGAL level is low because filtered NGAL is almost completely reabsorbed by the proximal tubular cells in megalin-dependent manner.[27] After tubular injury, NGAL can be detected within 2 hours to 3 hours with a dynamic dose-dependent response.[28] Due to the markedly up-regulation of monomeric NGAL expression with rapid kinetics related to the injury, both urinary NGAL and plasma have been extensively investigated as AKI biomarkers.[29]

Cystatin C
Cystatin C (CysC) is a 13-kDa nonglycosylated protein of the cystatin superfamily, which plays roles in intracellular catabolism of peptides and proteins.[30] It first was discovered and sequenced in 1981.[31] CysC has a function as a cysteine protease inhibitor and is produced by all human nucleated cells at stable production rates. Few circumstances can alter CysC production, including age, sex, systemic inflammation, and high doses of glucocorticoids.[32] Because CysC is freely filtered through the normal glomerulus and completely reabsorbed by proximal tubular cells, CysC has been studied as a marker of GFR. Elevated urinary CysC may indicate renal tubular damage, which can be utilized as a marker for AKI. Compared with serum creatinine, serum CysC is more sensitive to early renal dysfunction and urinary CysC may have some value to detect tubular injury.[33]

Kidney injury molecule-1
Kidney injury molecule-1 (KIM-1), a 38.7-kDa member of the immunoglobulin gene superfamily, is a cell transmembrane glycoprotein that functions as adhesion molecule and also serves as a receptor to facilitate the clearance of the apoptotic debris. Under normal conditions, KIM-1 is expressed at a low level absent in the kidneys. It is markedly up-regulated, however, in the tubular epithelial cells and shed its extracellular component into the tubular lumen, which can be detected in urine 24 hours to 48 hours after tubular injury.[34,35]

L-type fatty acid–binding protein
Liver-type fatty acid–binding protein (L-FABP) is a 14-kDA protein member of the superfamily of lipid-binding proteins. L-FABP binds fatty acids and transports them to the mitochondria and peroxisomes to produce energy for tubular epithelial cells. Urinary L-FABP was found to be up-regulated in correlation with tubular damage.[36]

Proenkephalin A 119 to 159
Proenkephalin amino acids 119 through 159 (penKid), a 5-kDa monomeric peptide, first was discovered in 1975.[37] It is a stable breakdown product used as a surrogate marker for the more unstable parent polypeptide, proenkephalin (PENK). Apart from penkid, another peptide product of PENK is enkephalin, which functions as an endogenous opioid. Enkephalin binds to opioid receptors, which are expressed throughout the body. Among these opioid receptors, the gamma-opioid receptors are found to be highly expressed in the kidney.[38] Although the mechanism of enkephalin in regulating renal function is unclear, it was proposed to involve neurohormonal activation under stress and inflammation.[39] Due to its low molecular weight, penkid is filtered freely through the glomerulus.[40] Hence, it has been further investigated as a novel filtration marker.[40,41]

Tissue inhibitor of metalloproteinases-2 and insulin like growth factor–binding protein 7
Tissue inhibitor of metalloproteinases-2 (TIMP2) and insulinlike growth factor–binding protein 7 (IGFBP7) are the first second-generation AKI biomarkers because they were discovered and validated to risk assess for AKI defined by widely accepted clinical criteria—KDIGO criteria.[42] TIMP2 is a 21-kDa multifunctional protein abundantly

expressed in many normal tissues and first identified as an natural inhibitor of MMP, enzyme that degrades extracellular matrix. IGFBP7 is a 29-kDa multifunctional protein with the primary role of regulating insulinlike growth factors in tissues and stimulates cell adhesion. In kidney, TIMP2 was found to be expressed and secreted predominantly by distal tubular cells, whereas IGFBP7 was expressed equally across the entire tubule yet secreted primarily by proximal tubular cells.[43] During the early stages of AKI, both proteins block the cyclin-dependent–protein kinase complexes, which results in G1 cell-cycle arrest to prevent further cell division with DNA damage (see **Fig. 3**).[44]

C-C motif chemokine ligand 14

C-C motif chemokine ligand 14 (CCL14) is a new third-generation AKI biomarker that was developed to risk assess for persistent AKI—that is, AKI that does not resolve for 3 days or more. Thus, CCL14 is a prognostic biomarker to be used in patients that already meet the diagnosis of stage 2 to stage 3 AKI. CCL14 is a member of the chemokine family that is constitutively expressed in several tissues, including kidney. CCL14 has been shown to be associated with proinflammatory chemotaxis by activating monocytes and macrophages in a variety of diseases, such as lupus, inflammatory bowel disease, multiple myeloma, rheumatoid arthritis, human immunodeficiency virus infection, and hepatitis.[45,46] The reason CCL14 has never been identified in animal models of AKI is that CCL14 is not expressed in mice. CCL14 is a human homolog of mouse CCL6, which was shown to be abundantly up-regulated in mouse kidney transitioning from acute to chronic injury.[47,48] The mechanism of CCL14 in AKI is not completely understood. It is proposed, however, that CCL14 was released from the injured tubular epithelial cells from the activation of inflammatory mediators. Binding of CCL14 to receptors on monocytes and T cells results in monocyte differentiation into macrophages and T-cell differentiation into proinflammatory type 1 helper T (T_H1) cells. Then, T_H1 cells stimulate macrophage polarity into M1 macrophages, which also have proinflammatory functions and can phagocytose injured renal epithelial cells (see **Fig. 3**).

Clinical Applications of Biomarkers in Acute Kidney Injury

Prediction of acute kidney injury

Neutrophil gelatinase–associated lipocalin NGAL has been found to be a fair predictor for AKI occurrence in critically ill patients, in kidney transplant patients, and after cardiac surgery. Ho and colleagues[49] have conducted a meta-analysis of predictive ability of NGAL for predicting AKI associated with cardiac surgery and found the area under the receiver operating characteristic curves (AUROCs) for urinary NGAL and plasma NGAL 0.72 and 0.71 respectively. Performance may be considerably better, however, in certain settings. For example, Srisawat and colleagues[50] demonstrated the ability of both urinary NGAL and plasma NGAL to predict AKI development in 206 patients with clinical suspicious of leptospirosis with AUROCs of 0.91 and 0.92, respectively.

Cystatin C Herget-Rosenthal and colleagues[51] have reported serum CysC increased by more than 50% to be 0.6 days earlier in detecting AKI (AUROC 0.92–0.98) compared with serum creatinine in a cohort of 85 intensive care unit (ICU) patients. In a primary cohort of 72 adults undergoing cardiac surgery, Koyner and colleagues[52] have reported the predictive index of urinary CysC obtained at 6 hours after postoperative ICU admission with an AUROC of 0.72 for AKI prediction. A subsequent larger cohort from the same study group, however, has indicated urinary CysC measured in the early postoperative period was unable to predict AKI in 1203 adults and 299 children undergoing cardiac surgery.[53]

Tissue inhibitor of metalloproteinases-2 and insulinlike growth factor–binding protein 7 In the first validation study, Kashani and colleagues[42] reported urinary

TIMP2-IGFBP7 to be superior to all existing biomarkers in prediction of AKI KDIGO stage 2 to stage 3 within 12 hours of sample collection with an AUROC of 0.80 in a heterogeneous group of patients, including sepsis, shock, trauma, and major surgery. Subsequently, the initial results have been confirmed by various cohorts. Although cardiac surgery remains the most common, urinary TIMP2-IGFBP7 has been shown to perform well in sepsis (AUROC 0.85), in surgery (AUROC 0.84), in patients with congestive heart failure (AUROC 0.89), and in patients with CKD (AUROC 0.91). The test has been shown to detect the stress rapidly, within 4 hours after exposures, and accurately predict subsequent AKI occurrence at the cutoff of 0.3 $(ng/mL)^2/1000$.

Prognosis of acute kidney injury

Neutrophil gelatinase–associated lipocalin Urinary NGAL can be used to distinguish so-called intrinsic AKI (ATN) from prerenal azotemia, which was defined by renal dysfunction responsive to fluid resuscitation and hemodynamic optimization, with an AUROC of 0.87 in hospitalized patients.[54] Recently, a prospective study in ICU patients reported the predictive ability for persistent AKI with AUROCs of 0.83 and 0.85 for urinary NGAL and plasma NGAL, respectively (a cutoff of 150 ng/mL for plasma NGAL and a cutoff of 80 ng/mL for urinary NGAL).[55] Furthermore, normalized urinary NGAL, obtained on the day of AKI diagnosis, has been reported to have the ability to differentiate between ATN, prerenal, and hepatorenal syndrome AKI) with an AUROC of 0.80 (at a cutoff of 110 ug/g creatinine) in a cohort of 320 hospitalized cirrhotic patients with AKI.[56]

C-C motif chemokine ligand 14 The first clinical study of CCL14 in AKI was reported by Hoste and colleagues,[57] in 2020. This was a multinational prospective observational study conducted in adult patients in medical and surgical ICU with moderate to severe AKI (KDIGO stage 2 or stage 3). Patients were enrolled within 36 hours of meeting the KDIGO criteria. Urinary CCL14 and other biomarkers were collected at time of enrollment. The primary outcome was the development of persistent AKI defined by KDIGO stage 3 AKI lasting for 72 hours or more. Patients not at stage 3 AKI at enrollment were required to reach stage 3 within 48 hours and then persist in stage 3 for at least 72 hours to be considered endpoint positive. In the analysis, the study included 331 participants from 21 ICU sites across United States and Europe. Persistent AKI occurred in 33% of the study population. The predictive ability of urinary CCL14 for persistent AKI was the highest among all biomarkers including plasma/urinary NGAL, urinary TIMP-2 and IGFBP7, and plasma CysC, with AUROC of 0.83 (95% CI, 0.78–0.97).

Prediction of renal replacement therapy

Neutrophil gelatinase–associated lipocalin The authors have investigated the performance of urinary NGAL measured on days 1, 7, and 14 to predict outcomes at day 60 after enrollment in critically ill patients with severe AKI requiring renal replacement therapy (RRT) and found the greatest odds of predicting by using the timepoint of largest relative reduction of urinary NGAL level compared with day 1 (AUROC 0.70).[58] Moreover, the authors have examined plasma NGAL in 181 patients with AKI following community-acquired pneumonia and found an AUROC of 0.74 for predicting death, need for RRT, and persistent AKI at hospital discharge.[59] Haase and colleagues[60] later determined the association between urinary NGAL by a multicenter pooled analysis of prospective studies and found that elevated urinary NGAL carried a risk for adverse outcomes, including RRT initiation, in-hospital death, and length of ICU and hospital stay similar to elevated serum creatinine. Moreover, results from De Loor and colleagues[61] and Parikh and colleagues[62] confirmed that urinary NGAL had inadequate predictive index, with AUROCs of 0.65 and 0.67, respectively, for predicting severe AKI after elective cardiac surgery. Matsuura and colleagues[63] reported an AUROC of 0.80 for using plasma NGAL collected at the time of admission, with a cutoff 142 ng/mL to predict 1-week AKI progression in 95 critically ill patients.

Regarding clinical implementation of NGAL, Srisawat and colleagues[64] recently published a feasibility study to examine the effect of early RRT in patients' plasma NGAL greater than or equal to 400 ng/mL. Although the early RRT intervention did not significantly reduce the primary endpoint of 28-day mortality compared with the standard RRT, the number of ventilator-free days were significantly higher in the early RRT group.[64]

Kidney injury molecule-1 Urinary KIM-1 has been reported to have significant association with short term adverse outcomes in a cohort of 201 patients with AKI from multifactorial causes. Compared with the lowest quintile of KIM-1, the fourth quartile group had 3.2-fold higher odds for dialysis requirement and hospital death.[65]

L-type fatty acid–binding protein Urinary L-FABP demonstrated an AUROC of 0.79 for predicting short-term outcomes, which include AKI progression, dialysis, and death within 7 days in 152 critically ill patients with early AKI. This study also tested urinary NGAL and urinary KIM-1 but discovered the AUROC of only 0.65 and 0.62, respectively.[66]

Cystatin C Serum CysC, when measured at preoperative visit and daily on postoperative days 1 to 5 in adult patients undergoing cardiac surgery, was not superior to serum creatinine in terms of short-term adverse outcomes prediction. Combining CysC with serum creatinine, however, seemed to add benefit for predicting adverse outcomes, including hospital mortality and dialysis, compared with serum creatinine alone.[67] On the other hand, urinary CysC has been shown to have good predictive performance with an AUROC of 0.92 for a need for RRT in a cohort of 73 patients with nonoliguric ATN.[68]

Proenkephalin A 119 to 159 Hollinger and colleagues[41] have conducted a prospective multinational study, The Kidney in Sepsis and Septic Shock (Kid-SSS) study, to validate plasma penkid as a marker for major adverse kidney event at day 7, which included death, need for RRT, and persistent AKI. This study enrolled 579 ICU patients with sepsis. Plasma penkid was measured within 24 hours after admission. The cutoff of 84 pmol/L was used in this study. The AUROC of plasma penkid for predicting MAKE day 7 was approximately 0.84.[41]

Tissue inhibitor of metalloproteinases-2 and insulinlike growth factor–binding protein 7 In a recent cohort of 719 critically ill patients, AKI patients with elevated urinary TIMP2-IGFBP7 more than 0.3 $(ng/mL)^2/1000$ were found to have increased risk of in-ICU mortality or initiation of CRRT (adjusted hazard ratio [HR] 2.04) compared with AKI patients with TIMP2-IGFBP7 less than or equal to 0.3 $(ng/mL)^2/1000$.[69] Using KDIGO bundle, an intervention consisting of hemodynamic optimization, avoiding nephrotoxic drugs, and preventing hyperglycemia, could significantly lower the occurrence of AKI within the first 72 hours after cardiac surgery in high risk patients defined by urinary TIMP2-IGFBP7 greater than 0.3 compared with controls (absolute risk reduction [ARR] 16.6%; 95% CI, 5.5%–27.9%; P = .004).[70] Implementing AKI care bundle, however, did not lower the incidence of moderate to severe AKI within the first 3 days after admission in a randomized controlled trial of 100 patients with systemic inflammatory response syndrome and elevated urinary TIMP2-IGFBP7 in the emergency department.[71]

Table 1
Summary of clinical applications of acute kidney injury biomarkers

	Type of Marker	Predict Acute Kidney Injury	Predict Persistent Acute Kidney Injury	Predict Short-term Outcomes	Predict Long-term Outcomes
Urinary CysC	Damage	–	NA	+	NA
Urinary NGAL	Damage	++	+	+	+
Plasma NGAL	Damage	++	+	+	+
Urinary KIM-1	Damage	+	NA	+	+
Urinary L-FABP	Damage	+	+	+	+
Urinary [TIMP-2]•[IGFBP7]	Stress	+++	+	+	+
Plasma penkid	Function	NA	++	++	NA
Urinary CCL14	Damage	NA	+++	NA	NA

Abbreviations: -, nonpredictive; +, fair prediction; ++, good prediction; +++, excellent prediction.

Prediction of Long-Term Outcomes

Neutrophil gelatinase–associated lipocalin, kidney injury molecule-1, and L-type fatty acid–binding protein Although the prognostic value of AKI biomarkers for long-term outcomes generally is less established, the Translational Research Investigating Biomarker Endpoints in AKI study, a prospective multicenter cohort of 1219 adults underwent cardiac surgery, has shown an independent association between long-term mortality (median 3-year follow-up) and elevated urinary biomarkers, including NGAL, KIM-1, L-FABP, interleukin 18, and albumin.[72]

Tissue inhibitor of metalloproteinases-2 and insulinlike growth factor–binding protein 7 A secondary analysis of the Sapphire study, a multinational prospective cohort of 744 critically ill patients without AKI at enrollment, has shown that elevated urinary TIMP2-IGFBP7 was associated with increased risk of long-term adverse outcomes, including mortality and receipt of RRT, with an HR of 1.44 (95% CI, 1.00–2.06) for levels greater than 0.3 to less than or equal to 2.0 and HR 2.16 (95% CI, 1.32–3.53) for levels greater than 2.0 compared with levels less than or equal to 0.3 at 9 months.[73]

SUMMARY

Although the continuum of AKI is highly complex, the advancement of biomarker development has been promising and brought about a deeper insight of the underlying mechanisms of AKI pathogenesis and renal recovery. Currently, biomarkers have become indispensable tools for clinicians to manage AKI with precision (**Table 1**). It is an ongoing quest, however, to search for better biomarkers and to validate the appropriate use and clinical significance of the existing biomarkers thoroughly through large clinical studies.

CLINICS CARE POINTS

- Current evidence showed that serum creatinine and urine output are inadequate for prompt diagnosis of AKI, because they represent only dysfunction of the kidney but not the damage to the kidney.

- AKI should not be diagnosed and managed based only on a single biomarker. Combining clinical contexts and serial measurements of proper biomarkers can improve the quality of care greatly.
- There still is limited evidence regarding the use of biomarker-guided interventions and improved outcomes in patients with AKI.

DISCLOSURE

N. Srisawat discloses grant support from Baxter. J.A. Kellum discloses grant support and consulting fees from Astute Medical, bioMérieux, and Baxter.

REFERENCES

1. Liebig J. Kreatin und Kreatinin, Bestandtheile des Harns der Menschen. Journal für Praktische Chemie 1847;40:288–92. https://doi.org/10.1002/prac.18470400170.
2. Kidney Disease: Improving Global Outcomes (KDIGO) Acute Kidney Injury Work Group. KDIGO clinical practice guideline for acute kidney injury. Kidney Int 2012; 2:1–138.
3. Bellomo R, Ronco C, Kellum JA, et al, Acute Dialysis Quality Initiative Workgroup. Acute renal failure - definition, outcome measures, animal models, fluid therapy and information technology needs: the Second International Consensus Conference of the Acute Dialysis Quality Initiative (ADQI) Group. Crit Care 2004;8: R204–12.
4. Mehta RL, Kellum JA, Shah SV, et al. Acute kidney injury network: report of an initiative to improve outcomes in acute kidney injury. Crit Care 2007;11:R31.
5. Star RA. Treatment of acute renal failure. Kidney Int 1998;54:1817–31.
6. Sise ME, Forster C, Singer E, et al. Urine neutrophil gelatinase-associated lipocalin identifies unilateral and bilateral urinary tract obstruction. Nephrol Dial Transplant 2011;26:4132–5.
7. Decoste R, Himmelman JG, Grantmyre J. Acute renal infarct without apparent cause: a case report and review of the literature. Can Urol Assoc J 2015;9: E237–9.
8. Ramcharan T, Matas AJ. Long-term (20-37 years) follow-up of living kidney donors. Am J Transplant 2002;2:959–64.
9. Molitoris BA. Therapeutic translation in acute kidney injury: the epithelial/endothelial axis. J Clin Invest 2014;124:2355–63.
10. Sharma A, Mucino MJ, Ronco C. Renal functional reserve and renal recovery after acute kidney injury. Nephron Clin Pract 2014;127:94–100.
11. Efstratiadis G, Voulgaridou A, Nikiforou D, et al. Rhabdomyolysis updated. Hippokratia 2007;11:129–37.
12. Moretti C, Frajese GV, Guccione L, et al. Androgens and body composition in the aging male. J Endocrinol Invest 2005;28:56–64.
13. Kimmel PL, Lew SQ, Bosch JP. Nutrition, ageing and GFR: is age-associated decline inevitable? Nephrol Dial Transplant 1996;11(Suppl 9):85–8.
14. Musso CG, Michelangelo H, Vilas M, et al. Creatinine reabsorption by the aged kidney. Int Urol Nephrol 2009;41:727–31.
15. Cockcroft DW, Gault MH. Prediction of creatinine clearance from serum creatinine. Nephron 1976;16:31–41.

16. Doi K, Yuen PS, Eisner C, et al. Reduced production of creatinine limits its use as marker of kidney injury in sepsis. J Am Soc Nephrol 2009;20:1217–21.

17. Siew ED, Peterson JF, Eden SK, et al. Use of multiple imputation method to improve estimation of missing baseline serum creatinine in acute kidney injury research. Clin J Am Soc Nephrol 2013;8:10–8.

18. Anderson RJ, Linas SL, Berns AS, et al. Nonoliguric acute renal failure. N Engl J Med 1977;296:1134–8.

19. Seguro AC, Lomar AV, Rocha AS. Acute renal failure of leptospirosis: nonoliguric and hypokalemic forms. Nephron 1990;55:146–51.

20. Ad-hoc working group of ERBP, Fliser D, Laville M, et al. A European Renal Best Practice (ERBP) position statement on the Kidney Disease Improving Global Outcomes (KDIGO) clinical practice guidelines on acute kidney injury: part 1: definitions, conservative management and contrast-induced nephropathy. Nephrol Dial Transplant 2012;27:4263–72.

21. Rifai N, Gillette MA, Carr SA. Protein biomarker discovery and validation: the long and uncertain path to clinical utility. Nat Biotechnol 2006;24:971–83.

22. Kjeldsen L, Johnsen AH, Sengelov H, et al. Isolation and primary structure of NGAL, a novel protein associated with human neutrophil gelatinase. J Biol Chem 1993;268:10425–32.

23. Cowland JB, Borregaard N. Molecular characterization and pattern of tissue expression of the gene for neutrophil gelatinase-associated lipocalin from humans. Genomics 1997;45:17–23.

24. Goetz DH, Holmes MA, Borregaard N, et al. The neutrophil lipocalin NGAL is a bacteriostatic agent that interferes with siderophore-mediated iron acquisition. Mol Cell 2002;10:1033–43.

25. Yang J, Goetz D, Li JY, et al. An iron delivery pathway mediated by a lipocalin. Mol Cell 2002;10:1045–56.

26. Cai L, Rubin J, Han W, et al. The origin of multiple molecular forms in urine of HNL/NGAL. Clin J Am Soc Nephrol 2010;5:2229–35.

27. Hvidberg V, Jacobsen C, Strong RK, et al. The endocytic receptor megalin binds the iron transporting neutrophil-gelatinase-associated lipocalin with high affinity and mediates its cellular uptake. FEBS Lett 2005;579:773–7.

28. Paragas N, Qiu A, Zhang Q, et al. The Ngal reporter mouse detects the response of the kidney to injury in real time. Nat Med 2011;17:216–22.

29. Mishra J, Ma Q, Prada A, et al. Identification of neutrophil gelatinase-associated lipocalin as a novel early urinary biomarker for ischemic renal injury. J Am Soc Nephrol 2003;14:2534–43.

30. Brzin J, Popovic T, Turk V, et al. Human cystatin, a new protein inhibitor of cysteine proteinases. Biochem Biophys Res Commun 1984;118:103–9.

31. Grubb A, Lofberg H. Human gamma-trace, a basic microprotein: amino acid sequence and presence in the adenohypophysis. Proc Natl Acad Sci U S A 1982;79:3024–7.

32. Knight EL, Verhave JC, Spiegelman D, et al. Factors influencing serum cystatin C levels other than renal function and the impact on renal function measurement. Kidney Int 2004;65:1416–21.

33. Coll E, Botey A, Alvarez L, et al. Serum cystatin C as a new marker for noninvasive estimation of glomerular filtration rate and as a marker for early renal impairment. Am J Kidney Dis 2000;36:29–34.

34. Bonventre JV. Kidney injury molecule-1 (KIM-1): a urinary biomarker and much more. Nephrol Dial Transplant 2009;24:3265–8.

35. Ichimura T, Bonventre JV, Bailly V, et al. Kidney injury molecule-1 (KIM-1), a putative epithelial cell adhesion molecule containing a novel immunoglobulin domain, is up-regulated in renal cells after injury. J Biol Chem 1998;273:4135–42.

36. Yokoyama T, Kamijo-Ikemori A, Sugaya T, et al. Urinary excretion of liver type fatty acid binding protein accurately reflects the degree of tubulointerstitial damage. Am J Pathol 2009;174:2096–106.

37. Hughes J, Smith TW, Kosterlitz HW, et al. Identification of two related pentapeptides from the brain with potent opiate agonist activity. Nature 1975;258:577–80.

38. Denning GM, Ackermann LW, Barna TJ, et al. Proenkephalin expression and enkephalin release are widely observed in non-neuronal tissues. Peptides 2008;29:83–92.

39. Beunders R, Struck J, Wu AHB, et al. Proenkephalin (PENK) as a novel biomarker for kidney function. J Appl Lab Med 2017;2:400–12.

40. Marino R, Struck J, Hartmann O, et al. Diagnostic and short-term prognostic utility of plasma pro-enkephalin (pro-ENK) for acute kidney injury in patients admitted with sepsis in the emergency department. J Nephrol 2015;28:717–24.

41. Hollinger A, Wittebole X, Francois B, et al. Proenkephalin A 119-159 (Penkid) is an early biomarker of septic acute kidney injury: the Kidney in Sepsis and Septic Shock (Kid-SSS) Study. Kidney Int Rep 2018;3:1424–33.

42. Kashani K, Al-Khafaji A, Ardiles T, et al. Discovery and validation of cell cycle arrest biomarkers in human acute kidney injury. Crit Care 2013;17:R25.

43. Emlet DR, Pastor-Soler N, Marciszyn A, et al. Insulin-like growth factor binding protein 7 and tissue inhibitor of metalloproteinases-2: differential expression and secretion in human kidney tubule cells. Am J Physiol Renal Physiol 2017; 312:F284–96.

44. Kellum JA, Chawla LS. Cell-cycle arrest and acute kidney injury: the light and the dark sides. Nephrol Dial Transplant 2016;31:16–22.

45. Charo IF, Ransohoff RM. The many roles of chemokines and chemokine receptors in inflammation. N Engl J Med 2006;354:610–21.

46. Vyshkina T, Sylvester A, Sadiq S, et al. CCL genes in multiple sclerosis and systemic lupus erythematosus. J Neuroimmunol 2008;200:145–52.

47. Kotarsky K, Sitnik KM, Stenstad H, et al. A novel role for constitutively expressed epithelial-derived chemokines as antibacterial peptides in the intestinal mucosa. Mucosal Immunol 2010;3:40–8.

48. Liu J, Kumar S, Dolzhenko E, et al. Molecular characterization of the transition from acute to chronic kidney injury following ischemia/reperfusion. JCI Insight 2017;2:e94716.

49. Ho J, Tangri N, Komenda P, et al. Urinary, plasma, and serum biomarkers' utility for predicting acute kidney injury associated with cardiac surgery in adults: a meta-analysis. Am J Kidney Dis 2015;66:993–1005.

50. Srisawat N, Praditpornsilpa K, Patarakul K, et al. Neutrophil Gelatinase Associated Lipocalin (NGAL) in leptospirosis acute kidney injury: a multicenter study in Thailand. PLoS One 2015;10:e0143367.

51. Herget-Rosenthal S, Marggraf G, Husing J, et al. Early detection of acute renal failure by serum cystatin C. Kidney Int 2004;66:1115–22.

52. Koyner JL, Bennett MR, Worcester EM, et al. Urinary cystatin C as an early biomarker of acute kidney injury following adult cardiothoracic surgery. Kidney Int 2008;74:1059–69.

53. Koyner JL, Garg AX, Shlipak MG, et al. Urinary cystatin C and acute kidney injury after cardiac surgery. Am J Kidney Dis 2013;61:730–8.

54. Singer E, Elger A, Elitok S, et al. Urinary neutrophil gelatinase-associated lipocalin distinguishes pre-renal from intrinsic renal failure and predicts outcomes. Kidney Int 2011;80:405–14.
55. Tecson KM, Erhardtsen E, Eriksen PM, et al. Optimal cut points of plasma and urine neutrophil gelatinase-associated lipocalin for the prediction of acute kidney injury among critically ill adults: retrospective determination and clinical validation of a prospective multicentre study. BMJ Open 2017;7:e016028.
56. Huelin P, Sola E, Elia C, et al. Neutrophil gelatinase-associated lipocalin for assessment of acute kidney injury in cirrhosis: a prospective study. Hepatology 2019;70:319–33.
57. Hoste E, Bihorac A, Al-Khafaji A, et al. Identification and validation of biomarkers of persistent acute kidney injury: the RUBY study. Intensive Care Med 2020;46(5): 943–53.
58. Srisawat N, Wen X, Lee M, et al. Urinary biomarkers and renal recovery in critically ill patients with renal support. Clin J Am Soc Nephrol 2011;6:1815–23.
59. Srisawat N, Murugan R, Lee M, et al. Plasma neutrophil gelatinase-associated lipocalin predicts recovery from acute kidney injury following community-acquired pneumonia. Kidney Int 2011;80:545–52.
60. Haase M, Devarajan P, Haase-Fielitz A, et al. The outcome of neutrophil gelatinase-associated lipocalin-positive subclinical acute kidney injury: a multicenter pooled analysis of prospective studies. J Am Coll Cardiol 2011;57: 1752–61.
61. De Loor J, Herck I, Francois K, et al. Diagnosis of cardiac surgery-associated acute kidney injury: differential roles of creatinine, chitinase 3-like protein 1 and neutrophil gelatinase-associated lipocalin: a prospective cohort study. Ann Intensive Care 2017;7:24.
62. Parikh CR, Coca SG, Thiessen-Philbrook H, et al. Postoperative biomarkers predict acute kidney injury and poor outcomes after adult cardiac surgery. J Am Soc Nephrol 2011;22:1748–57.
63. Matsuura R, Komaru Y, Miyamoto Y, et al. Response to different furosemide doses predicts AKI progression in ICU patients with elevated plasma NGAL levels. Ann Intensive Care 2018;8:8.
64. Srisawat N, Laoveeravat P, Limphunudom P, et al. The effect of early renal replacement therapy guided by plasma neutrophil gelatinase associated lipocalin on outcome of acute kidney injury: a feasibility study. J Crit Care 2017;43: 36–41.
65. Liangos O, Perianayagam MC, Vaidya VS, et al. Urinary N-acetyl-beta-(D)-glucosaminidase activity and kidney injury molecule-1 level are associated with adverse outcomes in acute renal failure. J Am Soc Nephrol 2007;18:904–12.
66. Parr SK, Clark AJ, Bian A, et al. Urinary L-FABP predicts poor outcomes in critically ill patients with early acute kidney injury. Kidney Int 2015;87:640–8.
67. Spahillari A, Parikh CR, Sint K, et al. Serum cystatin C- versus creatinine-based definitions of acute kidney injury following cardiac surgery: a prospective cohort study. Am J Kidney Dis 2012;60:922–9.
68. Herget-Rosenthal S, Poppen D, Husing J, et al. Prognostic value of tubular proteinuria and enzymuria in nonoliguric acute tubular necrosis. Clin Chem 2004;50: 552–8.
69. Xie Y, Ankawi G, Yang B, et al. Tissue inhibitor metalloproteinase-2 (TIMP-2) * IGF-binding protein-7 (IGFBP7) levels are associated with adverse outcomes in patients in the intensive care unit with acute kidney injury. Kidney Int 2019;95: 1486–93.

70. Meersch M, Schmidt C, Hoffmeier A, et al. Prevention of cardiac surgery-associated AKI by implementing the KDIGO guidelines in high risk patients identified by biomarkers: the PrevAKI randomized controlled trial. Intensive Care Med 2017;43(11):1551–61.
71. Schanz M, Wasser C, Allgaeuer S, et al. Urinary [TIMP-2].[IGFBP7]-guided randomized controlled intervention trial to prevent acute kidney injury in the emergency department. Nephrol Dial Transplant 2019;34:1902–9.
72. Coca SG, Garg AX, Thiessen-Philbrook H, et al. Urinary biomarkers of AKI and mortality 3 years after cardiac surgery. J Am Soc Nephrol 2014;25:1063–71.
73. Koyner JL, Shaw AD, Chawla LS, et al. Tissue Inhibitor Metalloproteinase-2 (TIMP-2)IGF-Binding Protein-7 (IGFBP7) levels are associated with adverse long-term outcomes in patients with AKI. J Am Soc Nephrol 2015;26:1747–54.

The Role of Renal Functional Reserve in Predicting Acute Kidney Injury

Dana Y. Fuhrman, DO, MS

KEYWORDS

- Renal functional reserve • Acute kidney injury • Acute protein load • Hyperfiltration
- Protein stimulation test • Glomerular filtration rate

KEY POINTS

- First described more than 20 years ago, renal functional reserve is not routinely quantified or applied in clinical practice.
- There are numerous proposed mechanisms explaining the change in glomerular filtration rate that occurs with a protein load, with the most accepted theories including the involvement of humoral mediators and resetting of tubuloglomerular feedback.
- There has been a recent renewed interest in the study of renal function reserve for the purpose of detecting patients more susceptible to clinical acute kidney injury and chronic kidney disease.
- Future investigations should focus on the impact of renal function reserve assessments on outcomes.

INTRODUCTION

First described in 1983 by Bosch and colleagues,[1] the concept of renal functional reserve (RFR) refers to the normal kidney's ability to increase its filtration rate in response to a stimulator such as a protein load. The numerical difference between a baseline and a protein-stimulated glomerular filtration rate (GFR) has been termed RFR. In healthy individuals, an increase in GFR after a protein load can range between 6% and 40% with a mean increase of 26% after a protein meal depending on the experimental conditions of the study.[2]

The kidney does not operate constantly at its maximum filtration capacity, but rather at approximately 75% of maximum GFR.[3] An individual may have an apparently

Pediatrics, Critical Care Medicine, and Nephrology, Department of Critical Care Medicine, The Center for Critical Care Nephrology, University of Pittsburgh School of Medicine, UPMC Children's Hospital of Pittsburgh, 4401 Penn Avenue, Children's Hospital Drive, Faculty Pavilion, Suite 2000, Pittsburgh, PA 15224, USA
E-mail address: dana.fuhrman@chp.edu
Twitter: @DanaFuhrman4 (D.Y.F.)

Crit Care Clin 37 (2021) 399–407
https://doi.org/10.1016/j.ccc.2020.11.008
0749-0704/21/© 2020 Elsevier Inc. All rights reserved.

criticalcare.theclinics.com

normal GFR, but a decreased RFR. A lack of GFR increase in response to a protein load has been shown in individuals with reduced nephron mass as a result of a single kidney,[1,4] type I diabetes mellitus,[5] high-grade vesicoureteral reflux,[6] hemolytic uremic syndrome,[7–9] obesity,[10] and hypertension.[11] Using amino acid infusions and plasma clearance of Tc99 m diethylene-triamine penta-acetic acid, Barai and colleagues[12] reported a decline in RFR with progression of chronic kidney disease.

Researchers have proposed that a kidney that has a history of injury may be operating at its maximal filtration capacity and, therefore, have reduced, or no available nephrons to increase GFR in response to a stimulus. Acute kidney injury (AKI) can result in a decrease in the number of functional nephrons in the kidney, whereby GFR measurements may not accurately represent the degree of structural injury. This can lead to an adaptive response such as glomerular hyperfiltration to maintain homeostasis. An increasing desire by investigators to uncover the silent loss of nephrons that can occur with AKI has led to a renewed interest in finding easily replicated, practical methods for quantifying RFR.

POSTULATED MECHANISMS FOR RENAL FUNCTIONAL RESERVE

Many mechanisms have been discussed in the literature regarding the changes in GFR that occur in response to a protein load with no single agreed on process (**Fig. 1**).

The most accepted mechanisms for a renal response to a protein load include the involvement of humoral mediators and resetting of tubuloglomerular feedback. It has been proposed that the mechanism may vary based on the disease process.[13] Animal models support an interplay of hemodynamic and structural changes. Simultaneous changes in renal plasma blood flow with changes in GFR in response to increases

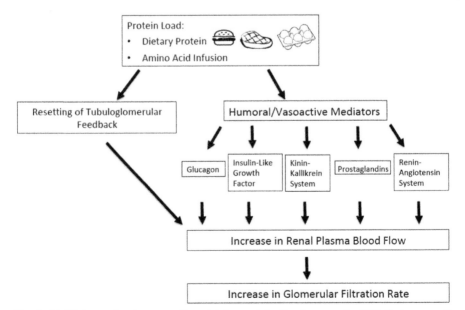

Fig. 1. Multiple mechanisms are thought to explain the increase in GFR that occurs in response to a protein load. The most commonly cited mechanisms include the involvement of humoral mediators and the resetting of tubuloglomerular feedback resulting in an increase in renal plasma blood flow.

in dietary protein have been demonstrated. Interestingly, rats fed high-protein diets have shown an increase in kidney size.[14]

The role of the deactivation of tubuloglomerular feedback in the GFR response to a protein load has been shown in animal models. In dogs using lithium clearance, Woods and colleagues[15] reported an increase in proximal tubular transport mediated by the sodium amino acid cotransport system after intravenous infusion of amino acids. This decreased distal sodium chloride delivery results in a deactivation of tubuloglomerular feedback and an accompanying increase in GFR. Likely there is a systemic effect of protein consumption, rather than simply a local effect acting on the kidney. Premen[16] infused serine, alanine, and proline into the intrarenal artery of dogs that led to a rise in renal blood flow when measured with p-aminohippuric acid, but did not increase GFR. However, an intravenous infusion of these amino acids led to significant elevations in renal blood flow and GFR, supporting the theory that a secondary systemic factor is likely needed before amino acids can cause a change in GFR.

The release of humoral factors at the time of protein consumption has been thought to explain the increase in GFR.[17–19] Several studies' results in both rats and humans support the role of glucagon in the renal response to a protein load by showing the inhibition of a renal hemodynamic response to amino acid infusion by somatostatin administration.[20,21] However, the increase in GFR with glucagon administration has been found to be moderate, suggesting that glucagon likely plays a facilitative role in the change in renal hemodynamics with amino acid infusion, rather than being the primary factor.[22] Insulinlike growth factor-1 has been shown to be higher in the glomeruli and liver of rats fed a high-protein verses low-protein diet.[23]

Investigators have explored the role of vasoactive mediators such as renal kallikrein and vasoactive kinins in the renal response to protein ingestion.[24] In humans, Bolin and colleagues[25] demonstrated that an oral protein load increases GFR concurrently with the urinary excretion of kinin. In a cohort of patients with hypertension, Pecly and colleagues[10] reported a lower RFR in obese patients when compared with patients without obesity. They found a lower increase in urinary kallikrein and an inability to elevate serum nitric oxide levels in the patients with obesity.

Ruilope and colleagues[26] reported evidence of the influence of angiotensin II and prostaglandin in the renal hemodynamic effects of amino acid infusions. Healthy human volunteers who received a low-sodium diet 3 days prior had a lack of increase in renal blood flow and GFR when given an amino acid infusion. However, the renal blood flow and GFR response with amino acid infusion was restored with treatment with an angiotensin-converting enzyme (ACE) inhibitor. They also reported in healthy human subjects a decrease in the change in renal blood flow and GFR with amino acid infusion in response to indomethacin administration. Investigations using nonsteroidal anti-inflammatory drugs (NSAIDs) to block prostaglandin synthesis have produced conflicting results regarding their impact on RFR. Some investigators have reported a loss of RFR with NSAID administration and others demonstrated a normal RFR after NSAID use.[18,19,27]

METHODS USED TO QUANTIFY RENAL FUNCTIONAL RESERVE

The percent change in GFR after a protein load varies from study to study depending on the type of protein used, dose of protein given, or other differences in experimental conditions.[2] Investigators commonly advise subjects to maintain a diet free of meat, fish, and fowl for 24 hours before testing. Most studies use an oral red meat protein load.[1,4,10] Researchers also have reported significant changes in GFR after giving subjects dairy products, egg white proteins, or baked goods.[28] Compared with other oral methods of protein loading, the use of beef has induced the largest response.

Investigators have used methods other than an oral protein load to elicit a change in GFR. The intravenous infusion of amino acids has been used[12,29]; however, not all amino acids elicit the same response. In rats, the infusion of non–branched chain amino acids has been shown to increase GFR, whereas the branched chain amino acid, leucine, does not modify GFR.[30] Amino acid infusions show a faster GFR response when compared with an oral protein load on average (30–60 minutes vs 60–180 minutes).[1,31] A dopamine infusion has been used in some studies.[31] The mechanism whereby dopamine increases GFR is thought to be different from a meat meal or the use of amino acids. Experimental results have shown a fall in filtration fraction with a dopamine infusion as a result of a coinciding greater increase in renal plasma blood flow when compared with GFR.[32]

The dose of protein given varies from study to study, with most investigators administering 1 to 2 g of protein per kilogram of body weight. Rodriguez-Iturbe and colleagues.[33] demonstrated an increased filtration fraction with protein loads of 1.1 and 1.3 g per kilogram of body weight but not with 0.55 g per kilogram of body weight. In 18 healthy adult volunteer subjects, Sharma and colleagues[13] tested the effect on GFR of ingesting 1 g/kg versus 2 g/kg of cooked red meat on the GFR response. They did not report a greater increase in GFR with the larger protein load.

Similar to the type of protein stimulus used, the method used to quantify GFR varies from study to study. Few investigators have reported using inulin or iohexol clearance.[4,34] Comparing creatinine clearance before and after a protein load is the most common method cited in the literature for quantifying RFR.[2,35] An important limitation with the use of creatinine clearance is the secretion of creatinine by renal tubular cells. The clearance of creatinine due to tubular secretion is lower in individuals with a normal GFR when compared with those with a moderately reduced GFR (40–80 mL/min per 1.73 m^2).[36] Given the concern that ingesting food containing preformed creatinine and creatinine precursors could lead to a wide variation in changes in creatinine clearance, some investigators have advocated for the use of milk, cheese, and baked goods to stimulate GFR, rather than use of meat products. Hellerstein and colleagues[37,38] have published on the use of cimetidine to successfully inhibit the tubular secretions of creatinine in RFR studies in children. Using cimetidine, they report a very close approximation of inulin clearance and creatinine clearance when they measured the 2 clearances simultaneously in pediatric patients.

Creatinine clearance studies are time-consuming, requiring multiple urine collections before and after a protein load, taking on average 6.5 to 7.0 hours to complete. Our group has previously shown that changes in cystatin C estimated GFR with cystatin C drawn 125 to 140 minutes after a protein load may be used to estimate RFR induced by a meat meal in healthy young adults (cystatin C estimated GFR peak vs baseline: 110.1 vs 98.1 mL/min per 1.73 m^2, $P<.003$).[39] This method has yet to be validated in any patient groups.

A RENEWED INTEREST IN RENAL FUNCTIONAL RESERVE

As a result of renal hyperfiltration, serum creatinine increases only after 50% of the nephrons are lost.[40] Initially, RFR and baseline GFR may remain intact after an injurious event; however, as a result of multiple renal insults, a patient may become more susceptible to clinical AKI and eventually chronic kidney disease (**Fig. 2**).[41] Patients with chronic medical conditions admitted to the intensive care unit are at a particularly greater risk of kidney function decline with repeat renal insults. Intrigued

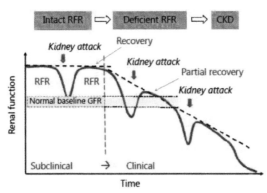

Fig. 2. After repeat episodes of AKI, a patient may have a deficient RFR, yet a normal baseline GFR. With partial recovery and subsequent renal injury, the patient may become more susceptible to AKI with minor insults, clinically evident AKI, and eventually chronic kidney disease. (*Reprinted from* Sharma A, Mucino MJ, Ronco C. Renal functional reserve and renal recovery after acute kidney injury. *Nephron Clin Practl.* 2014;127(1-4):94-100 by Karger. Reprinted with permission.)

by the use of RFR to detect the early functional decline in kidney function, investigators recently have focused on the use of RFR as a "stress test" for the kidney to be used to identify those individuals with a normal baseline GFR, but a deficient RFR.[41]

Before recent years, there have been very few studies describing the association of RFR with outcomes. The use of RFR in children with a history of hemolytic uremic syndrome has been explored, given the uncertainty of future renal health in these patients. Dieguez and colleagues[8] reported that children after hemolytic uremic syndrome with a low response to a protein load (less than a 36% increase) were more likely to develop proteinuria. Livi and colleagues[42] showed that in 28 patients with systemic sclerosis without a history of renal disease, lower baseline RFR is associated with a 9.5% decrease in RFR when evaluated 5 years later, whereas subjects with a higher baseline RFR had a 3.8% decrease in GFR when evaluated at 5 years.

Importantly, there has been a significant increase in the past 5 years in publications discussing the use of RFR for predicting outcomes. Husain-Syed and colleagues[43] explored the ability of preoperative RFR to predict AKI within 7 days after surgery in 110 patients undergoing elective cardiac surgery requiring cardiopulmonary bypass with a normal resting GFR. They stimulated GFR with a 1.2 mg per kilogram of body weight protein load in the form of an oral red meat meal and they calculated RFR using creatinine clearance before and after the protein meal. The investigators report that preoperative RFR was lower in patients who experienced AKI. In addition, RFR predicted AKI with an area under the receiver operator curve of 0.83 (confidence interval [CI] 0.70–0.96). Patients with an RFR $\leq$15 mL/min per 1.73 m^2 were 11.8 times more likely to experience AKI.

The same investigators studied the effect of repeat protein loading in 86 of the original subjects, again using an oral meat protein load and creatinine clearance.[44] Patients who met Kidney Disease Improving Global Outcomes (KDIGO) AKI criteria or had a rise in cell cycle arrest biomarkers (tissue inhibitor metalloproteinases-2 and insulinlike growth factor-binding protein 7) were more likely to show a decrease in RFR when repeated 3 months after surgery. No patients without AKI and low postoperative biomarker levels had a decrease in RFR greater than 4.7 mL/min per 1.73 m^2.

LIMITATIONS TO THE ROUTINE USE OF RENAL FUNCTIONAL RESERVE IN ROUTINE CLINICAL CARE

Despite its introduction into the literature more than 20 years ago, there is no routinely used method for quantifying RFR in clinical care. The wide variability of study results as a result of differing protocols and patient populations likely is playing a role in the lack of general acceptance of RFR as a routine method to measure kidney function. Importantly, patients of different ages and pathology are frequently grouped together in studies.[45] A decline in RFR has been shown to occur with age. Studies in humans have demonstrated a decline in GFR of approximately 0.8 mL/min per 1.73 m^2 per year after the age of 30 years.[46,47] Future investigations should include patients of similar ages and diagnoses.

There is a need for a simple reliable protocol that can be easily replicated. The most commonly cited method for quantifying RFR involves creatinine clearance methods, which are time-consuming and have the potential for error due to urine output measurements. In particular, in the pediatric population in which patients may not be toilet trained, there is a need for a method that does not rely on urine output determination. The use of other endogenous markers, like cystatin C, requires waiting for a change in the concentration of the marker to represent a change in GFR after a protein load is administered. Quantifying the disappearance rate of an exogenous marker, such as fluorescent molecules, has been proposed as a method to acquire real-time monitoring of GFR.[48] The use of real-time monitoring of GFR using fluorescent molecules and transdermal sensors have great promise for evaluating RFR accurately and efficiently.

Skepticism regarding the use of RFR may in part be due to a lack of evidence regarding the impact of RFR on outcomes or potential therapeutic implications of protein administration. Until recent years, few researchers have investigated the impact of RFR on outcomes. As discussed previously, Husain-Syed and colleagues[44] reported that in their patient cohort, individuals who met AKI criteria were more likely to a show decrease in RFR when repeated 3 months after cardiac surgery. Interestingly, no patients in this study met the criteria for AKI using KDIGO urine output criteria.[44] The investigators speculated that there might be a sustained impact of urine output after the protein load. Based on observations supporting the impact of protein on decreasing renal vascular resistance, Pu and colleagues[49] randomized 69 adult patients with estimated GFR values of 20 to 89 mL/min per 1.73 m^2 undergoing cardiac surgery requiring more than 1 hour of on-pump time to receive a continuous infusion of L-amino acids after anesthetic induction or standard of care. In the intervention arm, the amino acid infusion was continued until discharge from the intensive care unit. The duration of AKI defined by the KDIGO criteria was significantly reduced in the patients who received the amino acid infusion. Patients who received the supplementary amino acids demonstrated a significantly greater than baseline estimated GFR when compared with the patients who received standard of care (+10.8% difference, 95% CI, 1.0%–20%, $P = .033$). In addition, urine output was greater in the patient group that received the amino acid infusion.

Future investigations exploring therapeutic considerations if a lower RFR is found are important. Based on studies in animal models, ACE inhibitor and angiotensin II receptor blocker (ARB) medications have the potential to restore the response to a protein load in hyperfiltering states, such as diabetes and hypertension.[26,29] Given the proposed beneficial effects of ACE inhibitors and ARB medications in reducing intraglomerular pressure and proteinuria, an agreed on method to quantify RFR could lead to future investigations on the impact of these medications in patients with a declining RFR.[50–52]

SUMMARY

We can be falsely reassured by a normal GFR value when caring for the patients in the intensive care unit, particularly in the setting of decreased muscle mass or hyperfiltration. Future investigations should continue to explore the use of RFR in patients before kidney donation or before procedures carrying a higher risk of renal insult. Investigators are beginning to study the use of RFR for assessing renal recovery after AKI. There stands to be a benefit to quantifying RFR in certain patient groups, given the evidence that our patients may have a normal GFR, yet a decline in RFR associated with a greater risk of adverse kidney events.

CLINICS CARE POINTS

- When quantified before cardiac surgery, RFR has been found to be lower in patients who experience AKI postoperatively.
- Patients who experience AKI after cardiac surgery show a decrease in RFR when repeated 3 months after surgery.
- Providing an amino acid infusion before cardiopulmonary bypass has been shown to potentially decrease the duration of AKI after cardiac surgery.

DISCLOSURE

Dr Fuhrman is funded by a K23: DK116973.

REFERENCES

1. Bosch JP, Saccaggi A, Lauer A, et al. Renal functional reserve in humans. Effect of protein intake on glomerular filtration rate. Am J Med 1983;75(6):943–50.
2. Rodriguez-Iturbe B. The renal response to an acute protein load in man: clinical perspective. Nephrol Dial Transplant 1990;5(1):1–9.
3. Ronco C, Bellomo R, Kellum J. Understanding renal functional reserve. Intensive Care Med 2017;43(6):917–20.
4. Bosch JP, Lew S, Glabman S, et al. Renal hemodynamic changes in humans. Response to protein loading in normal and diseased kidneys. Am J Med 1986; 81(5):809–15.
5. Raes A, Donckerwolcke R, Craen M, et al. Renal hemodynamic changes and renal functional reserve in children with type I diabetes mellitus. Pediatr Nephrol 2007;22(11):1903–9.
6. Rahman RA, Bhatnagar V, Agarwala S, et al. Estimation of renal functional reserve in children with different grades of vesicoureteric reflux. J Indian Assoc Pediatr Surg 2018;23(2):74–80.
7. Tufro A, Arrizurieta EE, Repetto H. Renal functional reserve in children with a previous episode of haemolytic-uraemic syndrome. Pediatr Nephrol 1991;5(2):184–8.
8. Dieguez S, Ayuso S, Brindo M, et al. Renal functional reserve evolution in children with a previous episode of hemolytic uremic syndrome. Nephron Clin Pract 2004; 97(3):c118–22.
9. Perelstein EM, Grunfield BG, Simsolo RB, et al. Renal functional reserve compared in haemolytic uraemic syndrome and single kidney. Arch Dis Child 1990;65(7):728–31.
10. Pecly IM, Genelhu V, Francischetti EA. Renal functional reserve in obesity hypertension. Int J Clin Pract 2006;60(10):1198–203.

11. Zitta S, Stoschitzky K, Zweiker R, et al. Dynamic renal function testing by compartmental analysis: assessment of renal functional reserve in essential hypertension. Nephrol Dial Transplant 2000;15(8):1162–9.

12. Barai S, Gambhir S, Prasad N, et al. Functional renal reserve capacity in different stages of chronic kidney disease. Nephrology (Carlton) 2010;15(3):350–3.

13. Sharma A, Zaragoza JJ, Villa G, et al. Optimizing a kidney stress test to evaluate renal functional reserve. Clin Nephrol 2016;86(7):18–26.

14. MacKay E, MacKay LL, Addis T. Factors which determine renal weight: influence of age on the relation of renal weight to the protein intake and degree of renal hypertrophy produced by high protein diets. American Physiological Society 1928; 86(2):459–65.

15. Woods LL, Mizelle HL, Montani JP, et al. Mechanisms controlling renal hemodynamics and electrolyte excretion during amino acids. Am J Physiol 1986;251(2 Pt 2):F303–12.

16. Premen AJ. Nature of the renal hemodynamic action of amino acids in dogs. Am J Physiol 1989;256(4 Pt 2):F516–23.

17. Kleinman KS, Glassock RJ. Glomerular filtration rate fails to increase following protein ingestion in hypothalamo-hypophyseal-deficient adults. Preliminary observations. Am J Nephrol 1986;6(3):169–74.

18. Ruilope LM, Robles RG, Miranda B, et al. Renal effects of fenoldopam in refractory hypertension. J Hypertens 1988;6(8):665–9.

19. Hirschberg RR, Zipser RD, Slomowitz LA, et al. Glucagon and prostaglandins are mediators of amino acid-induced rise in renal hemodynamics. Kidney Int 1988; 33(6):1147–55.

20. Castellino P, Coda B, DeFronzo RA. Effect of amino acid infusion on renal hemodynamics in humans. Am J Physiol 1986;251(1 Pt 2):F132–40.

21. Meyer TW, Ichikawa I, Zatz R, et al. The renal hemodynamic response to amino acid infusion in the rat. Trans Assoc Am Physicians 1983;96:76–83.

22. Pitts R. The effects of infusing glycine and of varying the dietary protein intake on renal hemodynamics in the dog. Am J Physiol 1944;142:355–65.

23. Hirschberg R, Kopple JD. Response of insulin-like growth factor I and renal hemodynamics to a high- and low-protein diet in the rat. J Am Soc Nephrol 1991; 1(8):1034–40.

24. Jaffa AA, Harvey JN, Sutherland SE, et al. Renal kallikrein responses to dietary protein: a possible mediator of hyperfiltration. Kidney Int 1989;36(6):1003–10.

25. Bolin P, Jaffa AA, Rust PF, et al. Acute and chronic responses of human renal kallikrein and kinins to dietary protein. Am J Physiol 1989;257(5 Pt 2):F718–23.

26. Ruilope LM, Rodicio J, Garcia Robles R, et al. Influence of a low sodium diet on the renal response to amino acid infusions in humans. Kidney Int 1987;31(4): 992–9.

27. Brouhard BH, LaGrone L. Effect of indomethacin on the glomerular filtration rate after a protein meal in humans. Am J Kidney Dis 1989;13(3):232–6.

28. Hellerstein S, Berenbom M, Erwin P, et al. Measurement of renal functional reserve in children. Pediatr Nephrol 2004;19(10):1132–6.

29. De Nicola L, Blantz RC, Gabbai FB. Renal functional reserve in treated and untreated hypertensive rats. Kidney Int 1991;40(3):406–12.

30. Garcia GE, Hammond TC, Wead LM, et al. Effect of angiotensin II on the renal response to amino acid in rats. Am J Kidney Dis 1996;28(1):115–23.

31. Mansy H, Patel D, Tapson JS, et al. Four methods to recruit renal functional reserve. Nephrol Dial Transplant 1987;2(4):228–32.

32. McDonald RH Jr, Goldberg LI, McNay JL, et al. Effect of dopamine in man: augmentation of sodium excretion, glomerular filtration rate, and renal plasma flow. J Clin Invest 1964;43:1116–24.
33. Rodriguez-Iturbe B, Herrera J, Marin C, et al. Tubular stress test detects subclinical reduction in renal functioning mass. Kidney Int 2001;59(3):1094–102.
34. Rodenbach KE, Fuhrman DY, Maier PS, et al. Renal response to a protein load in healthy young adults as determined by iohexol infusion clearance, cimetidine-inhibited creatinine clearance, and cystatin C estimated glomerular filtration rate. J Ren Nutr 2017;27(4):275–81.
35. Molina E, Herrera J, Rodriguez-Iturbe B. The renal functional reserve in health and renal disease in school age children. Kidney Int 1988;34(6):809–16.
36. King AJ, Levey AS. Dietary protein and renal function. J Am Soc Nephrol 1993;3(11):1723–37.
37. Hellerstein S, Berenbom M, Alon US, et al. Creatinine clearance following cimetidine for estimation of glomerular filtration rate. Pediatr Nephrol 1998;12(1):49–54.
38. Hellerstein S, Berenbom M, Erwin P, et al. Creatinine for evaluation of glomerular filtration rate in children. Clin Pediatr (Phila) 2006;45(6):525–30.
39. Fuhrman DY, Maier PS, Schwartz GJ. Rapid assessment of renal reserve in young adults by cystatin C. Scand J Clin Lab Invest 2013;73(4):265–8.
40. Liu KD, Brakeman PR. Renal repair and recovery. Crit Care Med 2008;36(4 Suppl):S187–92.
41. Sharma A, Mucino MJ, Ronco C. Renal functional reserve and renal recovery after acute kidney injury. Nephron Clin Pract 2014;127(1–4):94–100.
42. Livi R, Guiducci S, Perfetto F, et al. Lack of activation of renal functional reserve predicts the risk of significant renal involvement in systemic sclerosis. Ann Rheum Dis 2011;70(11):1963–7.
43. Husain-Syed F, Ferrari F, Sharma A, et al. Preoperative renal functional reserve predicts risk of acute kidney injury after cardiac operation. Ann Thorac Surg 2018;105(4):1094–101.
44. Husain-Syed F, Ferrari F, Sharma A, et al. Persistent decrease of renal functional reserve in patients after cardiac surgery-associated acute kidney injury despite clinical recovery. Nephrol Dial Transplant 2019;34(2):308–17.
45. Fliser D, Zeier M, Nowack R, et al. Renal functional reserve in healthy elderly subjects. J Am Soc Nephrol 1993;3(7):1371–7.
46. Delanaye P, Schaeffner E, Ebert N, et al. Normal reference values for glomerular filtration rate: what do we really know? Nephrol Dial Transplant 2012;27(7):2664–72.
47. Davies DF, Shock NW. Age changes in glomerular filtration rate, effective renal plasma flow, and tubular excretory capacity in adult males. J Clin Invest 1950;29(5):496–507.
48. Solomon R, Goldstein S. Real-time measurement of glomerular filtration rate. Curr Opin Crit Care 2017;23(6):470–4.
49. Pu H, Doig GS, Heighes PT, et al. Intravenous amino acid therapy for kidney protection in cardiac surgery patients: a pilot randomized controlled trial. J Thorac Cardiovasc Surg 2019;157(6):2356–66.
50. Anderson S, Rennke HG, Brenner BM. Nifedipine versus fosinopril in uninephrectomized diabetic rats. Kidney Int 1992;41(4):891–7.
51. Tarif N, Bakris GL. Angiotensin II receptor blockade and progression of nondiabetic-mediated renal disease. Kidney Int Suppl 1997;63:S67–70.
52. Jafar TH, Stark PC, Schmid CH, et al. Proteinuria as a modifiable risk factor for the progression of non-diabetic renal disease. Kidney Int 2001;60(3):1131–40.

Starting Kidney Replacement Therapy in Critically Ill Patients with Acute Kidney Injury

Sean M. Bagshaw, MD, MSc, FRCPC[a],*, Ron Wald, MDCM, MPH, FRCPC[b]

KEYWORDS

- Acute kidney injury • Critical illness • Kidney • Renal replacement therapy
- Indications • Timing • Mortality • End-stage kidney disease

KEY POINTS

- Timing of kidney replacement therapy (KRT) initiation in critically ill patients with acute kidney injury (AKI), in the absence of urgent indications, has been a long-standing dilemma for clinicians.
- Numerous clinical trials have aimed to inform practice; however, they have found discrepant results, which has contributed to wide variations in practice.
- An earlier strategy has biological rationale, even in the absence of urgent indications; however, a conservative strategy can also prevent selected patients from ever receiving KRT.
- The recently published Standard Versus Accelerated Initiation of Renal Replacement Therapy in Acute Kidney Injury (STARRT-AKI) trial found no survival benefit to early compared with delayed strategies for KRT initiation; however, it showed an early strategy conferred risk for dialysis dependence.
- STARRT-AKI provides compelling evidence that a delayed strategy, characterized by watchful waiting and starting KRT when worsening, persistent, or medically refractory complications of AKI occur, should now be adopted as a standard approach.

INTRODUCTION

Acute kidney injury (AKI) continues to be a vexing clinical challenge for nephrologists, intensivists, and other health care professionals caring for critically ill patients.[1,2] Even mild and transient AKI seems to herald greater risk for short-term and long-term adverse events compared with patients not experiencing AKI, including new or

[a] Department of Critical Care Medicine, Faculty of Medicine and Dentistry, University of Alberta and Alberta Health Services, 2-124E, Clinical Sciences Building, 8440-112 ST Northwest, Edmonton, Alberta T6G 2B7, Canada; [b] Division of Nephrology, St. Michael's Hospital and University of Toronto, and Li Ka Shing Knowledge Institute of St. Michael's Hospital, 30 Bond Street, Toronto, Ontario M5B 1W8, Canada
* Corresponding author.
E-mail address: bagshaw@ualberta.ca

Crit Care Clin 37 (2021) 409–432
https://doi.org/10.1016/j.ccc.2020.11.005
0749-0704/21/© 2020 Elsevier Inc. All rights reserved.

worsened chronic kidney disease (CKD), progression to end-stage kidney disease (ESKD), cerebral and cardiovascular events,[3,4] new infections and sepsis,[5,6] gastrointestinal bleeding,[7] malignancy,[8] fracture risk,[9] and death.[10,11]

A substantial proportion of critically ill patients with AKI, defined by current consensus definitions,[12] particularly those who develop toxic, metabolic, or fluid-related complications caused by AKI,[11,13] are considered for and started on kidney replacement therapy (KRT).[1,14] KRT is used in 10% to 12% of critically ill patients with AKI; however, temporal trends imply use is growing.[15–18]

THE CLINICAL DILEMMA OF WHEN TO START KIDNEY REPLACEMENT THERAPY

The dilemma of whether and when to start KRT for critically ill patients with AKI, in the absence of clearly urgent clinical indications, is not new and has long been a vexing clinical issue for intensivists and nephrologists. This issue has been repeatedly identified as a high research priority for new evidence to better inform clinical practice guidelines and guide complex bedside care within nephrology and critical care. A recent Kidney Disease: Improving Global Outcomes (KDIGO) Conference on Controversies in Acute Kidney Injury revisited this issue and highlighted the existing uncertainty of when to start KRT in critically ill patients with AKI, particularly in patients without medically refractory complications of AKI.[19] The consensus document proposed consideration for starting KRT when a patient's metabolic and fluid demands exceed the kidneys' capacity during an episode of AKI such that complications would be inevitable. However, there are no reliable, validated, or widely available tools to simply quantify this kidney demand-supply relationship at the point of care.[20] Importantly, the document also acknowledged the dynamic and often rapidly evolving clinical context for patients with critical illness complicated by AKI, which can naturally affect decision making for when to start KRT.

In critically ill patients with complications of AKI that are refractory to medical management (eg, hyperkalemia, acidemia, fluid overload), there is generally consensus and little hesitancy about the role for urgent initiation of KRT (**Table 1**). However, the occurrence of some of these common urgent indications for KRT in critically ill patients with AKI are less commonly encountered in routine intensive care unit (ICU) practice.[21–23] As such, in the absence of such indications, KRT is likely started in response to trends in illness acuity, nonkidney organ dysfunction, coupled with the inherent subjective perception of benefit by health care professionals (ie, anticipation of worsening or low likelihood for kidney recovery).[23] The recent KDIGO Controversies Conference further proposed that decision making on starting KRT should be a shared process with patients and families and should routinely integrate the overall prognosis, the potential for kidney recovery, the patient-specific risks of KRT itself, and a clear understanding of patients' preferences[19] (**Fig. 1**).

KRT in ICU settings broadly aims to achieve and maintain fluid, electrolyte, acid-base, and uremic/metabolic solute homeostasis and to facilitate critically important life-support measures when indicated (eg, nutrition, parenteral medications, obligatory fluid intake, blood product transfusions). KRT can also mitigate the risk of life-threatening complications associated with AKI.[24,25] Moreover, given the importance of kidney-organ interaction in critical illness and the potential negative sequelae of AKI on distant organ function (eg, kidney-lung, kidney-heart, kidney-brain, kidney-liver interactions), KRT has been proposed as a platform of multiorgan support to further mitigate nonkidney organ dysfunction that may be exacerbated by the sequelae of AKI.[26]

Table 1
Summary of absolute and relative indications and contraindications for starting renal replacement therapy in critically ill patients with acute kidney injury

Urgent indications (in the absence of contraindications to KRT)	• Refractory hyperkalemia (eg, K^+ level $\geq$6.0 mmol/L, rapidly increasing, or cardiac toxicity) • Refractory acidemia and metabolic acidosis (eg, pH $\leq$ 7.2 or serum bicarbonate level $\leq$12 mmol/L despite normal or low arterial Pco_2) • Refractory hypoxemia (Pao_2/fraction of inspired oxygen ratio $\leq$200 and perception of volume overload; eg, diuretic-resistant pulmonary edema) • Symptoms or complications attributable to uremia (eg, bleeding, pericarditis, encephalopathy) • Overdose/toxicity from a dialyzable drug/toxin
Relative indications (in the absence of life-threatening complications of AKI)	• Limited physiologic reserve to tolerate the consequences of AKI (ie, demand-supply mismatch) • Advanced nonkidney organ dysfunction worsened or exacerbated by excessive fluid accumulation (ie, impaired respiratory function) • Anticipated solute burden (eg, tumor lysis syndrome, rhabdomyolysis, intravascular hemolysis) • Need for large-volume fluid administration (ie, nutrition, medications, or blood products) • Severity of the underlying disease • Concomitant accumulation of poisons or toxic drugs that can be removed by RRT (eg, salicylates, ethylene glycol, methanol, metformin)
Relative contraindications	• Low likelihood for benefit (ie, futile prognosis) • Patient receiving palliative care and/or approaching end of life • High likelihood of nonrecovery of renal function in patient who is not a candidate for long-term dialysis

Adapted from Ostermann, M., Wald, R. & Bagshaw, S. M. Timing of Renal Replacement Therapy in Acute Kidney Injury. Contrib Nephrol 2016; 187; 106-120; with permission; and Bagshaw, S. M. & Wald, R. Strategies for the optimal timing to start renal replacement therapy in critically ill patients with acute kidney injury. Kidney Int (2017); 91:1022-1032; with permission

Despite this, it must be acknowledged that KRT is an invasive organ support with the potential for complications from insertion and maintenance of a dedicated central venous catheter (eg, bloodstream infection[27]) and treatment-related complications (eg, hemodynamic instability, electrolyte abnormalities, nonrecovery of kidney function)[28](**Table 2**). Recent observations imply that a conservative approach to starting KRT, whereby KRT is started in response to worsening AKI and the development of

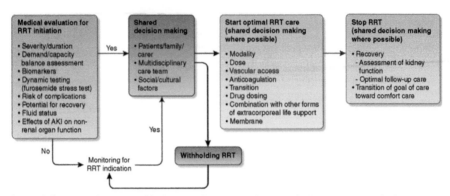

Fig. 1. Schematic diagram of kidney replacement therapy decisions in acute kidney injury. RRT, renal replacement therapy. (*Reproduced from* Ostermann, M. et al. Controversies in acute kidney injury: conclusions for a Kidney Disease: Improving Global Outcomes (KDIGO) Conference. Kidney Int 2020; 1-15; with permission.)

urgent indications, may be suitable for many critically ill patients.[27–30] However, the long-standing paucity of robust and widely generalizable evidence from randomized controlled trials (RCTs) had undoubtedly contributed to substantial variation in practice along with greater relative subjectivity among health care professionals for

Table 2
Benefits and drawbacks of early kidney replacement therapy in the absence of urgent indications in critically ill patients with severe acute kidney injury compared with delayed kidney replacement therapy

Benefits	Drawbacks
Avoid and/or control of volume accumulation and overload	Need for and complications associated with the dialysis catheter (eg, bleeding, pneumothorax, bloodstream infection)
Avoid and/or control of acid-base derangement	Need for and complications associated with anticoagulation regimens
Avoid and/or control of electrolyte/metabolic derangement and complication of uremia	Risk of iatrogenic episodes of hemodynamic instability that may exacerbate AKI and impede kidney repair/recovery
Avoid unnecessary or excess diuretic exposure	Risk of excess loss of unmeasured micronutrients and trace elements
Immunomodulation and clearance of inflammatory mediators	Risk of excess clearance or subtherapeutic levels of vital medications (ie, antimicrobials, anti-epileptics)
Platform to mitigate distant organ effects of AKI (eg, heart, lungs, liver, brain)	Unnecessary exposure to KRT in patients who had likelihood of kidney recovery with a conservative strategy
Restore demand-supply mismatch (eg, unloading or resting stressed and/or damaged kidneys)	Increased bedside workload for health care professionals, resource use, and direct health costs

Adapted from Ostermann, M., Wald, R. & Bagshaw, S. M. Timing of Renal Replacement Therapy in Acute Kidney Injury. Contrib Nephrol 2016; 187:106-120; with permission and Bagshaw, S. M. et al. Current state of the art for renal replacement therapy in critically ill patients with acute kidney injury. Intensive Care Med 2017; 43:841-854; with permission and Bagshaw, S. M. & Wald, R. Strategies for the optimal timing to start renal replacement therapy in critically ill patients with acute kidney injury. Kidney Int 2017; 91:1022-1032; with permission.

deciding when to start KRT in a given patient (ie, entrenched beliefs and behaviors).[15,22,31–33] This situation may also have contributed to variability in clinical practice.

This concise state-of-the art review critically appraises the current state of evidence, including the recently published Standard Versus Accelerated Initiation of Renal Replacement Therapy in Acute Kidney Injury (STARRT-AKI) trial, on strategies for initiating KRT in critically ill patients with AKI. It highlights current knowledge, provides a practical perspective for clinicians on existing clinical practice guidelines, and identifies additional evidence-care gaps for future research.

KIDNEY REPLACEMENT THERAPY AND CLINICAL OUTCOMES

KRT, along with mechanical ventilation, vasoactive therapy, and extracorporeal life support, is a core life-sustaining technology used in contemporary critical care practice. Although fewer patients typically receive KRT compared with mechanical ventilation, circulatory, or vasoactive support during a typical ICU course, the use of KRT has substantially grown.[1,15,16,18,22,33] This growth likely reflects evolving patient demographics, multimorbidity (eg, CKD), and innovations in medical therapies (eg, cancer therapeutics) and surgical interventions (eg, complex cardiac or hepatobiliary surgery, transplant). Although KRT adds complexity and costs to the bedside care of critically ill patients, temporal trends have shown modest reductions in mortality among those receiving KRT in selected clinical contexts.[11,34]

There has been genuine discourse on whether providing KRT in general significantly modifies patient outcomes or whether, as a supportive therapy in the setting of high illness acuity, KRT use is merely a surrogate for a patient's burden of preexisting illness (eg, CKD, cardiovascular disease, cancer) and the severity of critical illness. Select studies have implied that KRT per se may exert a hazard for death among patients with AKI[31,35,36] or, at minimum, not show association with improved outcome when comparing patients who do and do not receive KRT.[14] However, it is likely that many of these studies are susceptible to bias and limited ability to generalize caused by differences in populations (ie, case mix, illness acuity), confounding by indication and uncontrolled sources of bias (eg, practice variation, information bias).[37] Patient, clinician, and institutional-level factors may all interact to confound the association between KRT and outcome, including variation in decision making to even offer KRT.[14] In addition, there may be important effects of the type and size of ICU and volume of KRT performed on outcome, with smaller ICUs, those with less experience, and those treating fewer patients showing greater adjusted risk for mortality.[31,38]

In addition, it is vitally important to consider patient selection and suitability for KRT and its plausible association with outcome[39] (**Fig. 2**). It may be challenging to attribute an outcome benefit for KRT per se, because many patients may be likely to either survive or die with or without KRT. For example, high KRT use among patients with a low probability of survival (eg, frail, advanced chronic illness, and/or severe acute illness) can represent a plausible source of false-negative bias, because these patients shift the association to suggest KRT may mediate higher mortality.[40] Similarly, patients with lower illness acuity and less severe AKI who are started on KRT, where indications may be relative and where there was high a priori likelihood of kidney recovery, can also bias the association of KRT and mortality, because these patients may have survived regardless of whether KRT was provided.[41] In this circumstance, it is conceivable that the risk and/or harm associated with KRT per se could potentially outweigh benefit among those with a relative or marginal indication.[28] The focus

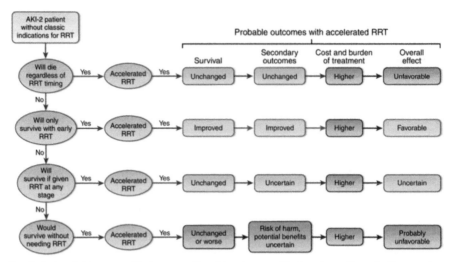

Fig. 2. Potential impact of heterogeneity of treatment effect and practice misalignment on outcome in a trial of timing of starting RRT in critically ill patients with AKI. (*Reproduced from* Prowle, J. R. & Davenport, A. Does early-start renal replacement therapy improve outcomes for patients with acute kidney injury? Kidney Int 2015 88:670-673; with permission.)

then is really on careful patient selection and the timely initiation of KRT for patients who are most likely to derive benefit and not experience greater attributable harm.[41] Selected observational studies in critically ill patients with AKI who develop urgent indications for KRT and/or persistent or worsening AKI imply that starting KRT may improve survival,[11,13,34] whereas recent data from the STARRT-AKI trial has implied that (too) early KRT can increase the risk for dialysis dependence.[28]

KIDNEY REPLACEMENT THERAPY AND CORONAVIRUS DISEASE 2019

Recent data have shown that KRT use in critically ill patients with coronavirus disease 2019 (COVID-19) has been substantially higher than historical use in comparable critically ill patients with AKI.[42,43] In the most recent report from the Intensive Care National Audit & Research Centre (ICNARC) Case Mix Programme Database, 26.5% (n = 2636 out of 9931) of patients received KRT for a median 7 days (interquartile range [IQR], 3–14) during ICU admission.[43] Patients receiving KRT support associated with COVID-19 were older, had greater prevalence of CKD, and were characterized by high illness acuity and greater nonkidney organ support (ie, invasive mechanical ventilation) compared with historical controls.[43] ICU mortality among patients receiving any KRT was 42.5%. Although there were data suggesting high KRT use in COIVD-19, it remains unclear what specifically is triggering the start of KRT and whether this high use is driven by patient-specific or clinician-specific factors.

DEFINITIONS OF TIMING FOR STARTING KIDNEY REPLACEMENT THERAPY

There is little consensus on how to define timing relative to the start of KRT in AKI. Observational studies and clinical trials have used a wide spectrum of arbitrary definitions for early, delayed, or late initiation of KRT.[44,45] Definitions have integrated physiologic parameters (eg, urine output), biochemical parameters (eg, serum creatinine, urea), inflammatory or novel biomarker thresholds (eg, neutrophil gelatinase-associated lipocalin

[NGAL], cystatin C, tissue inhibitor of metalloproteinase-2 and insulin growth factor binding protein-7 [TIMP-2*IGFBP-7]),[46,47] timing relative to AKI onset, timing relative to hospital or ICU admission, timing relative to the development of a recognized clinical or biochemical complication of AKI or urgent indication for KRT,[11,13,44,45,48] and the dynamic response to a standardized furosemide stress test (FST).[49–52] The terms early, delayed, and late are relative and subjective. Across the spectrum of clinical circumstances, what may represent early KRT in one setting may represent delayed in another, where the constellation of clinical characteristics, diagnoses, and acuity differ. The heterogeneity in operational definitions for timing has clearly been a challenge for clinicians trying to make inferences of the literature and has likely compounded uncertainty in recommendations in clinical practice guidelines.

RATIONALE FOR AN EARLY STRATEGY TO STARTING KIDNEY REPLACEMENT THERAPY

There is strong physiologic rationale for why earlier initiation of KRT in critically ill patients with severe AKI, even in the absence of urgent indications, should confer benefit for selected patients, in particular in circumstances where there is a perception that recovery from AKI may not be imminent.[53] Earlier KRT can theoretically facilitate more rapid correction of electrolyte and acid-base derangements and control of uremia, and mitigate fluid accumulation (see **Table 2**). Earlier KRT can prevent the occurrence of complications of AKI and may facilitate weaning from mechanical ventilation.[11,54] The role of KRT to modulate inflammation and immune function in septic and other vasoplegic states (eg, after cardiac surgery) is hypothetically attractive but remains controversial.[55,56] The practice of earlier KRT initiation in critically ill patients with AKI seems to confer numerous benefits, but this approach is largely supported by observational data and small randomized clinical trials.[30,44,45,57,58]

RATIONALE FOR A CONSERVATIVE STRATEGY TO KIDNEY REPLACEMENT THERAPY INITIATION

A substantial proportion of patients with severe AKI recover kidney function, so it is reasonable to conclude that a conservative strategy can prevent selected patients from ever receiving KRT. This approach may translate into health resource and cost savings, but such delays can conceivably predispose to prolonged exposure to the fluid and metabolic hazards of AKI. In the Artificial Kidney Initiation in Kidney Injury (AKIKI) trial, patients allocated to the delayed KRT strategy had biochemical evidence of worsening AKI (eg, higher serum creatinine, urea, and potassium levels; lower serum bicarbonate level and pH) at the time of starting KRT compared with patients allocated to the early strategy.[27] Moreover, patients in the delayed strategy also received significantly more interventions to manage the fluid and metabolic complications of AKI (eg, hyperkalemia and metabolic acidosis).[27] Similarly, in the STARRT-AKI trial, patients allocated to the standard (delayed) strategy showed biochemical evidence of worsening AKI and a greater toxic milieu when starting KRT compared with those in the accelerated (early) strategy.[28] Although observational data have suggested such complications of AKI exert incremental hazard for death,[11] the attributable harm from such complications is unclear.

There are also potential consequences of earlier start to KRT in the absence of urgent indications. Such patients require dedicated central venous dialysis catheter access, have their blood exposed to an extracorporeal circuit, and receive anticoagulation to maintain circuit patency (eg, systemic heparin, regional citrate). The potential for exposure to episodes of hemodynamic instability caused by excessive ultrafiltration or rapid changes in osmolality may represent an underappreciated mechanism that disrupts and contributes to iatrogenic delay in kidney recovery.[28,59] This risk is particularly relevant for patients who have been started on KRT for marginal indications, where the risk exceeds benefit.[41] In addition, starting a critically ill patient on KRT adds to bedside workload. Several studies have suggested that these issues can be avoided in selected patients if a conservative approach (delayed strategy) is adopted.[27–30] Many RCTs have failed to show incremental improvement in outcomes with early KRT in the absence of urgent indications,[27,30,60–62] a finding reaffirmed in the STARRT-AKI trial.[28] These data now strongly imply that a conservative approach with watchful waiting is warranted for patients without urgent indications. Naturally, any perceived benefit for early start of KRT would have to be balanced with the clinical context, specifically the risk for potential harm, the added resource implications, and within the context of the patient's and family's preferences for care.[19,41]

CURRENT CLINICAL PRACTICE GUIDELINE RECOMMENDATIONS

Several organizations have published clinical practice guideline statements focused on timing of initiation of KRT in critically ill settings; however, many are dated and require revision[12,63,64](Table 3). In 2012, the Kidney Disease Improving Global Outcomes (KDIGO) consortium made 2 statements regarding the timing of KRT initiation in AKI, based on expert opinion.[12] The first was to start KRT emergently when life-threatening changes in fluid, electrolyte, and acid-base balance exist. The second asked clinicians to consider the broader clinical context, the presence of conditions that can be modified with renal replacement therapy (RRT), and trends of laboratory tests, rather than single blood urea nitrogen and creatinine thresholds alone, when making the decision to start RRT. Although the second statement may be perceived as vague and provide clinicians with a wide scope of subjective parameters to inform their decision making, it was a reasonable reflection of contemporary bedside practice given the available evidence. In 2013, the National Institute for Health and Care Excellence (NICE) in the United Kingdom published recommendations that are similar to KDIGO.[63] The NICE guidelines acknowledged the paucity of evidence from RCTs on when to start KRT in both critically ill children and adults and emphasized the need to develop and evaluate tools, such as clinical risk prediction scores or novel point-of-care tests (eg, novel kidney damage biomarkers). In 2015, the French Intensive Care Society (SRLF) published recommendations for KRT in ICU settings, including statements on when to start KRT.[64] Each of these organizations acknowledged the limitations in current evidence and associated clinical uncertainty and each called for additional evidence from RCTs to inform practice and update guidelines. Since their publication, several RCTs have now been reported.[27–30,65] Future iterations of these and any other clinical practice guidelines should also integrate the importance of shared decision making with patients and families in decisions on whether and when to escalate support with KRT[19](see **Fig. 1**).

CLINICAL TRIAL EVIDENCE ON TIMING OF STARTING KIDNEY REPLACEMENT THERAPY

Several randomized trials have aimed to inform practice by understanding the ideal circumstances for commencing KRT in critically ill patients with AKI.[27,29,47,52,61,62,66] Three large and recently published trials[27,29,66] found discrepant results and have generated uncertainty on the best approach to starting KRT for critically ill patients with AKI.[65]

Table 3
Summary of clinical practice guideline statements for timing of initiation of kidney replacement therapy in critically ill patients with acute kidney injury

Organization	Recommendations
KDIGO[12]	1. Initiate KRT emergently when life-threatening changes in fluid, electrolyte, and acid-base balance exist (not rated) 2. Consider the broader clinical context, the presence of conditions that can be modified with KRT, and trends of laboratory tests, rather than single blood urea nitrogen and creatinine thresholds alone, when making the decision to start KRT (not rated)
NICE[63]	1. Discuss any potential indications for RRT with a nephrologist, pediatric nephrologist, and/or critical care specialist immediately to ensure that the therapy is started as soon as needed 2. Refer adults, children, and young people immediately for KRT if any of the following are not responding to medical management: • Hyperkalemia • Metabolic acidosis • Complications of uremia (ie, pericarditis, encephalopathy) • Fluid overload • Pulmonary edema 3. Base the decision to start KRT on the condition of the adult, child, or young person as a whole and not on an isolated urea, creatinine, or potassium value
SRLF[64]	1. KRT should be initiated without delay in life-threatening situations (hyperkalemia, metabolic acidosis, tumor lysis syndrome, refractory pulmonary edema). (Expert opinion; strong agreement) 2. The available data are insufficient to define optimal timing of initiation of KRT outside life-threatening situations. (Expert opinion; strong agreement) 3. In children, fluid and sodium overload probably of >10%, and very probably of >20% should be considered as one of the criteria for initiation of RRT. (Expert opinion; poor agreement) 4. Early initiation of KRT means at KDIGO stage 2 or within 24 h after onset of acute renal failure that seems unlikely to be reversible. (Expert opinion; poor agreement) 5. Late initiation of KRT means >48 h after onset of acute renal failure, KDIGO stage 3, or when a life-threatening situation arises because of acute renal failure. (Expert opinion; poor agreement)

Abbreviations: NICE, National Institute for Health and Care Excellence; SRLF, French Intensive Care Society.

The AKIKI trial was a French multicenter RCT that tested whether a delayed strategy of KRT initiation would confer improved survival in 620 critically ill patients with severe AKI who were receiving mechanical ventilation and/or vasoactive support compared with an early strategy[27] (**Table 4**). Patients allocated to the early strategy started KRT within 6 hours of fulfilling KDIGO stage 3 AKI, and those receiving the delayed strategy only commenced KRT when patients developed medically refractory complications of worsening AKI (eg, oliguria or anuria for $\geq$72 hours following randomization, uremia, hyperkalemia, metabolic acidosis, and/or pulmonary edema caused by volume overload). The delayed strategy did not improve 60-day all-cause mortality (49.7% vs 48.5%, $P = .79$). Receipt of KRT occurred in only 51% of patients in the delayed strategy compared with 98% in the early strategy. The median difference for starting KRT between strategies was 57 hours (IQR, 25–83 hours) among those

Table 4
Summary of recently completed randomized clinical trials evaluating the timing of initiation of kidney replacement therapy in intensive care unit settings

Feature	ELAIN[66]	AKIKI[27]	IDEAL-ICU[29]	STARRT-AKI[28]
Country	Germany	France	France	Multinational
Sites (N)	1	31	24	168
Participants (N)	231	620	488[a]	3019
Setting/Population	Mixed medical/surgical ICU (94.8% surgical)	Mixed medical/surgical ICU (79.7% medical)	Mixed medical/surgical ICU (septic shock)	Mixed medical/surgical ICU
ARR for Sample Size Calculation (%)	18	15	10	6
Control Group Mortality (%)	55	55	55	44
Interventions:				
Early (Accelerated)	KDIGO stage 2 (within 8 h)	KDIGO stage 3 (within 6 h)	RIFLE-Failure (within 12 h)	KDIGO stage 2 (within 12 h)
Delayed (Conservative)	KDIGO stage 3 (within 12 h)	Specific criteria/emergent indications	Specific criteria 48–60 h after eligibility or emergent indications	Specific criteria/emergent indications
Time Difference (h)	25.5	57.0	43.9	25.0
Received KRT in Delayed (%)	90.8	51.0	62.0	61.8
KRT Modality	CRRT	Physician discretion (initial IHD 55%)	Physician discretion	Physician discretion
SOFA Score at Enrollment	~16.0	~10.9	~12.3	~11.7
Primary End Point	90-d mortality	60-d mortality	90-d mortality	90-d mortality
Early (Accelerated) (%)	39.3	48.5	58.0	43.9
Delayed (Conservative) (%)	54.7	49.7	54.0	43.7
Effect Estimate	HR, 0.66 (95% CI, 0.45–0.97)	HR, 1.03 (95% CI, 0.82–1.29)	RR, 1.08[b] (95% CI, 0.90–1.30)	RR, 1.00 (95% CI, 0.93–1.09)

Kidney Recovery	KRT dependence at 90 d	KRT dependence at 60 d	KRT dependence at 90 d	KRT dependence at 90 d
Early (Accelerated) (%)	53.6	2.0	2.0	10.4
Delayed (Conservative) (%)	38.7	5.0	3.0	6.0
Effect Estimate	OR, 0.55 (95% CI, 0.32–0.93)	RR, 0.53[b] (95% CI, 0.20–1.41)	RR, 0.83[b] (95% CI, 0.28–2.46)	RR, 1.74 (95% CI, 1.24–2.43)
Adverse Events	Aggregate	CRBSI	Indication for emergent KRT[c]	Aggregate
Early (Accelerated) (%)	75.0	10.0	—	23.0
Delayed (Conservative) (%)	68.5	3.0	17	16.5
Effect Estimate	RR, 1.18[b] (95% CI, 0.86–1.61)	RR, 1.35[b] (95% CI, 1.08–1.68)	—	RR, 1.40 (95% CI, 1.21–1.62)

Abbreviations: CI, confidence interval; CRBSI, catheter-related bloodstream infection; CRRT, continuous RRT; ELAIN, Early Versus Late Initiation of Renal Replacement Therapy In Critically Ill Patients With Acute Kidney Injury; IDEAL-ICU, Initiation of Dialysis Early Versus Late in the Intensive Care Unit; HR, hazard ratio; IHD, intermittent hemodialysis; OR, odds ratio; RIFLE, risk, injury, failure, loss of kidney function, and ESKD; RR, risk ratio; SOFA, Sequential Organ Failure Assessment.

[a] Terminated prematurely because of futility.

[b] Calculated; not provided in primary publication.

[c] Reported for patients allocated to the delayed KRT strategy only.

who received KRT. KRT-free days were greater (19 vs 17 days, $P<.001$) and the occurrence of catheter-related bloodstream infections was lower (5% vs 10%, $P = .03$) in the delayed compared with the early strategy. There were no differences in secondary outcomes including ventilator and vasoactive-free days through day 28, lengths of stay in ICU and hospital, and dialysis dependence at 60 days. AKIKI also reported an analysis comparing the 2 strategies for starting KRT in subgroups with acute respiratory distress syndrome (ARDS) (n = 207; 33%) and sepsis (n = 348; 56%).[67] Findings of these post hoc secondary analyses supported the main trial findings, showing no substantial differences in 60-day mortality between strategies and similar proportions in the delayed strategy not receiving KRT. In another AKIKI post hoc analysis focused on the 60 (10%) patients with premorbid CKD, defined as a prehospital estimated glomerular filtration rate (eGFR) 30 to 60 mL/min/1.73 m^2, there was suggestion of heterogeneity in treatment effect on 60-day mortality, with those allocated to early KRT having a greater risk of death.[68]

The Early Versus Late Initiation of Renal Replacement Therapy In Critically Ill Patients with Acute Kidney Injury (ELAIN) trial was a single-center German RCT of 231 critically ill patients that tested whether early KRT, defined as starting KRT within 8 hours of fulfilling KDIGO stage 2 AKI, would improve patient survival compared with delayed KRT, defined as starting KRT within 12 hours of developing KDIGO stage 3 AKI or on the development of an urgent indication (eg, hyperkalemia, oligoanuria, hypermagnesemia, organ edema resistant to diuretics)[69](see **Table 4**). Eligible patients were predominantly surgical; were required to have a plasma NGAL level greater than 150 ng/mL; and at least 1 of sepsis, volume overload, worsening Sequential Organ Failure Assessment (SOFA) score, or receipt of vasoactive support. All patients allocated to the early strategy started KRT, as well as 91% in the delayed strategy, where the primary trigger to start KRT was progression to stage 3 AKI.[66] The median difference from randomization to starting KRT was less than 1 day (21 hours; IQR, 18–24 hours). Mortality at 90 days was reduced by 15.4% in the early compared with delayed strategy (39.3% vs 54.7%; hazard ratio, 0.66; 95% confidence interval [CI], 0.45–0.97). ELAIN also found that the early strategy conferred a greater likelihood of kidney recovery and dialysis independence, and shorter duration of ICU stay and hospitalization compared with a delayed strategy. ELAIN also measured several inflammatory mediators to provide biological and mechanistic insights into outcome differences between the strategies. Two proinflammatory mediators (interleukin [IL]-6, IL-8) showed greater reduction in those allocated to the early compared with those receiving the delayed strategy. In a post hoc analysis at 1 year, ELAIN found the benefits of the early strategy on a composite of major adverse kidney events to be durable.[70]

The Initiation of Dialysis Early Versus Late in the Intensive Care Unit (IDEAL-ICU) was a French multicentre randomized trial of early versus delayed KRT strategies that aimed to enroll 864 patients with septic shock and AKI.[71] Patients fulfilling RIFLE (risk, injury, failure, loss of kidney function, and ESKD)–Failure AKI criteria within the first 48 hours of onset of septic shock were eligible. The early strategy was defined as starting KRT within 12 hours of eligibility, whereas the delayed strategy was defined by KRT being deferred for greater than or equal to 48 hours (but no more than 60 hours) from the onset of RIFLE-Failure AKI, unless patients developed AKI complications and urgent indications to start KRT (see **Table 4**). The trial was terminated prematurely because of futility after randomization of only 488 patients (56.5%). Death at 90 days was no different between strategies: 58% in the early and 54% in the delayed strategy.[29] Almost all (97%) patients in the early strategy received KRT versus 62% in the delayed strategy. In 17% of patients allocated to the delayed strategy, AKI complications ensued and emergent KRT was started before 48 hours. Mortality at 90 days in these patients was 68.2% (n = 28/41), perhaps supporting prior data implying there may be some hazard to the expectant follow-up of AKI and the protocolized delay of KRT initiation in selected patients.[11,27]

These trials have been further evaluated in a series of meta-analyses over the last decade.[44,45,57,58,72–76] Most recently, Gaudry and colleagues[30] reported an individual-patient data meta-analysis that pooled 10 trials (2143 patients). Patient-level data were available from 9 trials (2083 patients), of which 933 (50%) were randomly allocated to receive early KRT and 946 (50%) to delayed KRT. The prevalence of baseline CKD was 18% and 68% had sepsis. Pooled patient-level analysis showed no significant different in mortality at 28 days (43% for early vs 44% for delayed; risk ratio [RR] 1.01; 95% CI, 0.91–1.13) **(Fig. 3)** or other secondary end points.[30]

Recently, the main phase of STARRT-AKI trial was published.[28] The STARRT-AKI trial was a large multinational collaboration across 15 countries and 168 sites designed to compare a strategy of accelerated (early) with standard (delayed) KRT initiation in 3019 critically ill patients with severe AKI (aligned with KDIGO stage 2) who did not have an urgent indication for starting KRT.[77] Patients allocated to the accelerated strategy were to commence KRT within 12 hours of full eligibility. The standard strategy comprised a watchful-waiting approach whereby KRT was discouraged unless patients fulfilled one of the following urgent indications: serum potassium level greater than or equal to 6.0 mmol/L, pH less than or equal to 7.20, or serum bicarbonate less than or equal to 12 mmol/L; evidence of severe hypoxemia (Pao_2/fraction of inspired oxygen $\leq$200) perceived to be attributed to volume overload; or the persistence of AKI for greater than or equal to 72 hours following randomization.[77] The primary outcome was 90-day all-cause mortality.

STARRT-AKI was pragmatic in its approach to starting KRT and was unique among trials by integrating clinician equipoise into the eligibility criteria.[77] This approach helped to ensure that STARRT-AKI only enrolled patients for whom the dilemma about when to start KRT was most relevant.[62] This approach has been increasingly adopted

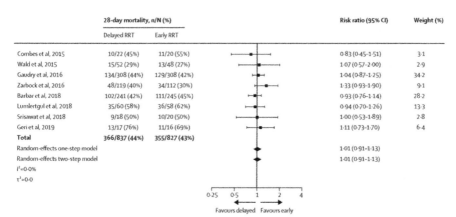

Fig. 3. Twenty-eight-day mortality among studies included by RRT initiation strategy in the intention-to-treat population among the overall sample. (*From* Gaudry S, et al. Delayed versus early initiation of renal replacement therapy for severe acute kidney injury: a systematic review and individual patient data meta-analysis of randomised clinical trials. Lancet 2020;395:1506-15; Reproduced with permission of Elsevier.)

in large, pragmatic, real-world randomized trials.[78,79] For a patient to be fully eligible, the most responsible clinician (ie, intensivist and/or nephrologist) was required to affirm clinical equipoise. If clinicians perceived that immediate KRT was warranted or that imminent kidney recovery was probable and that KRT should be deferred, the patient was excluded. Although the integration of equipoise into the eligibility algorithm may have led to some variability in the types of patients enrolled, this rationale better reflected real-world decision making. Moreover, this design innovation honors the uncertainty principle when conducting clinicals trials and respects the boundaries of current standards of practice. Many trials in ICU settings, particularly those that are unblinded, likely have clinicians who object to their patients being enrolled, which likely represents an unmeasured source of selection bias not captured in most Consolidated Standards of Reporting Trials (CONSORT) figures. Importantly, there is also an ethical argument to this approach. Excluding patients who are perceived by their clinicians to need immediate KRT or who are expected to soon recover kidney function is ethically necessary and clinically sound. In STARRT-AKI, there were 2196 (24.9%) provisionally eligible patients excluded because of clinicians mandating immediate KRT. Follow-up data were available for 32%, and these showed that 89% started KRT and that their in-hospital mortality was 47%. Alternatively, 5690 (64.4%) provisionally eligible patients were excluded because of clinicians mandating deferral because of anticipation of kidney recovery. Follow-up data were available for 49% and showed that only 13% subsequently started KRT with an in-hospital mortality of only 23%. This percentage was substantially lower than the aggregate in-hospital mortality for the total randomized population (38%; n = 1098 out of 2917). The integration of clinician equipoise was thus effective in excluding patients from the trial for whom the study question was not relevant.

The baseline characteristics of patients were similar between strategies. Of note, the prevalence of baseline CKD was 44%, substantially greater than the 18% across prior trials.[30] In addition, 67% had a medical reason for ICU admission, 58% had sepsis, mean SOFA score was 11.7 (standard deviation, 3.6), and 77% and 70% were receiving mechanical ventilation and vasoactive support at the time of randomization, respectively (see **Table 4**).

Among patients randomized to the accelerated strategy, 97% started KRT a median of 6.1 hours (IQR, 3.9–8.8 hours) after full eligibility, whereas, in the standard strategy, 61.8% started KRT after a median of 31.1 hours (IQR, 19.0–71.8 hours). This finding implies that more than one-third of patients either died or recovered kidney function without ever starting KRT; however, patients in the standard strategy who received KRT also showed worsening parameters of AKI, specifically higher serum creatinine level, serum urea level, serum potassium level, SOFA score, and fluid accumulation, and lower bicarbonate level and pH at the time KRT was started compared with the accelerated strategy, as similarly shown[27] (**Fig. 4**). For those who started KRT in the standard strategy, only 66% fulfilled a trial-specific indication for KRT, the most common being PaO2/FiO2 (P/F) ratio less than or equal to 200 and strong clinical perception of volume overload (44%), and AKI duration of greater than or equal to 72 hours from randomization (24%). Among those initiating KRT, continuous RRT was the most common initial modality (69%), followed by conventional intermittent hemodialysis (26%) and slow low-efficiency hemodialysis (4%).

STARRT-AKI found that the accelerated strategy did not confer a reduction in 90-day all-cause mortality (43.9% vs 43.7% in the standard strategy: RR, 1.00; 95% CI, 0.93–1.09) (**Fig. 5**). This finding was robust across several preplanned sensitivity analyses, including an adjusted analysis (adjusted odds ratio [OR], 1.05; 95% CI, 0.90–1.23) and an as-treated analysis, where patients who crossed over between

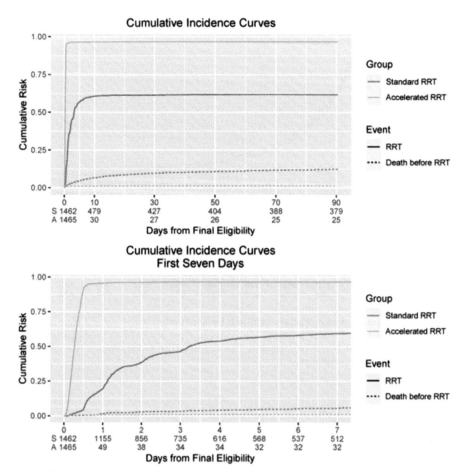

Fig. 4. Time to RRT initiation accounting for the competing risk of death from the STARRT-AKI trial. (*Reproduced from* STARRT-AKI Investigators et al. Timing of Initiation of Renal-Replacement Therapy in Acute Kidney Injury. N Engl J Med 2020; 383:240-251; with permission.)

treatment arms were analyzed according to the KRT treatment strategy that was received (RR, 1.01; 95% CI, 0.87–1.17). In prespecified subgroups (sex, baseline eGFR, Simplified Acute Physiology Score (SAPS) II, sepsis, surgical status, and geographic region) there was no substantial heterogeneity of treatment effect on 90-day mortality. As opposed to the secondary analysis of the AKIKI trial, STARRT-AKI did not find a higher death rate among patients with CKD treated with an accelerated strategy.[30,68] Similarly, there was no heterogeneity of treatment effect on 90-day mortality by illness acuity, defined by deciles of SAPS II score (**Fig. 6**).

Dialysis dependence among survivors at 90 days, a key secondary end point, was found to be more frequent among patients in the accelerated compared with standard strategy (10.4% vs 6.0%; RR, 1.74; 95% CI, 1.24–2.43). This finding was robust in preplanned inverse-probability–weighted (adjusted OR, 1.75; 95% CI, 1.33–2.30) and multinominal analyses (adjusted OR, 1.82; 95% CI, 1.26–2.63). The mechanisms responsible for this dialysis dependence are uncertain but may relate to dialysis-induced kidney

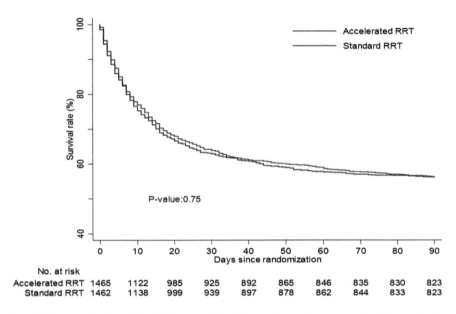

Fig. 5. Time to death within 90 days stratified by accelerated and standard strategies for starting KRT from the STARRT-AKI trial. (*Reproduced from* STARRT-AKI Investigators et al. Timing of Initiation of Renal-Replacement Therapy in Acute Kidney Injury. N Engl J Med 2020; 383:240-251; with permission.)

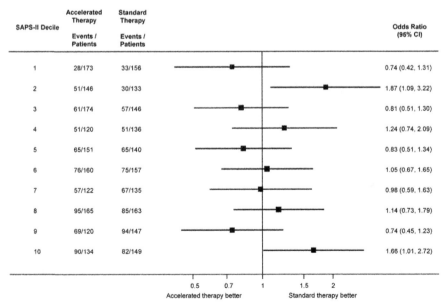

Fig. 6. Heterogeneity of treatment effect by deciles of SAPS II score, a fully adjusted model from the STARRT-AKI trial. (*Reproduced from* STARRT-AKI Investigators et al. Timing of Initiation of Renal-Replacement Therapy in Acute Kidney Injury. N Engl J Med 2020; 383:240-251; with permission.)

injury, potentially exacerbated by iatrogenic episodes of hemodynamic instability, impaired repair, and delayed recovery.[80,81] There were no substantial differences in KRT-free days at 90 days, ventilator-free or vasoactive-free days at 28 days, or hospital-free days at 90 days. Patients in the accelerated strategy had fewer days of KRT, ICU stay, and hospitalization; however, they also showed higher risk for rehospitalization at 90 days (20.9% vs 17.0%; RR, 1.23; 95% CI, 1.02–1.49) compared with the standard strategy. It is unclear whether higher rehospitalization rates are specifically associated with the ongoing need for dialysis.

Adverse events occurred more commonly among patients in the accelerated strategy (23.0% vs 16.5%; RR, 1.40; 95% CI, 1.21–1.62) compared with the standard strategy, driven largely by more episodes of hypotension and hypophosphatemia. Catheter-related bloodstream infections occurred with greater frequency in the accelerated strategy (7 events vs 1 event, $P = .07$), as shown previously, implying treatment with KRT may portend greater infection risk.[27] STARRT-AKI largely focused on adverse events associated with dialysis catheter placement and KRT. As such, it may be logical to expect more adverse events related to these with the accelerated strategy considering there were more days at risk compared with the standard strategy.

STARRT-AKI was a large, suitably powered, widely generalizable trial with robustly reported patient-centered outcomes that will inform bedside clinical practice and future iterations of clinical practice guidelines.[28] The trial definitively proves that accelerated initiation of KRT does not improve patient survival compared with a more conservative approach. STARRT-AKI showed a higher risk of dialysis dependence among 90-day survivors (number needed to harm, 23) and a higher occurrence of adverse events (number needed to harm, 16) with an accelerated strategy, findings that are certain to have importance to patients, along with use of health resources.

IMPLICATIONS FOR CLINICIANS

STARRT-AKI provides compelling evidence that a standard (delayed) strategy to starting KRT, characterized by watchful waiting and starting KRT when confronted with worsening, persistent, or medically refractory complications of AKI, should now be recommended as the default standard and adopted (**Fig. 7**). However, such evidence does not obfuscate the importance of sound patient-centered bedside practice. Clinicians should not only adopt a shared approach to decision making for starting KRT, considering prognosis, potential for recovery and/or harm, and patient/family preferences for care,[19] but should naturally consider the evolving and dynamic nature of critical illness and AKI.

EXISTING KNOWLEDGE GAPS

There have been substantial advances in the understanding of when to consider starting KRT in critically ill patients with severe AKI; however, there remain numerous existing knowledge gaps that should be the nidus of future investigation. Potential themes of work should consider focus on (1) improved understanding of strategies for starting KRT in critically ill children, recognizing that fewer children routinely receive KRT and die in ICU compared with adults[82,83]; (2) continued development and evaluation of clinical risk prediction leveraging electronic alerting and machine learning, and novel markers (ie, NGAL, TIMP-2*IGFBP-7, urinary C-C motif chemokine ligand 14 [CCL14]) to improve precision in the selection of patients most likely to benefit from starting KRT; (3) evaluation of the interaction between KRT strategies and the course of support, weaning, and outcome among patients receiving mechanical ventilation,

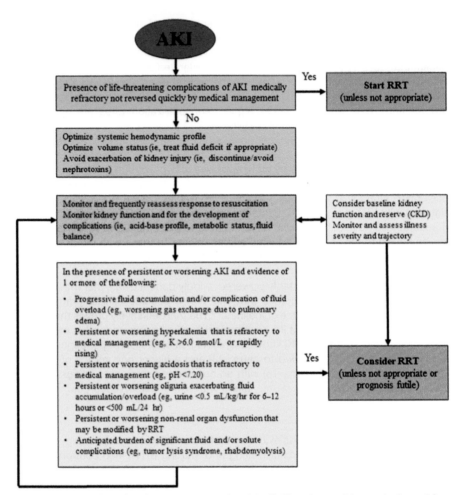

Fig. 7. Proposed algorithm for initiation RRT in critically ill patients with AKI. (*Adapted from* Ostermann, M., Wald, R. & Bagshaw, S. M. Timing of Renal Replacement Therapy in Acute Kidney Injury. Contrib Nephrol 2016; 187; 106-120; with permission; and Bagshaw, S. M. & Wald, R. Strategies for the optimal timing to start renal replacement therapy in critically ill patients with acute kidney injury. Kidney Int (2017); 91:1022-1032; with permission.)

despite no substantial differences in ventilator-free days shown in STARRT-AKI and AKIKI[28,67]; (4) evaluation of the interaction between fluid balance, accumulation, and KRT strategies and organ support and outcomes; and (5) evaluation of the interaction between the potential hazard of untreated AKI, treatments of managing AKI complications, and KRT strategy on KRT use and outcomes.[54,84–86]

SUMMARY

The long-standing questions surrounding the optimal timing of KRT initiation in critically ill patients with AKI seem to have been largely answered following publication of STARRT-AKI.[28] Clinicians should now recognize that starting KRT may be avoidable in many patients without an adverse impact on survival.[41] In some cases, KRT may not be appropriate given a patient's or family's preferences for care or because of the perception of being nonbeneficial in the context of the overall prognosis for a patient nearing the end of life, where KRT will clearly not modify outcome.[14] For now, a conservative approach to starting KRT, characterized by watchful waiting and initiating KRT when confronted with worsening, persistent, or medically refractory complications of AKI, is supported by high-quality evidence and should be recommended in updated iterations of clinical practice guidelines.

CLINICS CARE POINTS

- Timing of KRT initiation in critically ill patients with AKI, in the absence of urgent indications, has been a long-standing dilemma for clinicians.

- Numerous clinical trials have aimed to inform practice; however, they have found discrepant results, and this has contributed to wide variations in practice.

- An earlier strategy has biological rationale, even in the absence of urgent indications; however, a conservative strategy can also prevent selected patients from ever receiving KRT.

- The recently published STARRT-AKI found no survival benefit to early compared with delayed strategies for KRT initiation; however, it showed that an early strategy conferred greater risk for dialysis dependence.

- STARRT-AKI provides compelling evidence that a delayed strategy, characterized by watchful waiting and starting KRT when worsening, persistent, or medically refractory complications of AKI occur, should now be adopted as a standard approach.

ACKNOWLEDGMENTS

S.M. Bagshaw is supported by a Canada Research Chair in Critical Care Nephrology.

DISCLOSURE

S.M. Bagshaw has received fees for scientific advisory from Baxter and CNA Diagnostics, speaking fees from Baxter and Spectral Medical, and study adjudication from BioPorto. R. Wald has received fees for scientific advisory and speaking fees from Baxter. S.M. Bagshaw and R. Wald also received unrestricted grant support from Baxter, in partnership with the Canadian Institutes of Health Research (CIHR), to fund the STARRT-AKI trial. The authors declare no further conflicts of interest.

REFERENCES

1. Hoste EA, Bagshaw SM, Bellomo R, et al. Epidemiology of acute kidney injury in critically ill patients: the multinational AKI-EPI study. Intensive Care Med 2015; 41(8):1411–23.
2. Melo FDAF, Macedo E, Fonseca Bezerra AC, et al. A systematic review and meta-analysis of acute kidney injury in the intensive care units of developed and developing countries. PLoS One 2020;15(1):e0226325.
3. Wu VC, Wu CH, Huang TM, et al. Long-term risk of coronary events after AKI. J Am Soc Nephrol 2014;25(3):595–605.
4. Wu VC, Wu PC, Wu CH, et al. The impact of acute kidney injury on the long-term risk of stroke. J Am Heart Assoc 2014;3(4). https://doi.org/10.1161/JAHA.114.000933.

5. Lai TS, Wang CY, Pan SC, et al. Risk of developing severe sepsis after acute kidney injury: a population-based cohort study. Crit Care 2013;17(5):R231.

6. Wu VC, Wang CY, Shiao CC, et al. Increased risk of active tuberculosis following acute kidney injury: a nationwide, population-based study. PLoS One 2013;8(7): e69556.

7. Wu PC, Wu CJ, Lin CJ, et al, National Taiwan University. Long-term risk of upper gastrointestinal hemorrhage after advanced AKI. Clin J Am Soc Nephrol 2015; 10(3):353–62.

8. Chao CT, Wang CY, Lai CF, et al. Dialysis-requiring acute kidney injury increases risk of long-term malignancy: a population-based study. J Cancer Res Clin Oncol 2014;140(4):613–21.

9. Wang WJ, Chao CT, Huang YC, et al. The impact of acute kidney injury with temporary dialysis on the risk of fracture. J Bone Miner Res 2014;29(3):676–84.

10. Vaara ST, Pettilä V, Kaukonen KM, et al. The attributable mortality of acute kidney injury: a sequentially matched analysis*. Crit Care Med 2014;42(4):878–85.

11. Liborio AB, Leite TT, Neves FM, et al. AKI complications in critically ill patients: association with mortality rates and RRT. Clin J Am Soc Nephrol 2015;10(1):21–8.

12. Kidney Disease: Improving Global Outcomes (KDIGO) Acute Kidney Injury Work Group. KDIGO clinical practice guideline for acute kidney injury. Kidney Int 2012; 2:1–138.

13. Vaara ST, Reinikainen M, Wald R, et al. Timing of RRT based on the presence of conventional indications. Clin J Am Soc Nephrol 2014;9(9):1577–85.

14. Bagshaw SM, Adhikari NKJ, Burns KEA, et al. Selection and receipt of kidney replacement in critically ill older patients with AKI. Clin J Am Soc Nephrol 2019;14(4):496–505.

15. Hsu RK, McCulloch CE, Ku E, et al. Regional variation in the incidence of dialysis-requiring AKI in the United States. Clin J Am Soc Nephrol 2013;8(9):1476–81.

16. Kolhe NV, Fluck RJ, Muirhead AW, et al. Regional variation in acute kidney injury requiring dialysis in the English national health service from 2000 to 2015 - a national epidemiological study. PLoS One 2016;11(10):e0162856.

17. Siddiqui NF, Coca SG, Devereaux PJ, et al. Secular trends in acute dialysis after elective major surgery–1995 to 2009. CMAJ 2012;184(11):1237–45.

18. Wald R, McArthur E, Adhikari NK, et al. Changing incidence and outcomes following dialysis-requiring acute kidney injury among critically ill adults: a population-based cohort study. Am J Kidney Dis 2015;65(6):870–7.

19. Ostermann M, Bellomo R, Burdmann EA, et al. Controversies in acute kidney injury: conclusions for a kidney disease: improving Global outcomes (KDIGO) conference. Kidney Int 2020;98(2):294–309.

20. Ostermann M, Wald R, Bagshaw SM. Timing of renal replacement therapy in acute kidney injury. Contrib Nephrol 2016;187:106–20.

21. Bagshaw SM, Wald R, Barton J, et al. Clinical factors associated with initiation of renal replacement therapy in critically ill patients with acute kidney injury-a prospective multicenter observational study. J Crit Care 2012;27(3):268–75.

22. Clark E, Wald R, Levin A, et al. Timing the initiation of renal replacement therapy for acute kidney injury in Canadian intensive care units: a multicentre observational study. Can J Anaesth 2012;59(9):861–70.

23. Clark E, Wald R, Walsh M, et al. Timing of initiation of renal replacement therapy for acute kidney injury: a survey of nephrologists and intensivists in Canada. Nephrol Dial Transplant 2012;27(7):2761–7.

24. Bagshaw SM, Darmon M, Ostermann M, et al. Current state of the art for renal replacement therapy in critically ill patients with acute kidney injury. Intensive Care Med 2017;43(6):841–54.
25. Bagshaw SM, Wald R. Strategies for the optimal timing to start renal replacement therapy in critically ill patients with acute kidney injury. Kidney Int 2017;91(5): 1022–32.
26. Ronco C, Ricci Z, De Backer D, et al. Renal replacement therapy in acute kidney injury: controversy and consensus. Crit Care 2015;19:146.
27. Gaudry S, Hajage D, Schortgen F, et al. Initiation strategies for renal-replacement therapy in the intensive care Unit. N Engl J Med 2016;375(2):122.
28. STARRT-AKI Investigators; Canadian Critical Care Trials Group; Australian and New Zealand Intensive Care Society Clinical Trials Group; United Kingdom Critical Care Research Group; Canadian Nephrology Trials Network; Irish Critical Care Trials Group, Bagshaw SM, Wald R, Adhikari NKJ, et al. Timing of initiation of renal-replacement therapy in acute kidney injury. N Engl J Med 2020;383: 240–51.
29. Barbar SD, Clere-Jehl R, Bourredjem A, et al. Timing of renal-replacement therapy in patients with acute kidney injury and sepsis. N Engl J Med 2018; 379(15):1431–42.
30. Gaudry S, Hajage D, Benichou N, et al. Delayed versus early initiation of renal replacement therapy for severe acute kidney injury: a systematic review and individual patient data meta-analysis of randomised clinical trials. Lancet 2020; 395(10235):1506–15.
31. Elseviers MM, Lins RL, Van der Niepen P, et al. Renal replacement therapy is an independent risk factor for mortality in critically ill patients with acute kidney injury. Crit Care 2010;14(6):R221.
32. Gaudry S, Ricard JD, Leclaire C, et al. Acute kidney injury in critical care: experience of a conservative strategy. J Crit Care 2014;29(6):1022–7.
33. Srisawat N, Sileanu FE, Murugan R, et al. Variation in risk and mortality of acute kidney injury in critically ill patients: a multicenter study. Am J Nephrol 2015; 41(1):81–8.
34. Wilson FP, Yang W, Machado CA, et al. Dialysis versus nondialysis in patients with AKI: a propensity-matched cohort study. Clin J Am Soc Nephrol 2014;9(4): 673–81.
35. Clec'h C, Darmon M, Lautrette A, et al. Efficacy of renal replacement therapy in critically ill patients: a propensity analysis. Crit Care 2012;16(6):R236.
36. Guerin C, Girard R, Selli JM, et al. Initial versus delayed acute renal failure in the intensive care unit. A multicenter prospective epidemiological study. Rhône-Alpes Area Study Group on Acute Renal Failure. Am J Respir Crit Care Med 2000;161(3 Pt 1):872–9.
37. Bagshaw SM, Uchino S, Kellum JA, et al. Association between renal replacement therapy in critically ill patients with severe acute kidney injury and mortality. J Crit Care 2013;28(6):1011–8.
38. Vaara ST, Reinikainen M, Kaukonen KM, et al. Association of ICU size and annual case volume of renal replacement therapy patients with mortality. Acta Anaesthesiol Scand 2012;56(9):1175–82.
39. Prowle JR, Davenport A. Does early-start renal replacement therapy improve outcomes for patients with acute kidney injury? Kidney Int 2015;88(4):670–3.
40. Kawarazaki H, Uchino S, Tokuhira N, et al. Who may not benefit from continuous renal replacement therapy in acute kidney injury? Hemodial Int 2013;17(4): 624–32.

41. Clark EG, Bagshaw SM. Unnecessary renal replacement therapy for acute kidney injury is harmful for renal recovery. Semin Dial 2015;28(1):6–11.

42. Chan L, Chaudhary K, Saha A, et al. Acute kidney injury in hospitalized patients with COVID-19. medRxiv 2020. https://doi.org/10.1101/2020.05.04.20090944.

43. ICNARC. INCARC report on COVID-19 in critical care (10 July 2020). 2020. Available at: https://www.icnarc.org/Our-Audit/Audits/Cmp/Reports. Accessed July 12, 2020.

44. Karvellas CJ, Farhat MR, Sajjad I, et al. A comparison of early versus late initiation of renal replacement therapy in critically ill patients with acute kidney injury: a systematic review and meta-analysis. Crit Care 2011;15(1):R72.

45. Wierstra BT, Kadri S, Alomar S, et al. The impact of "early" versus "late" initiation of renal replacement therapy in critical care patients with acute kidney injury: a systematic review and evidence synthesis. Crit Care 2016;20(1):122.

46. Klein SJ, Brandtner AK, Lehner GF, et al. Biomarkers for prediction of renal replacement therapy in acute kidney injury: a systematic review and meta-analysis. Intensive Care Med 2018;44(3):323–36.

47. Srisawat N, Laoveeravat P, Limphunudom P, et al. The effect of early renal replacement therapy guided by plasma neutrophil gelatinase associated lipocalin on outcome of acute kidney injury: a feasibility study. J Crit Care 2018;43: 36–41.

48. Liu KD. Therapeutic strategies for clinical trials targeting renal recovery. Nephron Clin Pract 2014;127(1–4):113–6.

49. Rewa OG, Bagshaw SM, Wang X, et al. The furosemide stress test for prediction of worsening acute kidney injury in critically ill patients: a multicenter, prospective, observational study. J Crit Care 2019;52:109–14.

50. Chawla LS, Davison DL, Brasha-Mitchell E, et al. Development and standardization of a furosemide stress test to predict the severity of acute kidney injury. Crit Care 2013;17(5):R207.

51. Koyner JL, Davison DL, Brasha-Mitchell E, et al. Furosemide stress test and biomarkers for the prediction of AKI severity. J Am Soc Nephrol 2015;26(8):2023–31.

52. Lumlertgul N, Peerapornratana S, Trakarnvanich T, et al. Early versus standard initiation of renal replacement therapy in furosemide stress test non-responsive acute kidney injury patients (the FST trial). Crit Care 2018;22(1):101.

53. Bagshaw SM, Lamontagne F, Joannidis M, et al. When to start renal replacement therapy in critically ill patients with acute kidney injury: comment on AKIKI and ELAIN. Crit Care 2016;20(1):245.

54. Vieira JM Jr, Castro I, Curvello-Neto A, et al. Effect of acute kidney injury on weaning from mechanical ventilation in critically ill patients. Crit Care Med 2007;35(1): 184–91.

55. Combes A, Bréchot N, Amour J, et al. Early High-volume hemofiltration versus standard care for post-cardiac surgery shock. The HEROICS Study. Am J Respir Crit Care Med 2015;192(10):1179–90.

56. Payen D, Mateo J, Cavaillon JM, et al. Impact of continuous venovenous hemofiltration on organ failure during the early phase of severe sepsis: a randomized controlled trial. Crit Care Med 2009;37(3):803–10.

57. Seabra VF, Balk EM, Liangos O, et al. Timing of renal replacement therapy initiation in acute renal failure: a meta-analysis. Am J Kidney Dis 2008;52(2):272–84.

58. Xiao L, Jia L, Li R, et al. Early versus late initiation of renal replacement therapy for acute kidney injury in critically ill patients: a systematic review and meta-analysis. PLoS One 2019;14(10):e0223493.

59. Augustine JJ, Sandy D, Seifert TH, et al. A randomized controlled trial comparing intermittent with continuous dialysis in patients with ARF. Am J Kidney Dis 2004; 44(6):1000–7.

60. Bouman CS, Oudemans-Van Straaten HM, Tijssen JG, et al. Effects of early high-volume continuous venovenous hemofiltration on survival and recovery of renal function in intensive care patients with acute renal failure: a prospective, randomized trial. Crit Care Med 2002;30(10):2205–11.

61. Jamale TE, Hase NK, Kulkarni M, et al. Earlier-start versus usual-start dialysis in patients with community-acquired acute kidney injury: a randomized controlled trial. Am J Kidney Dis 2013;62(6):1116–21.

62. Wald R, Adhikari NK, Smith OM, et al. Comparison of standard and accelerated initiation of renal replacement therapy in acute kidney injury. Kidney Int 2015; 88(4):897–904.

63. National Institute for Health and Care Excellence (NICE). Acute kidney injury: prevention, detection and management. 2019. Available at: https://www.nice.org.uk/guidance/ng148. Accessed July 12, 2020.

64. Vinsonneau C, Allain-Launay E, Blayau C, et al. Renal replacement therapy in adult and pediatric intensive care : recommendations by an expert panel from the French intensive care Society (SRLF) with the French Society of Anesthesia intensive care (SFAR) French Group for pediatric intensive care Emergencies (GFRUP) the French dialysis Society (SFD). Ann Intensive Care 2015;5(1):58.

65. Zarbock A, Mehta RL. Timing of kidney replacement therapy in acute kidney injury. Clin J Am Soc Nephrol 2019;14(1):147–9.

66. Zarbock A, Kellum JA, Schmidt C, et al. Effect of early vs delayed initiation of renal replacement therapy on mortality in critically ill patients with acute kidney injury: the ELAIN Randomized Clinical Trial. JAMA 2016;315(20):2190–9.

67. Gaudry S, Hajage D, Schortgen F, et al. Timing of renal support and outcome of septic shock and acute respiratory distress syndrome. A Post Hoc Analysis of the AKIKI Randomized Clinical Trial. Am J Respir Crit Care Med 2018;198(1):58–66.

68. Gaudry S, Verney C, Hajage D, et al. Hypothesis: early renal replacement therapy increases mortality in critically ill patients with acute on chronic renal failure. A post hoc analysis of the AKIKI trial. Intensive Care Med 2018;44(8):1360–1.

69. Zarbock A, Gerß J, Van Aken H, et al. Erratum to: 'Early versus late initiation of renal replacement therapy in critically ill patients with acute kidney injury (The ELAIN-Trial): study protocol for a randomized controlled trial'. Trials 2016; 17(1):260.

70. Meersch M, Küllmar M, Schmidt C, et al. Long-term clinical outcomes after early initiation of RRT in critically ill patients with AKI. J Am Soc Nephrol 2018;29(3): 1011–9.

71. Barbar SD, Binquet C, Monchi M, et al. Impact on mortality of the timing of renal replacement therapy in patients with severe acute kidney injury in septic shock: the IDEAL-ICU study (initiation of dialysis early versus delayed in the intensive care unit): study protocol for a randomized controlled trial. Trials 2014;15:270.

72. Lai TS, Shiao CC, Wang JJ, et al. Earlier versus later initiation of renal replacement therapy among critically ill patients with acute kidney injury: a systematic review and meta-analysis of randomized controlled trials. Ann Intensive Care 2017;7(1):38.

73. Chen JJ, Lee CC, Kuo G, et al. Comparison between watchful waiting strategy and early initiation of renal replacement therapy in the critically ill acute kidney injury population: an updated systematic review and meta-analysis. Ann Intensive Care 2020;10(1):30.

74. Fayad AII, Buamscha DG, Ciapponi A. Timing of renal replacement therapy initiation for acute kidney injury. Cochrane Database Syst Rev 2018;(12):CD010612.

75. Li Y, Li H, Zhang D. Timing of continuous renal replacement therapy in patients with septic AKI. Medicine 2019;98(33):e16800.

76. Zhang L, Chen D, Tang X, et al. Timing of initiation of renal replacement therapy in acute kidney injury: an updated meta-analysis of randomized controlled trials. Ren Fail 2020;42(1):77–88.

77. STARRT-AKI Investigators. STandard versus accelerated initiation of renal replacement therapy in acute kidney injury: study protocol for a multi-national, multi-center, randomized controlled trial. Can J Kidney Health Dis 2019;6. 2054358119852937.

78. CRASH-3 Trial Collaborators. Effects of tranexamic acid on death, disability, vascular occlusive events and other morbidities in patients with acute traumatic brain injury (CRASH-3): a randomised, placebo-controlled trial. Lancet 2019; 394(10210):1713–23.

79. Horby P, Lim WS, Emberson J, et al. Effect of dexamethasone in hospitalized patients with COVID-19: preliminary report. 2020. Available at: https://www.medrxiv.org/content/10.1101/2020.06.22.20137273v1.

80. Mahmoud H, Forni LG, McIntyre CW, et al. Myocardial stunning occurs during intermittent haemodialysis for acute kidney injury. Intensive Care Med 2017; 43(6):942–4.

81. Marants R, Qirjazi E, Grant CJ, et al. Renal perfusion during hemodialysis: intradialytic blood flow decline and effects of dialysate cooling. J Am Soc Nephrol 2019;30(6):1086–95.

82. Alobaidi R, Morgan C, Goldstein SL, et al. Population-based epidemiology and outcomes of acute kidney injury in critically ill children. Pediatr Crit Care Med 2020;21(1):82–91.

83. Kaddourah A, Basu RK, Bagshaw SM, et al. Epidemiology of acute kidney injury in critically ill children and young adults. N Engl J Med 2017;376(1):11–20.

84. Murugan R, Balakumar V, Kerti SJ, et al. Net ultrafiltration intensity and mortality in critically ill patients with fluid overload. Crit Care 2018;22(1):223.

85. Murugan R, Kerti SJ, Chang CH, et al. Association of net ultrafiltration rate with mortality among critically ill adults with acute kidney injury receiving continuous venovenous hemodiafiltration: a secondary analysis of the randomized evaluation of normal vs Augmented level (renal) of renal replacement therapy trial. JAMA Netw Open 2019;2(6):e195418.

86. Naorungroj T, Neto AS, Zwakman-Hessels L, et al. Early net ultrafiltration rate and mortality in critically ill patients receiving continuous renal replacement therapy. Nephrol Dial Transplant 2020. https://doi.org/10.1093/ndt/gfaa032.

Kidney Replacement Therapy for Fluid Management

Vikram Balakumar, MD[a,b,1],
Raghavan Murugan, MD, MS, FRCP, FCCM[b,c],*

KEYWORDS

- Acute kidney injury • Continuous renal replacement therapy • Fluid overload
- Net ultrafiltration • Renal replacement therapy • Mortality

KEY POINTS

- Fluid overload is present in two-third of critically ill patients with acute kidney injury and is associated with long-term risk of death.
- Fluid removal using net ultrafiltration during kidney replacement therapy provides adequate volume control and is supported by clinical practice guidelines.
- Net ultrafiltration prescription should be based on patient body weight (ie, milliliters per kilogram per hour) rather than absolute volumes (ie, milliliters per hour).
- Emerging studies suggest that higher ultrafiltration rates are associated with mortality caused by cardiovascular stress.
- Future research is required on dialysate cooling, ultrafiltration, and sodium profiling for preventing hemodynamic instability during ultrafiltration in critically ill patients.

INTRODUCTION

Fluid overload (FO) is a common complication in critically ill patients with acute kidney injury (AKI) in the intensive care unit (ICU). FO occurs because of dysregulation of kidney's ability to maintain fluid homeostasis in the face of administration of intravenous fluids, blood products, nutrition, and other medications required to support acutely ill

Source of support: Partial support for this work was provided by the National Institute of Diabetes and Digestive and Kidney Diseases (5R01DK106256).

[a] Department of Critical Care Medicine, Mercy Hospitals, Springfield, MO, USA; [b] Department of Critical Care Medicine, Center for Critical Care Nephrology, University of Pittsburgh School of Medicine, Pittsburgh, PA, USA; [c] Department of Critical Care Medicine, The Clinical Research, Investigation, and Systems Modeling of Acute Illness (CRISMA) Center, University of Pittsburgh School of Medicine, University of Pittsburgh, 3347 Forbes Avenue, Suite 220, Room 206, Pittsburgh, PA 15261, USA

[1] Present address: 1235 E Cherokee Street, Springfield, MO 65804.

* Corresponding author.

E-mail address: murdganr@upmc.edu

Twitter: @vikrambalakumar (V.B.); @RagiCCM (R.M.)

Crit Care Clin 37 (2021) 433–452
https://doi.org/10.1016/j.ccc.2020.11.006
0749-0704/21/© 2020 Elsevier Inc. All rights reserved.

patients. Among critically ill patients, intravenous fluids are frequently prescribed for treatment of hypovolemia, hypotension, and oliguria.[1] However, following intravenous fluid administration, a large portion of the given volume is rapidly redistributed in the extravascular space, particularly in inflammatory conditions such as sepsis, which is associated with capillary leak.[2] Thus, as a result of iatrogenic fluid administration, underlying critical illness, and decreased kidney excretion of extracellular volume, ICU patients with AKI are at risk for FO. Clinically, FO is recognized by weight gain from baseline, examination findings, radiographic features and complications such as respiratory insufficiency and increasing oxygen requirements, inability to wean from ventilator, and intra-abdominal hypertension.[3]

Conceptually, FO could be defined as an absolute increase in total body volume or relative increase in percentage of extracellular volume over the isovolemic status of the patient. However precise quantification of fluid status requires the gold standard for measuring volume by using radioisotopic tracer dilution techniques.[4,5] However this technique is time consuming, expensive, and not readily available for clinicians in routine clinical practice. Thus, for practical and epidemiologic purposes, FO is most frequently defined as a positive value of total fluid intake minus total fluid output and expressed as a percentage of patient hospital admission body weight.[6] Although this definition is simplistic and does not account for the premorbid volume status or weight of the patient, both of which are influenced by underlying disease processes, this definition has been widely validated to predict risk of death both in critically ill adults and children.[7–11] Using this definition, more than two-third of critically ill adults with AKI have an FO at the time of initiation of kidney replacement therapy (KRT),[7] and, despite fluid removal, mortality remains greater than 40% in this patient population.[7,12–15]

When a patient develops oliguric AKI and FO, clinicians frequently prescribe diuretics. However, when critically ill patients fail a trial of diuretic therapy, extracorporeal net fluid removal (net ultrafiltration [UF_{NET}]) from the patient is frequently initiated to achieve adequate volume control.[6] The practice of mechanical removal of extracellular volume from the patient is recommended by international clinical practice guidelines that suggest emergent initiation of ultrafiltration when life-threatening changes in fluid exist.[6,16,17] However, in critically ill children, ultrafiltration is frequently used for prevention or to prevent worsening of FO while allowing for simultaneous administration of fluids associated with medications, blood products, and nutrition.[9,18] However, there remains a wide variation in clinical practice on timing of initiation, indication, dosing, and discontinuation of ultrafiltration.[19]

Emerging evidence suggests a J-shaped association between UF_{NET} rate and mortality among critically ill patients. Both slower and faster UF_{NET} rates are associated with increased morbidity and mortality compared with moderate UF_{NET} rates.[20] Slower UF_{NET} rates are associated with prolonged tissue exposure to FO and organ edema,[15,21,22] whereas faster UF_{NET} rates are frequently complicated by cardiac arrhythmias, prolonged dependence on KRT, and death.[23,24] This article discusses the association between fluid balance and outcomes, principles of volume management using KRT, vascular refill during UF_{NET}, hemodynamic monitoring during UF_{NET}, association of UF_{NET} rate with clinical outcomes, areas of uncertainty, and directions for future research.

FLUID BALANCE AND OUTCOMES

Several observational studies have examined the association between positive fluid balance and outcomes in critically ill patients (**Table 1**). Most of these studies found that survivors had higher volumes of fluid removed during KRT and greater negative

Table 1
Observational studies examining association between fluid balance and outcomes among critically ill patients receiving kidney replacement therapy

Author, Year	FO Definition	Patients with FO	Patients Requiring KRT (%)	Mortality (%)
Murugan et al,[23] 2019	Organ edema	44.2	100	44.2
Murugan et al,[15] 2019	≥5% VRWG	100%	10	64.1
Bagshaw,[87] 2019	>5%–10% VRWG or clinical diagnosis	35% of KRT patients; 16.2% of total	46	50
Woodward et al,[88] 2019	>10% VRWG	49.5%	100	60.3
Dill et al,[89] 2018	Clinical diagnosis	75%	96	56
Albino et al,[90] 2018	Not reported	Not reported	100	81.7
Silversides et al,[91] 2018	Positive cumulative FB	87.3%	10	31
Kim et al,[92] 2017	≥10% VRWG	36.4%	100	53.4
Balakumar et al,[7] 2017	≥5% VRWG	45.3%	8.5	27.4
Kellum et al,[93] 2016	≥10% VRWG	EGDT 9.8%, PSC 6.8%, usual care 6.3%	EGDT 6.1, PSC 7.7, usual care 4.3	EGDT 38.9, PSC 37, usual care 38.6
Garzotto et al,[94] 2016	% VRWG	Not reported	11.4	12.75
Xu et al,[95] 2015	≥7.2% VRWG	Not reported	100	65
Chen et al,[36] 2015	BIVA, NT-pro-BNP level	50.6%	100	48.3
Rhee et al,[38] 2015	MF-BIA	Not reported	100	40.4
Silversides et al,[46] 2014	Mean daily FB	Not reported	100	51
Vaara et al,[11] 2012	≥10% VRWG	26.9%	100	39.2
Heung et al,[96] 2012	>10% VRWG	42.4%	100	65.3
Fulop et al,[97] 2010	≥10% VRWG	46.9%	100	50.6

Abbreviations: BIVA, bioelectrical impedance vector analysis; EGDT, early goal directed therapy; FB, fluid balance; MF-BIA, multifrequency bioimpedance analysis; NT-pro-BNP, N-terminal pro–brain natriuretic peptide; PSC, protocol-based standard care; VRWG, volume-related weight gain.

daily fluid balance compared with nonsurvivors.[8,12] For instance, in the secondary analysis of the Randomized Evaluation of the Normal Versus Augmented Level (RENAL) trial of renal replacement therapy in patients with severe AKI,[12] survivors had negative fluid balance compared with nonsurvivors. A negative mean daily fluid balance during KRT was independently associated with a decreased risk of death, increased dialysis-free days, and increased hospital-free days.

In another study using the Program to Improve Care in Acute Renal Disease (PIC-ARD) cohort of critically ill patients with AKI and greater than 10% FO, survivors had less fluid accumulation at the initiation of KRT compared with nonsurvivors.[8] Among critically ill children with FO, several observational studies have also found that earlier use of ultrafiltration to prevent worsening of FO attenuated the risk of death.[9,10,18] However, observational studies are prone to confounding because fluid could only be removed in patients who can tolerate fluid removal. Thus, it could be that this tolerance and ability to regulate fluid homeostasis, rather than fluid removal per se, is associated with better outcomes, suggesting that the ability to remove fluid and consequent negative fluid balance is just a marker for better physiologic reserve. To date, no randomized trial has been conducted to establish causality between fluid removal and survival.

FO is associated with organ dysfunction, which is mediated by interstitial edema resulting in impaired metabolite diffusion, distorted tissue architecture, decreased organ perfusion, venous and lymphatic drainage, and impaired cell-cell interactions.[25] Although the effects of tissue edema are more pronounced in encapsulated organs such as liver and kidneys, which lack the accommodative capacity to hold additional volume, nearly every organ system is affected by interstitial edema. For example, myocardial edema can worsen left ventricular function and may also precipitate cardiac arrhythmias. Poor surgical wound healing and anastomotic dehiscence may occur because of tissue edema. Importantly, abdominal visceral edema increases risk for intra-abdominal hypertension, which further perpetuates AKI by renal venous congestion and FO.[26]

Among patients receiving KRT, positive fluid balance has been hypothesized to impair kidney recovery by causing kidney edema and distortion of kidney architecture, predisposing to persistent kidney injury and dependence on dialysis.[27] However, negative fluid balance has been associated with earlier independence from KRT compared with positive fluid balance.[12] In our prior work,[7] we found that KRT attenuated the relationship between positive fluid balance and long-term risk of mortality. We found that only exposure to positive fluid balance more than 72 hours was associated with mortality, suggesting that the association between fluid balance and mortality may be time dependent.[7] Fluid used to rescue patients from hypotension and shock during early resuscitation may attenuate the risk of death associated with such conditions (eg, septic shock). However, a more persistent exposure to FO was associated with harm and supports the concept of deresuscitation as soon as hypovolemia and shock have resolved. Taken together, these findings suggest that, once FO has occurred, early pharmacologic or extracorporeal fluid removal using ultrafiltration to obtain euvolemia may reduce the long-term risk of death.

Fluid balance should be considered a target for management in patients receiving KRT. For many, if not most, critically ill patients, fluid balance is as important or more important than solute control because the indications for KRT in critically ill patients are often related to fluid management rather than solute control. Continuous kidney replacement therapy (CKRT), in particular, is often initiated for FO (either for prevention or to prevent worsening of FO). Recently, the Acute Disease Quality Initiative (ADQI) recommended monitoring of FO after resuscitation and initiating CKRT at 10% to 20% to prevent further worsening of FO while allowing for simultaneous fluid administration volumes associated with medications, blood products, and nutrition.[17,28]

Various evolving technologies are being used to monitor FO in the ICU. Bioimpedance analysis is a noninvasive technology that assesses the electrical properties of tissues by measuring the reactance and resistance of an alternating current passed through the body through an electrode placed on the skin. Bioimpedance values can be plotted on reactance-resistance graphs to derive a vector length, which is associated with the individual's overall volume status.[29] Using bioimpedance, total body, extracellular, and intracellular water could be measured. Several studies have evaluated the feasibility of bioimpedance in critically ill patients,[30–35] and volume status assessed by bioimpedance has been associated with mortality in patients treated with CKRT.[36–38] However, 1 study found that the sensitivity of repeated bioimpedance measurement to detect fluid accumulation or changes in fluid balance less than 2 L was low.[32] Moreover, bioimpedance has not been compared with the gold standard of tracer dilution methods to accurately assess volume status,[4,5] and has not been validated for fluid removal in critically ill patients.

Another promising evolving technology, called peripheral intravenous analysis (PIVA), uses spectral analysis of the peripheral venous waveform to assess intravascular volume.[39–42] This method continuously measures peripheral venous pressure through a sidearm of a standard intravenous catheter, and then uses fast Fourier transformation to assess the amplitude of the waveform, which, through a proprietary algorithm, is transformed into a metric that, in animal and human experiments, seems to be a surrogate for intravascular blood volume.[39,41,42] Preliminary studies in a porcine model of hemorrhagic shock,[42] as well as in humans undergoing hemodialysis,[39] have provided a correlation between PIVA values and volume status. Changes in volume status caused by blood removal in humans or pigs led to changes in the venous waveform signal before changes in blood pressure or pulse rate, suggesting that the venous waveform signal is more sensitive to changes in intravascular volume than standard vital signs.[42] Nevertheless, PIVA has not been evaluated in critically ill patients.

PRINCIPLES OF VOLUME MANAGEMENT USING KIDNEY REPLACEMENT THERAPY

Clinical assessment of overall volume status and the optimal UF_{NET} requirements are determined in part by physical examination, patient fluid balance, weight, hemodynamics, evidence of organ edema (eg, pulmonary edema), as well as adequate perfusion. Other noninvasive methods, such as lung ultrasonography, inferior vena cava (IVC) collapsibility, and bioimpedance, can also be used to diagnose and assess the severity of FO (**Table 2**). A patient's need for volume management using KRT is determined by the underlying patient characteristics, clinical goals, type of disease, severity of illness, and comorbidities. Ultrafiltration can be used in conjunction with fluids administered to maintain precise fluid balance in critically ill patients with oliguric AKI.[43]

The decision to use KRT for fluid removal should be made by taking into account (1) the total volume of fluid that needs to be removed to achieve clinical goals; (2) ongoing fluid administration needs as well as ongoing net input and output; (3) hemodynamic status (blood pressure, need for vasopressors); (4) rate at which fluid needs to be removed from the patient; (5) need for solute removal, electrolyte correction, or control of uremia; (6) resources available at a particular institution; and (7) patient response to fluid removal.

Multiple techniques for delivering KRT and ultrafiltration are currently in practice (**Table 3**). In critically ill patients, CKRT is often prescribed as the initial modality of choice[19] for several reasons: (1) slower fluid removal making negative fluid balance more achievable with hemodynamic stability[8]; (2) slower control of solute concentration avoids large fluctuations and fluid shifts; (3) greater flexibility in responding to the patient's changing fluid removal needs and hemodynamic status; and (4) simple operability with user-friendly machines.[44]

In order to achieve precision in fluid balance using CKRT, it is critical to understand the differences between machine balance and net patient fluid balance. The balance of anticoagulation, UF_{NET}, and replacement fluid rates determines the CKRT machine balance. This machine balance can then be added and adjusted to net patient inputs and outputs to influence patient fluid balance. It is important to recognize that precise

Table 2
Tools used for assessing volume status in critically ill patients

Assessment Tool	Invasive or Noninvasive	Comments
Physical examination	Noninvasive	Serial examinations more useful in detecting edema
Chest radiograph	Noninvasive	Standardized vascular pedicular width and cardiothoracic ratio correlate well with hypervolemia; used in assessing clinical response to diuresis
CVP	Invasive	Higher CVP is a marker of extrathoracic organ dysfunction
BIVA	Noninvasive	Simple, rapid, and reproducible method to determine body fluid composition in critically ill; demographic specific and dependent on body position
Ultrasonography assessment of IVC; IVC-CI	Noninvasive	Simple, reliable, validated bedside tool to diagnose hypervolemic states such as CHF and increased RA pressures
Ultrasonography lung assessment	Noninvasive	Simple, quick method; B profile detects EVLW in critically ill; helpful in guiding fluid removal
BVM	Noninvasive	Entirely extracorporeal, can be used with intermittent or continuous dialysis, real-time hematocrit monitoring can inform UF rates

Abbreviations: BVM, blood volume monitoring; CHF, congestive heart failure; CVP, central venous pressure; EVLW, extravascular lung water; IVC-CI, IVC Collapsibility Index; RA, right atrium; UF, ultrafiltration.

fluid regulation using CKRT needs not only to consider the dynamic changes in machine fluid balance but also to integrate machine fluid balance with dynamic changes in patient fluid balance.

For instance, if the clinician considered just the inputs and outputs in the CKRT but did not take into account the various inputs (such as intravenous fluids) and outputs (such as drain outputs) in the patient, then the balance of fluid therapy would be inadequate and the patient could be at risk for either FO or excessive fluid losses. Both the machine and patient fluid balance should be assessed at fixed intervals and should be combined to estimate the machine-patient integrated fluid balance (ibalance).[43] Recent evidence suggests that only one-third of critical care practitioners reported evaluating the net machine-patient fluid balance frequently during CKRT.[19] Quality initiatives have been proposed to identify and initiate CKRT in patients at 10% to 20% FO, quantifying how often daily fluid balance goals are met, and removal of greater than 80% of daily prescribed ultrafiltrate as a quality metric.[17,28]

Hemodynamic stability usually dictates the rate of UF_{NET} in critically ill patients, and clinical discretion is essential.[6] As the fluid is removed, clinicians should monitor the patient's hemodynamic status and slow or suspend UF_{NET} if there are signs of intolerance (eg, decreasing cardiac output, tachycardia, vasopressor requirement to maintain mean arterial pressure) (**Fig. 1**). Several strategies, such as cooling of dialysate and slowing UF_{NET} rates, may be useful to reduce risks. In general, UF_{NET} should not be commenced during the resuscitation phase in a hemodynamically unstable patient with hypovolemic shock requiring vasopressor support. However, UF_{NET} may be initiated at a slower rate during the stabilization and deresuscitation phases in patients who are on a low and stable dose of a vasopressor with careful monitoring.

Table 3
Modalities of kidney replacement therapy used for volume management in critically ill patients

KRT Modality	Mechanisms of Clearance	Blood Flow (mL/min)	Ultrafiltration Rate (mL/h)	Advantages	Disadvantages
IHD	Concurrent diffusion and convection	250–400	0–1000	Rapid solute and volume control	Hypotension, requires specialized equipment
SLED	Concurrent diffusion and convection	100–200	0–1000	Flexible scheduling, cost-effective	Hemodynamic intolerance in unstable patients
SCUF	Predominantly convection	<100	100–300	Low-intensity procedure	Unable to obtain solute removal
CVVH	Convection	200–400	1000–4000	Aggressive volume control	RF required to optimize plasma chemistry
CVVHD	Diffusion	100–200	80–200	No RF required	Lesser volume removal
CVVHDF	Diffusion and convection	100–200	1000–2000	Balance of solute control and volume removal	Nursing intensive procedure, high cost

Abbreviations: CVVH, continuous venovenous hemofiltration; CVVHD, continuous venovenous hemodialysis; CVVHDF, continuous venovenous hemodiafiltration; IHD, intermittent hemodialysis; RF, replacement fluid; SCUF, slow continuous ultrafiltration; SLED, sustained low-efficiency dialysis.

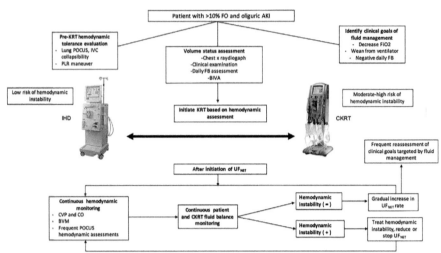

Fig. 1. Fluid management algorithm in patients requiring UF$_{NET}$. Before initiation of UF$_{NET}$, clinical goals of fluid management must be identified. An assessment of FO severity must be made along with evaluating hemodynamic tolerance of the patient. Subsequently, choice of KRT is determined based on risk of hemodynamic instability. If risk is high, CKRT is preferred. Once fluid removal has been initiated, careful monitoring of hemodynamic parameters along with frequent assessment of fluid intake and outputs of the patient is recommended. If hemodynamic instability occurs during fluid removal, it must be addressed expeditiously. If no instability occurs, fluid removal rate can be titrated carefully to achieve the clinical goals previously identified while continuing to monitor fluid balance and hemodynamic tolerance of the patient. FO is expressed as percentage of body weight gain from baseline. BIVA, bioimpedance vector analysis; BVM, blood volume monitoring; CO, cardiac output; CVP, central venous pressure; FB, fluid balance; Fio$_2$, fractional inspiration of oxygen concentration; IHD, intermittent hemodialysis; PLR, passive leg raise; POCUS, point-of-care ultrasonography.

The authors suggest keeping UF$_{NET}$ rates low in critically ill patients until the safety of higher rates is confirmed in randomized trials because emerging evidence suggests that faster UF$_{NET}$ rates are associated with increased mortality, especially in patients who are hemodynamically unstable.[23] However, in some patients, such as those with life-threatening and severe left ventricular failure and acute respiratory distress syndrome with FO and refractory hypoxemia, higher UF$_{NET}$ rates may need to be used in the short term and prioritized over the use of, or increase in the dose of, vasopressors, to prevent sudden death, and must be guided by clinical response.

If hemodynamic instability and hypotension occur, fluid removal should be temporarily withheld and the patient evaluated immediately for causes of hypotension, such as increased dose of sedation or use of new sedatives, initiation of a new medication that causes hypotension, hemorrhage, loss of vasomotor tone caused by sepsis, or adrenal insufficiency. Sedatives and new medications should be withheld temporarily. If hypotension persists, fluids or vasopressors can be administered based on the likely cause of hypotension. Clinician discretion must be used in the timing of restarting of fluid removal once the patient has become hemodynamically stable.

VASCULAR REFILL DURING NET ULTRAFILTRATION

An important principle governing fluid removal is the concept of plasma refilling rate. During extracorporeal fluid removal, fluid is primarily removed from the intravascular compartment. Plasma refilling rates from the interstitial compartment determine the rate of change of the intravascular blood volume. If the ultrafiltration rate exceeds the plasma refilling rate, decreased blood volume ensues and contributes to hemodynamic instability. However, there is no way to easily predict the plasma refilling and, thus, a cautious trial-and-error approach to fluid removal starting with low fluid removal rates and titrating upward as tolerated is a reasonable approach.

A crucial aspect of volume management is detection and management of hemodynamic instability during UF_{NET}. At least 2 out of 5 patients undergoing CKRT have an episode of hypotension within the first hour of its initiation.[45] Hemodynamic instability increases the risk of in-hospital death[46] and nonrecovery of kidney function.[47] Several mechanisms may be contributing to the occurrence of hemodynamic instability. These mechanisms include decreased cardiac output either from hypovolemia and/or pump failure, decreased peripheral vascular resistance, coupled with an inability to mount a compensatory physiologic response.[48] Hypovolemia precipitated by UF_{NET} is seen in clinical conditions characterized by capillary leak, such as sepsis,[49] where rate of ultrafiltration exceeds plasma refilling rate and hemodynamic instability ensues.

Hypotension has been reported during ultrafiltration with all modalities of kidney replacement therapies used in the ICU. Although clinicians frequently use CKRT for the management of hemodynamically unstable patients, hypotensive episodes have been reported in 19% to 97% of patients during treatment with CKRT depending on the definition used to define intradialytic hypotension.[45,50–52] Among critically ill patients treated with intermittent hemodialysis, hypotension has been reported in 10% to 70% of patients.[53–56] Although the attributable risk of UF_{NET} per se on hemodynamic instability is difficult to quantify precisely, intradialytic hypotension is an independent predictor of mortality among critically ill patients.[46]

One small randomized trial conducted among critically ill patients treated with prolonged intermittent KRT found that cooling of dialysate temperature to 35°C compared with 37°C was associated with less intradialytic hypotension and ability to achieve prescribed target ultrafiltration.[57] Another trial in patients treated with CKRT found improved hemodynamic stability.[58] However, further studies are required in critically ill patients to confirm safety and efficacy. Sodium modeling is another method in which higher dialysate sodium concentration is used at the beginning of intermittent hemodialysis and gradually decreased over time to avoid abrupt decrease of plasma osmolarity.[59,60] One small randomized trial showed that sodium modeling might decrease hemodynamic instability during acute hemodialysis.[61] However, other studies found no such association.[62] However the impact of sodium modeling during CKRT remains unexplored and it is unclear whether sodium modeling will increase overall sodium load in critically ill patients.[48]

Observational studies have also explored what hemodynamic characteristics before initiation of UF_{NET} predict an increased risk of hypotension. For instance, 1 study evaluated the ability of the passive leg raise maneuver done before initiation of hemodialysis to predict intradialytic hypotension,[63] and found that 9% increase in cardiac index with passive leg raise test before hemodialysis predicted intradialytic hypotension with a sensitivity of 77% and specificity of 96%.

Another study evaluated the IVC Collapsibility Index (IVC-CI) [defined as ($IVC_{max} - IVC_{min}$)/$IVC_{max}*100$], which is a dynamic hemodynamic parameter based on measurements of IVC collapsibility seen during respiration/ventilation obtained via limited echocardiography. IVC diameter greater than 2.1 cm with a collapse of less than 50% with sniff or collapse of less than 20% (when sniff is unable to be performed) is a sign of high right atrial pressures.[64] It is not only reliable in diagnosing hypervolemic states[65] but can be used effectively by nurses and clinicians to guide fluid removal in patients with heart failure.[66] Nevertheless its predictive value in other critically ill patients remains uncertain.

One observational study examined the correlation of IVC-CI in ICU patients with AKI, AKI on chronic kidney disease, and kidney failure who underwent hemodialysis within 24 hours after assessment of IVC-CI.[67] Before dialysis, IVC-CI less than 20% had a sensitivity of 70% in predicting ultrafiltration volume greater than or equal to 0.5 L. Notably, they observed that predialysis mean central venous pressure, pulmonary artery occlusion pressure, and cardiac output were poor predictors of ultrafiltration volume per session.

Similarly, using point-of-care ultrasonography, a prospective single-center study[68] assessed the ability of predialytic hemodynamic profile of 248 ICU patients with AKI undergoing intermittent hemodialysis for ultrafiltration to predict intradialytic hypotension. The investigators combined ultrasonography assessments of IVC[69] and lung profiles[70] to stratify patients into 4 distinct groups: A, pulmonary congestion (B profile on lung ultrasonography) and hypervolemia (noncollapsible IVC); B, no pulmonary congestion (A profile on lung ultrasonography) and hypervolemia (noncollapsible IVC); C, pulmonary congestion and no hypervolemia (collapsible IVC); D, no pulmonary congestion and no hypervolemia. Intradialytic hypotension was seen in 79 patients (31%). Among these 4 groups, the risk for hypotension and dialysis discontinuation was lowest in group A (ie, patients with ultrasonography evidence of hypervolemia and pulmonary congestion). The risk was highest in groups B and C (ie, patients with hypervolemia and no pulmonary congestion and those without hypervolemia and with pulmonary congestion).

ASSOCIATION OF NET ULTRAFILTRATION RATE WITH OUTCOMES

Among critically ill patients requiring fluid removal, the optimal rate of UF_{NET} remains uncertain and there is a wide variation in clinical practice.[19] Typically, clinicians carefully set UF_{NET} rate based on target fluid balance, severity of FO, and the hemodynamic stability of the patient. Despite careful titration by clinicians, emerging evidence from observational studies suggests a J-shaped association between the rate of UF_{NET} and mortality among critically ill patients.

In a single-center retrospective study, the authors examined the association of UF_{NET} rate with 1-year mortality among 1075 critically ill patients with AKI and FO greater than 5% of patient body weight (**Table 4**).[15] The UF_{NET} rate was calculated as the net volume of fluid removed per day from initiation of either CKRT or intermittent hemodialysis until the end of ICU stay adjusted for patient hospital admission body weight. After accounting for confounders, the UF_{NET} rates less than or equal to 20 mL/kg/d compared with UF_{NET} rates greater than 25 mL/kg/d were associated with higher mortality. Among the subgroup of patients only treated with CRRT, UF_{NET} rates less than 0.5 mL/kg/h compared with rates greater than 1.0 mL/kg/h were associated with higher odds of death. Another study among 1398 patients treated with CKRT also found UF_{NET} rate less than 35 mL/kg/d was associated with higher odds of 30-day mortality compared with rate greater than or equal to 35 mL/kg/d[22] These findings suggest that a slower UF_{NET} rate is associated with an increased risk of death.

In a secondary analysis of the RENAL cohort, Murugan and colleagues[23] examined the association between the UF_{NET} rate and risk-adjusted 90-day mortality in 1434 critically ill patients treated with CKRT. UF_{NET} rate was defined as the volume of fluid removed per hour adjusted for patient body weight. Using tertiles of UF_{NET} rates, rates greater than 1.75 mL/kg/h compared with rates less than 1.01 mL/kg/h, as well as rates 1.01 to 1.75 mL/kg/h, were associated with lower risk-adjusted 90-

Table 4
Studies showing association between net ultrafiltration rates and outcomes in critically ill patients with acute kidney injury

Author	Patients (N)	Type of KRT	Exposure UF_{NET} Rate	Comparator UF_{NET} Rate	Finding
Gleeson,[98] 2015	157	CKRT	Higher rate	Lower rate	↑ Dialysis dependence in survivors
Pajewski et al,[99] 2018	100	IHD and CKRT	Higher rate	Lower rate	↑ Dialysis dependence at 90 d among survivors
Murugan et al,[15] 2018	1075	IHD and CKRT	>25 mL/kg/d	<20 mL/kg/d and 20–25 mL/kg/d	↓ 1-y mortality
Murugan et al,[23] 2019	1434	CVVHDF	>1.75 mL/kg/h	<1.01 and 1.01–1.75 mL/kg/h	↑ 90-d mortality
Tehranian et al,[22] 2019	1398	CKRT	≥35 mL/kg/d	<35 mL/kg/d	↓ 30-d mortality
Naorungroj et al,[71] 2020	347	CKRT	>1.75 mL/kg/h	<1.01 and 1.01–1.75 mL/kg/h	↑ 28-d hospital mortality
Murugan et al,[23] 2019	1433	CKRT	>1.75 mL/kg/h	<1.01 and 1.01–1.75 mL/kg/h	↑ dialysis dependence at day 90 and progression to kidney failure
Naorungroj, 2020	347	CKRT	>1.75 mL/kg/h	<1.01 and 1.01–1.75 mL/kg/h	Risk of death not mediated by negative fluid balance, vasopressor, or hypotension
Naorungroj, 2020	1434	CKRT	>1.75 mL/kg/h	<1.01 and 1.01–1.75 mL/kg/h	Heterogeneity of treatment effect

day survival. Every 0.5-mL/kg/h increase in the UF_{NET} rate was associated with a 7% increased mortality. Patients with UF_{NET} rates greater than 1.75 mL/kg/h had higher rates of organ dysfunction, mechanical ventilation, and organ edema, and longer ICU stays compared with patients with UF_{NET} rate less than 1.01 mL/kg/h and 1.01 to 1.75 mL/kg/h. Patients with UF_{NET} rates greater than 1.75 mL/kg had more negative median daily and cumulative fluid balances. Furthermore, UF_{NET} rates greater than 1.75 mL/kg/h were also associated with a greater trend toward cardiac arrhythmias. UF_{NET} rates greater than 1.75 mL/kg/h were associated with dialysis dependence at day 90 and progression to kidney failure compared with rates less than 1.01 mL/kg/h.[24]

Using cluster and bayesian heterogeneity of treatment effect analysis, the probability of harm associated with UF_{NET} rate greater than 1.75 mL/kg/h was 99.6% compared with UF_{NET} rate group of 1.01 to 1.75 mL/kg/h, and 32.5% compared with UF_{NET} rate less than 1.01 mL/kg/h among severely ill patients who have sepsis, metabolic acidosis, and organ edema, and those treated with mechanical ventilation and vasopressors (Naorungroj TSN, A, Murugan R, Kellum JA, Gallagher M, Bellomo R. Heterogeneity of mortality effect of net ultrafiltration rate among critically ill adults receiving continuous renal replacement therapy. Submitted for publication). However, the moderate UF_{NET} rate group between 1.01 and 1.75 mL/kg/h was consistently associated with the lowest risk of death compared with UF_{NET} rates less than 1.01 mL/kg/h or rates greater than 1.75 mL/kg/h.

Among patients with organ edema at study enrollment, the probability of harm associated with UF_{NET} rates greater than 1.75 mL/kg/h compared with rates less than 1.01 mL/kg/h was only 35.4%, suggesting that higher UF_{NET} rates in patients with isolated edema may be associated with a lower risk of death (Naorungroj TSN, A, Murugan R, Kellum JA, Gallagher M, Bellomo R. Heterogeneity of mortality effect of net ultrafiltration rate among critically ill adults receiving continuous renal replacement therapy. Submitted for publication). However, among patients who are hemodynamically unstable, both UF_{NET} rates greater than 1.75 mL/kg/h and rates less than 1.01 mL/kg/h were associated with mortality compared with rates less than 1.01 to 1.75 mL/kg/h (Naorungroj TSN, A Murugan R Kellum JA Gallagher M Bellomo R. Heterogeneity of mortality effect of net ultrafiltration rate among critically ill adults receiving continuous renal replacement therapy. Submitted for publication). This association of UF_{NET} rate greater than 1.75 mL/kg/h with mortality was also validated in an independent cohort of 347 patients treated with CKRT.[71] A subsequent mediation analysis suggested that UF_{NET} rates greater than 1.75 mL/kg/h were independently associated with risk of death and were not mediated through negative fluid balance, lower blood pressure, vasopressor use, or electrolyte abnormalities such as hypokalemia or hypophosphatemia.[72]

Several observational studies conducted among patients with kidney failure treated with intermittent hemodialysis have also found that higher ultrafiltration rates are associated with increased mortality.[73–77] In an analysis of 110,880 incident hemodialysis patients, ultrafiltration rates greater than or equal to 10 mL/kg/h compared with rates between 6 to 8 mL/kg/h were associated with increased risk-adjusted mortality.[75] Using the international Dialysis Outcomes and Practice Patterns (DOPPS) cohort of 22,000 prevalent hemodialysis patients, 1 study reported increased all-cause mortality among patients treated with ultrafiltration rate greater than or equal to 10 versus less than 10 mL/kg/h.[77] In addition, using the Hemodialysis (HEMO) cohort, 1 study reported that ultrafiltration rates greater than 13 mL/kg/h were associated with both all-cause and cardiovascular mortality in 1846 prevalent hemodialysis patients.[74]

The Centers for Medicare and Medicaid Services in the United States have proposed that ultrafiltration rates should be limited to less than 13 mL/kg/h among patients with kidney failure treated with hemodialysis based on the studies mentioned earlier.[78] However, randomized trials establishing causality between ultrafiltration rates and clinical outcomes among patients with kidney failure have not been conducted. Note that UF_{NET} rate greater than 1.75 mL/kg/h associated with mortality in critically ill patients treated with CKRT is considerably lower than the ultrafiltration rates of greater than 13 mL/kg/h that are associated with mortality in outpatients with kidney failure treated with hemodialysis. This association of lower UF_{NET} rates with mortality among patients treated with CKRT might be caused by increased susceptibility of critically ill patients to low UF_{NET} rates compared with non–critically ill outpatients. However, it is impossible to exclude confounding by unmeasured factors, and thus randomized clinical trials are required to confirm these findings.

AREAS OF UNCERTAINTY AND DIRECTIONS FOR FUTURE RESEARCH

Despite the use of UF_{NET} in the treatment of FO since the advent of dialysis for more than 7 decades, many aspects of volume management remain unclear. For instance, no randomized clinical trial has evaluated whether UF_{NET} is associated with lower mortality in critically ill patients. Although it may not be feasible to randomize patients to fluid removal versus no fluid removal, future studies should examine different rates of UF_{NET} on organ function and patient outcomes (**Table 5**). Although many clinicians believe that an ultrafiltration protocol would be beneficial, whether a protocol-based approach compared with an individualized ultrafiltration approach is associated with better outcomes is uncertain.[19] Furthermore, the optimal timing of initiation of UF_{NET} also remains unclear. Although many clinicians favor early fluid removal,[19] whether such an intervention improves outcome is uncertain. Although FO was the main reason for starting KRT among patients allocated to delayed KRT in several randomized trials that examined the timing of initiation of KRT,[79–81] none exclusively examined timing with respect to the initiation of ultrafiltration. Moreover, fluid balance at the end of the intervention was not reported in these trials.[82] Furthermore, there is increasing

Table 5
Areas of uncertainty and directions for further research involving net ultrafiltration

Directions for Further Research	Comments
Optimal rate of UF_{NET}	Randomized trials are needed to examine whether moderate compared with faster UF_{NET} rates are associated with lower rates of hypotension, ischemic organ injury, and mortality
Optimal monitoring technology during UF_{NET}	Further research is required to examine whether bioimpedance and PIVA accurately reflect intravascular volume
Timing of initiation	Whether earlier and preemptive initiation of UF_{NET} for prevention of FO is associated with improved outcomes is uncertain
Optimal modality	Which modality of UF_{NET} is associated with outcomes needs further research
Sodium modeling	Studies in critically ill patients treated with CKRT should evaluate whether sodium modeling is associated with improved hemodynamic stability
Dialysate cooling	Larger studies are required to examine whether dialysate cooling is associated with hemodynamic stability and organ protection
Sequential ultrafiltration and dialysis	Studies should evaluate whether UF_{NET} followed by dialysis is associated with improved outcomes compared with dialysis followed by UF_{NET} or dialysis with concurrent UF_{NET}
Remote ischemia preconditioning	Whether remote ischemia preconditioning before KRT and UF_{NET} is associated with less organ dysfunction/injury needs to be examined
Passive intradialytic exercise	Whether passive intradialytic exercise is associated with organ protection requires further research
Individualized UF_{NET} guided by artificial intelligence approaches	Whether artificial intelligence–based approaches and individualized UF_{NET} approaches improve outcomes requires evaluation

recognition that exposure of patients to longer duration of KRT is associated with poor outcomes. Whether early discontinuation of KRT and ultrafiltration following emergent management of life-threatening FO followed by a wait-and-watch approach is associated with improved outcomes is uncertain.

Monitoring technologies to accurately and continuously assess intravascular volume are needed. Although emerging newer technologies, such as bioimpedance and PIVA, are promising, whether UF_{NET} rate titration based on such monitoring devices is associated with improved outcomes also needs to be evaluated. Furthermore, studies are required to examine whether a sequential approach to ultrafiltration in which ultrafiltration is done first without removing solutes followed by combined dialysis and ultrafiltration is associated with improved outcomes.

Priority should be given to mechanistic studies to understand how UF_{NET} rates and dialysis are associated with organ dysfunction and to disentangle which component of intradialytic organ injury is potentially modifiable. For instance, ongoing research, such as cooling the dialysate,[83] remote ischemic preconditioning,[84,85] sodium modeling,[59,60] and intradialytic exercise,[86] has shown promising results in preventing dialysis-associated organ injury. However, its implications for critically ill patients are uncertain. The results of mechanistic studies and the use of artificial intelligence approaches in the near future may aid with precise and individualized titration of UF_{NET} in critically ill patients.

SUMMARY

Despite the widespread use of ultrafiltration for the treatment of FO, whether the use of ultrafiltration is associated with improved outcomes in critically ill patients remains unclear. Emerging evidence suggests that faster UF_{NET} rates are associated with ischemic organ injury and mortality, whereas slower UF_{NET} rates are associated with prolonged exposure to FO and mortality in critically ill patients. Randomized trials are urgently required to determine optimal UF_{NET} rates that are associated with improved patient-centered clinical outcomes, and further research should focus on interventions to reduce risks associated with UF_{NET}.

CLINICS CARE POINTS

- Minimize fluid administration to patients with oliguric AKI to prevent FO.
- The rate of UF_{NET} should be set based on patient body weight (mL/kg/h) rather than on absolute volumes (mL/h).
- Cool dialysate to less than or equal to 36°C.
- Careful attention should be paid to patient hemodynamics with frequent assessment of end-organ perfusion and function.
- Avoid intradialytic hypoxemia.
- Moderate UF_{NET} rates between 1.01 and 1.75 mL/kg/h of patient body weight are associated with the lowest risk of death in critically ill patients.
- Patient fluid balance and machine fluid balance must be assessed frequently and integrated.
- Avoid or minimize exposure to high UF_{NET} rates, if feasible. Use high rates only to treat immediate life-threatening FO and terminate once the life-threatening event resolves.

DISCLOSURE

Dr R. Murugan received grants and personal fees from La Jolla Inc; grants from Bioporto, Inc and the National Institute of Diabetes and Digestive and Kidney Diseases; and personal fees from Beckman Coulter and AM Pharma, Inc, outside the submitted work.

REFERENCES

1. Miller TE, Bunke M, Nisbet P, et al. Fluid resuscitation practice patterns in intensive care units of the USA: a cross-sectional survey of critical care physicians. Perioper Med (Lond) 2016;5:15.
2. Sánchez M, Jiménez-Lendínez M, Cidoncha M, et al. Comparison of fluid compartments and fluid responsiveness in septic and non-septic patients. Anaesth Intensive Care 2011;39(6):1022–9.
3. O'Connor ME, Jones SL, Glassford NJ, et al. Defining fluid removal in the intensive care unit: a national and international survey of critical care practice. J Intensive Care Soc 2017;18(4):282–8.
4. Recommended methods for measurement of red-cell and plasma volume: international Committee for Standardization in Haematology. J Nucl Med 1980;21(8): 793–800.
5. Dworkin HJ, Premo M, Dees S. Comparison of red cell and whole blood volume as performed using both chromium-51-tagged red cells and iodine-125-tagged albumin and using I-131-tagged albumin and extrapolated red cell volume. Am J Med Sci 2007;334(1):37–40.
6. Rosner MH, Ostermann M, Murugan R, et al. Indications and management of mechanical fluid removal in critical illness. Br J Anaesth 2014;113(5):764–71.
7. Balakumar V, Murugan R, Sileanu FE, et al. Both positive and negative fluid balance may be associated with reduced long-term survival in the critically ill. Crit Care Med 2017;45(8):e749–57.
8. Bouchard J, Soroko SB, Chertow GM, et al. Fluid accumulation, survival and recovery of kidney function in critically ill patients with acute kidney injury. Kidney Int 2009;76(4):422–7.
9. Goldstein SL, Somers MJ, Baum MA, et al. Pediatric patients with multi-organ dysfunction syndrome receiving continuous renal replacement therapy. Kidney Int 2005;67(2):653–8.
10. Sutherland SM, Zappitelli M, Alexander SR, et al. Fluid overload and mortality in children receiving continuous renal replacement therapy: the prospective pediatric continuous renal replacement therapy registry. Am J Kidney Dis 2010;55(2): 316–25.
11. Vaara ST, Korhonen AM, Kaukonen KM, et al. Fluid overload is associated with an increased risk for 90-day mortality in critically ill patients with renal replacement therapy: data from the prospective FINNAKI study. Crit Care 2012;16(5):R197.
12. Renal Replacement Therapy Investigators, Bellomo R, Cass A, et al. An observational study fluid balance and patient outcomes in the Randomized Evaluation of Normal vs. Augmented Level of Replacement Therapy trial. Crit Care Med 2012; 40(6):1753–60.
13. Renal Replacement Therapy Investigators, Bellomo R, Cass A, et al. Intensity of continuous renal-replacement therapy in critically ill patients. N Engl J Med 2009; 361(17):1627–38.

14. Veterans Affairs Acute Renal Failure Trial Network (ATN), Palevsky PM, Zhang JH, et al. Intensity of renal support in critically ill patients with acute kidney injury. N Engl J Med 2008;359(1):7–20.

15. Murugan R, Balakumar V, Kerti SJ, et al. Net ultrafiltration intensity and mortality in critically ill patients with fluid overload. Crit Care 2018;22(1):223.

16. Kidney Disease: Improving Global Outcomes (KDIGO) Working Group. Clinical practice guideline for acute kidney injury. Kidney Int Suppl 2012;2:1–138.

17. Rewa OG, Tolwani A, Mottes T, et al. Quality of care and safety measures of acute renal replacement therapy: Workgroup statements from the 22nd acute disease quality initiative (ADQI) consensus conference. J Crit Care 2019;54:52–7.

18. Modem V, Thompson M, Gollhofer D, et al. Timing of continuous renal replacement therapy and mortality in critically ill children*. Crit Care Med 2014;42(4): 943–53.

19. Murugan R, Ostermann M, Peng Z, et al. Net ultrafiltration prescription and practice among critically ill patients receiving renal replacement therapy: a multinational survey of critical care practitioners. Crit Care Med 2020;48(2):e87–97.

21. Serpa Neto A, Naorungroj T, Murugan R, et al. Heterogeneity of effect of net ultrafiltration rate among critically ill adults receiving continuous renal replacement therapy. Blood Purif 2020;1–11.

20. Murugan R, Kellum JA. Fluid balance and outcome in acute kidney injury: is fluid really the best medicine? Crit Care Med 2012;40(6):1970–2.

22. Tehranian S, Shawwa K, Kashani KB. Net ultrafiltration rate and its impact on mortality in patients with acute kidney injury receiving continuous renal replacement therapy. Clin Kidney J 2019;1–6. https://doi.org/10.1093/ckj/sfz179.

23. Murugan R, Kerti SJ, Chang CH, et al. Association of net ultrafiltration rate with mortality among critically ill adults with acute kidney injury receiving continuous venovenous hemodiafiltration: a secondary analysis of the randomized evaluation of normal vs augmented level (RENAL) of renal replacement therapy trial. JAMA Netw Open 2019;2(6):e195418.

24. Murugan R, Kerti SJ, Chang CH, et al. Net ultrafiltration rate and renal recovery among critically ill adults with acute kidney injury receiving continuous renal replacement therapy: a competing risk secondary analysis of the randomized evaluation of normal versus augmented level of renal replacement therapy trial. J Am Soc Nephrol 2020. This article is in peer review.

25. O'Connor ME, Prowle JR. Fluid overload. Crit Care Clin 2015;31(4):803–21.

26. Prowle JR, Echeverri JE, Ligabo EV, et al. Fluid balance and acute kidney injury. Nat Rev Nephrol 2010;6(2):107.

27. Wald R, Quinn RR, Luo J, et al. Chronic dialysis and death among survivors of acute kidney injury requiring dialysis. JAMA 2009;302(11):1179–85.

28. Mottes TA, Goldstein SL, Basu RK. Process based quality improvement using a continuous renal replacement therapy dashboard. BMC Nephrol 2019;20(1):17.

29. Piccoli A, Rossi B, Pillon L, et al. A new method for monitoring body fluid variation by bioimpedance analysis: the RXc graph. Kidney Int 1994;46(2):534–9.

30. Basso F, Berdin G, Virzi GM, et al. Fluid management in the intensive care unit: bioelectrical impedance vector analysis as a tool to assess hydration status and optimal fluid balance in critically ill patients. Blood Purif 2013;36(3–4):192–9.

31. Hise A, Gonzalez MC. Assessment of hydration status using bioelectrical impedance vector analysis in critical patients with acute kidney injury. Clin Nutr 2018; 37(2):695–700.

32. Jones SL, Tanaka A, Eastwood GM, et al. Bioelectrical impedance vector analysis in critically ill patients: a prospective, clinician-blinded investigation. Crit Care 2015;19:290.

33. Razzera EL, Marcadenti A, Rovedder SW, et al. Parameters of bioelectrical impedance are good predictors of nutrition risk, length of stay, and mortality in critically ill patients: a prospective cohort study. JPEN J Parenter Enteral Nutr 2019;44(5):849–54.

34. Rochwerg B, Cheung JH, Ribic CM, et al. Assessment of postresuscitation volume status by bioimpedance analysis in patients with sepsis in the intensive care unit: a pilot observational study. Can Respir J 2016;2016:8671742.

35. Samoni S, Vigo V, Resendiz LI, et al. Impact of hyperhydration on the mortality risk in critically ill patients admitted in intensive care units: comparison between bioelectrical impedance vector analysis and cumulative fluid balance recording. Crit Care 2016;20:95.

36. Chen H, Wu B, Gong D, et al. Fluid overload at start of continuous renal replacement therapy is associated with poorer clinical condition and outcome: a prospective observational study on the combined use of bioimpedance vector analysis and serum N-terminal pro-B-type natriuretic peptide measurement. Crit Care 2015;19:135.

37. Park KH, Shin JH, Hwang JH, et al. Utility of volume assessment using bioelectrical impedance analysis in critically ill patients receiving continuous renal replacement therapy: a prospective observational study. Korean J Crit Care Med 2017;32(3):256–64.

38. Rhee H, Jang KS, Shin MJ, et al. Use of multifrequency bioimpedance analysis in male patients with acute kidney injury who are undergoing continuous venovenous hemodiafiltration. PLoS One 2015;10(7):e0133199.

39. Hocking KM, Alvis BD, Baudenbacher F, et al. Peripheral i.v. analysis (PIVA) of venous waveforms for volume assessment in patients undergoing haemodialysis. Br J Anaesth 2017;119(6):1135–40.

40. Miles M, Alvis BD, Hocking K, et al. Peripheral intravenous volume analysis (PIVA) for quantitating volume overload in patients hospitalized with acute decompensated heart failure-a pilot study. J Card Fail 2018;24(8):525–32.

41. Sileshi B, Hocking KM, Boyer RB, et al. Peripheral venous waveform analysis for detecting early hemorrhage: a pilot study. Intensive Care Med 2015;41(6):1147–8.

42. Hocking KM, Sileshi B, Baudenbacher FJ, et al. Peripheral venous waveform analysis for detecting hemorrhage and iatrogenic volume overload in a porcine model. Shock 2016;46(4):447–52.

43. Murugan R, Hoste E, Mehta RL, et al. Precision fluid management in continuous renal replacement therapy. Blood Purif 2016;42(3):266–78.

44. Kellum JA, Lameire N, Aspelin P, et al. Kidney disease: improving global outcomes (KDIGO) acute kidney injury work group. KDIGO clinical practice guideline for acute kidney injury. Kidney Int supplements 2012;2(1):1–138.

45. Akhoundi A, Singh B, Vela M, et al. Incidence of adverse events during continuous renal replacement therapy. Blood Purif 2015;39(4):333–9.

46. Silversides JA, Pinto R, Kuint R, et al. Fluid balance, intradialytic hypotension, and outcomes in critically ill patients undergoing renal replacement therapy: a cohort study. Crit Care 2014;18(6):624.

47. Augustine JJ, Sandy D, Seifert TH, et al. A randomized controlled trial comparing intermittent with continuous dialysis in patients with ARF. Am J kidney Dis 2004;44(6):1000–7.

48. Douvris A, Zeid K, Hiremath S, et al. Mechanisms for hemodynamic instability related to renal replacement therapy: a narrative review. Intensive Care Med 2019;45(10):1333–46.

49. Backer DD, Creteur J, Preiser J-C, et al. Microvascular blood flow is altered in patients with sepsis. Am J Respir Crit Care Med 2002;166(1):98–104.

50. Shawwa K, Kompotiatis P, Jentzer JC, et al. Hypotension within one-hour from starting CRRT is associated with in-hospital mortality. J Crit Care 2019;54:7–13.

51. Uchino S, Bellomo R, Morimatsu H, et al. Continuous renal replacement therapy: a worldwide practice survey. The beginning and ending supportive therapy for the kidney (B.E.S.T. kidney) investigators. Intensive Care Med 2007;33(9): 1563–70.

52. Vinsonneau C, Camus C, Combes A, et al. Continuous venovenous haemodiafiltration versus intermittent haemodialysis for acute renal failure in patients with multiple-organ dysfunction syndrome: a multicentre randomised trial. Lancet 2006;368(9533):379–85.

53. Bitker L, Bayle F, Yonis H, et al. Prevalence and risk factors of hypotension associated with preload-dependence during intermittent hemodialysis in critically ill patients. Crit Care 2016;20:44.

54. Schortgen F, Soubrier N, Delclaux C, et al. Hemodynamic tolerance of intermittent hemodialysis in critically ill patients: usefulness of practice guidelines. Am J Respir Crit Care Med 2000;162(1):197–202.

55. Tanguay TA, Jensen L, Johnston C. Predicting episodes of hypotension by continuous blood volume monitoring among critically ill patients in acute renal failure on intermittent hemodialysis. Dynamics 2007;18(3):19–24.

56. Tonelli M, Astephen P, Andreou P, et al. Blood volume monitoring in intermittent hemodialysis for acute renal failure. Kidney Int 2002;62(3):1075–80.

57. Edrees FY, Katari S, Baty JD, et al. A pilot study evaluating the effect of cooler dialysate temperature on hemodynamic stability during prolonged intermittent renal replacement therapy in acute kidney injury. Crit Care Med 2019;47(2): e74–80.

58. Robert R, Mehaud JE, Timricht N, et al. Benefits of an early cooling phase in continuous renal replacement therapy for ICU patients. Ann Intensive Care 2012;2(1):40.

59. Oliver MJ, Edwards LJ, Churchill DN. Impact of sodium and ultrafiltration profiling on hemodialysis-related symptoms. J Am Soc Nephrol 2001;12(1):151–6.

60. Song JH, Lee SW, Suh CK, et al. Time-averaged concentration of dialysate sodium relates with sodium load and interdialytic weight gain during sodium-profiling hemodialysis. Am J Kidney Dis 2002;40(2):291–301.

61. Paganini EP, Sandy D, Moreno L, et al. The effect of sodium and ultrafiltration modelling on plasma volume changes and haemodynamic stability in intensive care patients receiving haemodialysis for acute renal failure: a prospective, stratified, randomized, cross-over study. Nephrol Dial Transplant 1996;11(Suppl 8):32–7.

62. Lynch KE, Ghassemi F, Flythe JE, et al. Sodium modelling to reduce intradialytic hypotension during haemodialysis for acute kidney injury in the intensive care unit. Nephrology (Carlton). 2016;21(10):870–7.

63. Monnet X, Cipriani F, Camous L, et al. The passive leg raising test to guide fluid removal in critically ill patients. Ann Intensive Care 2016;6(1):46.

64. Rudski LG, Lai WW, Afilalo J, et al. Guidelines for the echocardiographic assessment of the right heart in adults: a report from the American Society of Echocardiography: Endorsed by the European Association of Echocardiography, a

registered branch of the European Society of Cardiology, and the Canadian Society of Echocardiography. J Am Soc Echocardiography 2010;23(7):685–713.

65. Blehar DJ, Dickman E, Gaspari R. Identification of congestive heart failure via respiratory variation of inferior vena cava diameter. Am J Emerg Med 2009; 27(1):71–5.

66. Gundersen GH, Norekval TM, Haug HH, et al. Adding point of care ultrasound to assess volume status in heart failure patients in a nurse-led outpatient clinic. A randomised study. Heart 2016;102(1):29–34.

67. Kaptein MJ, Kaptein JS, Oo Z, et al. Relationship of inferior vena cava collapsibility to ultrafiltration volume achieved in critically ill hemodialysis patients. Int J Nephrol Renovasc Dis 2018;11:195–209.

68. da Hora Passos R, Caldas J, Ramos JGR, et al. Ultrasound-based clinical profiles for predicting the risk of intradialytic hypotension in critically ill patients on intermittent dialysis: a prospective observational study. Crit Care 2019;23(1):389.

69. Cheriex EC, Leunissen KML, Janssen JHA, et al. Echography of the inferior vena cava is a simple and reliable tool for estimation of 'Dry weight' in haemodialysis patients. Nephrol Dial Transplant 1989;4(6):563–8.

70. Gargani L. Lung ultrasound: a new tool for the cardiologist. Cardiovasc Ultrasound 2011;9(1):6.

71. Naorungroj T, Neto AS, Zwakman-Hessels L, et al. Early net ultrafiltration rate and mortality in critically ill patients receiving continuous renal replacement therapy. Nephrol Dial Transplant 2020. https://doi.org/10.1093/ndt/gfaa032.

72. Naorungroj TSN A, Zawkman-Hessels L, Yanase F, et al. Mediators of the impact of hourly net ultrafiltration rate on mortality in critically ill patients receiving continuous renal replacement therapy. Crit Care Med 2020;48(10):e934–42.

73. Flythe JE, Curhan GC, Brunelli SM. Shorter length dialysis sessions are associated with increased mortality, independent of body weight. Kidney Int 2013; 83(1):104–13.

74. Flythe JE, Kimmel SE, Brunelli SM. Rapid fluid removal during dialysis is associated with cardiovascular morbidity and mortality. Kidney Int 2011;79(2):250–7.

75. Kim TW, Chang TI, Kim TH, et al. Association of ultrafiltration rate with mortality in incident hemodialysis patients. Nephron 2018;139(1):13–22.

76. Movilli E, Gaggia P, Zubani R, et al. Association between high ultrafiltration rates and mortality in uraemic patients on regular haemodialysis. A 5-year prospective observational multicentre study. Nephrol Dial Transplant 2007;22(12):3547–52.

77. Saran R, Bragg-Gresham JL, Levin NW, et al. Longer treatment time and slower ultrafiltration in hemodialysis: associations with reduced mortality in the DOPPS. Kidney Int 2006;69(7):1222–8.

78. Kramer H, Yee J, Weiner DE, et al. Ultrafiltration rate thresholds in maintenance hemodialysis: an NKF-KDOQI controversies report. Am J Kidney Dis 2016; 68(4):522–32.

79. Barbar SD, Clere-Jehl R, Bourredjem A, et al. Timing of renal-replacement therapy in patients with acute kidney injury and sepsis. N Engl J Med 2018; 379(15):1431–42.

80. Gaudry S, Hajage D, Schortgen F, et al. Initiation strategies for renal-replacement therapy in the intensive care unit. N Engl J Med 2016;375(2):122–33.

81. Zarbock A, Kellum JA, Schmidt C, et al. Effect of early vs delayed initiation of renal replacement therapy on mortality in critically ill patients with acute kidney injury: the ELAIN randomized clinical trial. JAMA 2016;315(20):2190–9.

82. Canaud B, Cohen EP. Initiation of renal-replacement therapy in the intensive care unit. N Engl J Med 2016;375(19):1901.

83. Eldehni MT, Odudu A, McIntyre CW. Randomized clinical trial of dialysate cooling and effects on brain white matter. J Am Soc Nephrol 2015;26(4):957–65.

84. Crowley LE, McIntyre CW. Remote ischaemic conditioning-therapeutic opportunities in renal medicine. Nat Rev Nephrol 2013;9(12):739–46.

85. Salerno FR, Crowley LE, Odudu A, et al. Remote ischemic preconditioning protects against hemodialysis-induced cardiac injury. Kidney Int Rep 2020;5(1):99–103.

86. Penny JD, Salerno FR, Brar R, et al. Intradialytic exercise preconditioning: an exploratory study on the effect on myocardial stunning. Nephrol Dial Transplant 2019;34(11):1917–23.

87. Bagshaw SM, Adhikari NKJ, Burns KEA, et al. Selection and receipt of kidney replacement in critically ill older patients with AKI. Clin J Am Soc Nephrol 2019;14(4):496–505.

88. Woodward CW, Lambert J, Ortiz-Soriano V, et al. Fluid overload associates with major adverse kidney events in critically ill patients with acute kidney injury requiring continuous renal replacement therapy. Crit Care Med 2019;47(9):e753–60.

89. Dill J, Bixby B, Ateeli H, et al. Renal replacement therapy in patients with acute respiratory distress syndrome: a single-center retrospective study. Int J Nephrol Renovasc Dis 2018;11:249–57.

90. Ballarin Albino B, Gobo-Oliveira M, Balbi AL, et al. Mortality and recovery of renal function in acute kidney injury patients treated with prolonged intermittent hemodialysis sessions lasting 10 versus 6 hours: results of a randomized clinical trial. Int J Nephrol 2018;2018:4097864.

91. Silversides JA, Fitzgerald E, Manickavasagam US, et al. Deresuscitation of patients with iatrogenic fluid overload is associated with reduced mortality in critical illness. Crit Care Med 2018;46(10):1600–7.

92. Kim IY, Kim JH, Lee DW, et al. Fluid overload and survival in critically ill patients with acute kidney injury receiving continuous renal replacement therapy. PLoS One 2017;12(2):e0172137.

93. Kellum JA, Chawla LS, Keener C, et al. The effects of alternative resuscitation strategies on acute kidney injury in patients with septic shock. Am J Respir Crit Care Med 2016;193(3):281–7.

94. Garzotto F, Ostermann M, Martín-Langerwerf D, et al. The dose response multicentre investigation on fluid assessment (DoReMIFA) in critically ill patients. Crit Care 2016;20(1):196.

95. Xu J, Shen B, Fang Y, et al. Postoperative fluid overload is a useful predictor of the short-term outcome of renal replacement therapy for acute kidney injury after cardiac surgery. Medicine (Baltimore) 2015;94(33):e1360.

96. Heung M, Wolfgram DF, Kommareddi M, et al. Fluid overload at initiation of renal replacement therapy is associated with lack of renal recovery in patients with acute kidney injury. Nephrol Dial Transplant 2012;27(3):956–61.

97. Fülöp T, Pathak MB, Schmidt DW, et al. Volume-related weight gain and subsequent mortality in acute renal failure patients treated with continuous renal replacement therapy. ASAIO J 2010;56(4):333–7.

98. Gleeson PJC IA, Sexton DJ, Fontana V, et al. Determinants of renal recovery and mortality in patients undergoing continuous renal replacement therapy in the ICU. Intensive Care Med Exp 2015;3(Suppl 1):A54.

99. Pajewski R, Gipson P, Heung M. Predictors of post-hospitalization recovery of renal function among patients with acute kidney injury requiring dialysis. Hemodial Int 2018;22(1):66–73.

Acute Kidney Disease to Chronic Kidney Disease

Javier A. Neyra, MD, MSCS[a],*, Lakhmir S. Chawla, MD[b]

KEYWORDS

- Acute kidney injury • AKI • Acute kidney disease • AKD • Chronic kidney disease
- CKD • Kidney recovery

KEY POINTS

- Acute kidney injury (AKI) and chronic kidney disease (CKD) are common interconnected syndromes that represent a public health problem. AKI and CKD predispose to each other in a vicious circle and may exert negative impacts independently or synergistically.
- The term AKD has emerged and is defined as the post-AKI status of acute or subacute kidney damage/dysfunction manifested by persistence of AKI stage 1 or greater (Kidney Disease: Improving Global Outcomes criteria) beyond 7 to 90 days after the initial AKI diagnosis. If criteria of AKI persist beyond 90 days, it is considered incident or progressive CKD according to baseline kidney function.
- Pathways of maladaptive repair predisposing to inflammation and fibrosis leading to CKD have been identified and include cell cycle arrest, endothelial injury followed by capillary regression and rarefaction, mitochondrial dysfunction, fibroblast/macrophage-aberrant differentiation and function, and the immune response with imbalance of more proinflammatory injury and less anti-inflammatory repair.
- Limited clinical data exist with regard to AKD epidemiology. Studies published after AKD was formally defined have limited generalizability as they represent heterogeneous populations with distinct timeframes of observation to define AKD. At least 1 of 4 AKI survivors developed AKD by 90 days of follow-up.
- Useful risk-stratification tools to predict risk of AKD and its prognosis are needed. Timely kidney-protective approaches centered in aspects such as fluid management, exposure to nephrotoxic agents, and follow-up care may have a big impact in AKD management and outcomes.

[a] Department of Internal Medicine, Division of Nephrology, Bone and Mineral Metabolism, University of Kentucky Medical Center, 800 Rose Street, MN668, Lexington, KY 40536, USA;
[b] Department of Medicine, Veterans Affairs Medical Center, 3350 La Jolla Village Drive, San Diego, CA 92161, USA
* Corresponding author.
E-mail address: javier.neyra@uky.edu

Crit Care Clin 37 (2021) 453–474
https://doi.org/10.1016/j.ccc.2020.11.013
0749-0704/21/© 2020 Elsevier Inc. All rights reserved.

INTRODUCTION

Chronic kidney disease (CKD) represents an enormous public health problem due to its high prevalence, economic impact, and strong association with morbidity and mortality.[1–3] Acute kidney injury (AKI) is a common complication during hospitalization that occurs in approximately 1 of 5 hospitalized patients and in 1 of 2 critically ill patients in the intensive care unit (ICU).[4–6] These 2 clinical syndromes are interconnected, as survivors of AKI have increased risk of CKD and end-stage kidney disease (ESKD),[7,8] as well as cardiovascular disease.[9–14] Conversely, patients with underlying CKD have an increased risk of AKI, so that AKI and CKD predispose to each other in a vicious circle and may exert negative impacts independently or synergistically.[4,15–17]

The heterogeneity in AKI definitions from different etiologies and practice variations for AKI diagnosis and management precluded, for many years, the development of robust epidemiologic data that clearly delineated the interplay between AKI and CKD. To overcome these barriers, the Kidney Disease: Improving Global Outcomes (KDIGO) Clinical Practice Guidelines emerged to standardize criteria for AKI diagnosis and management.[18] Although the main goals of promoting early AKI recognition and standardizing AKI diagnosis were fulfilled, the period of transition from AKI to CKD (also known as acute kidney disease [AKD]) was poorly defined and seldom characterized in clinical practice. In this context, the Acute Disease Quality Initiative (ADQI) 16 Workgroup proposed a consensus and more practical definition of AKD to promote its widespread application in clinical research and direct patient care.[19]

In this article, we review the AKD definition and the challenges of its recognition, emerging epidemiologic data of AKD, key pathophysiological concepts of the AKI-to-AKD-to-CKD interplay, and important aspects of AKD management for reducing the burden of CKD.

EPIDEMIOLOGY OF CHRONIC KIDNEY DISEASE

CKD is a major public health problem that affects more than 20 million individuals in the United States ($\sim$15% of the US population) and carries devastating human and economic burden.[1] CKD is a major cause of disproportionate morbidity and mortality, ranking as the ninth leading cause of death in the United States.[2] The financial cost of CKD care accounts for 20% of total Medicare spending with the most costly care related to ESKD.[3] Therefore, there is an urgent need to identify public health interventions that can mitigate the incidence and progression of CKD.

To mitigate the burden of CKD and its devastating complications, such as cardiovascular disease and death, identification of modifiable risk factors for development and progression of CKD is necessary. A critical contributor to the prevalence of CKD is AKI, which increases the risk of development of CKD by as much as 10-fold, and strongly associates with cardiovascular disease, poor health-related quality of life, rehospitalizations, and death.[4,8–11,20–24]

EPIDEMIOLOGY OF ACUTE KIDNEY INJURY

AKI affects up to 20% of hospitalized patients and up to 50% of patients admitted to the ICU.[4–6] The incidence of AKI is growing by 10% per year,[25–27] whereas the morbidity and mortality associated with its occurrence remain exceedingly high.[28,29] AKI is associated with increased length of ICU and hospital stay, and disproportionate increased resource utilization and health care costs.[30] Furthermore, complications after an episode of AKI are also common and include cardiovascular disease,[9–13] hypertension,[14] and the development or progression of CKD or ESKD.[7,23,24] Estimates of 10-fold higher risk of CKD and 3-fold higher risk of ESKD following an episode of AKI have been determined from multiple observational studies.[7,8] Importantly, ESKD due to AKI carries higher 6-month mortality risk than ESKD related to other causes.[31] Therefore, early AKI recognition and risk-stratification are needed for implementation of timely interventions that can mitigate further kidney damage and complications of AKI.[32]

Survivors of AKI, especially those with severe AKI, are at high risk for developing CKD, and this is compounded by concerns of inequitable access to health care or inadequate postdischarge processes of health care.[33] This is particularly important because survivors of AKI frequently experience recurrence of AKI and rehospitalizations at rates of up to 25% and 50% within a year after discharge, respectively.[34] Hence, improving care following AKI has been recognized as critical to reducing AKI to CKD transition and CKD progression and importantly, to improving patient-centered quality-of-life outcomes.[35]

There is a bidirectional interplay between AKI and CKD and recognized risk factors of kidney disease, such as age, diabetes, hypertension, and proteinuria beget both conditions.[14,36,37] Therefore, there was a dire need to systematically differentiate patients with ongoing acute kidney pathology versus those in the recovery phase of AKI, specifically in the period of 7 to 90 days following AKI diagnosis. This context nurtured the concept of AKD, which was formally proposed and defined by the ADQI Workgroup 16 in 2017.[19] This new concept is critically important, as AKD represents a period in which tailored interventions both in inpatient and outpatient settings can be potentially instituted to favorably alter the natural history of kidney disease (**Fig. 1**).

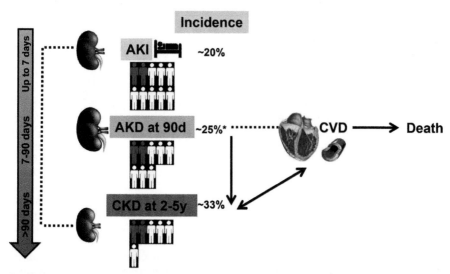

Fig. 1. Conceptual interplay and epidemiology of AKI, AKD, and CKD. The incidence of AKI in hospitalized patients is approximately 20% and AKD occurs in 1 of 4 survivors of AKI by 90-days post-AKI onset, albeit epidemiologic data of AKD are still limited. It is estimated that 1 of 3 patients surviving an episode of AKI may develop incident or progressive CKD within the subsequent 2 to 5 years. An important consequence of AKI is cardiovascular disease, which carries a great burden of morbidity and mortality in these patients. CVD, cardiovascular disease.

ACUTE KIDNEY DISEASE AFTER ACUTE KIDNEY INJURY
Definition of Acute Kidney Injury

The KDIGO Clinical Practice Guideline defined AKI as an absolute increase in serum creatinine (SCr) by 0.3 mg/dL (26.5 μmol/L) within 48 hours; or a relative increase in SCr 1.5 times baseline within 7 days; or urine volume less than 0.5 mL/kg per hour for 6 hours.[18] However, one should recognize that despite the urine volume criterion is known to be informative of AKI incidence and prognosis[38] and is now more commonly used and monitored in clinical practice given the recognition of the detrimental effects of fluid overload,[39–41] it has seldom been examined in observational studies of AKI. Therefore, the epidemiology and characterization of AKI are mostly based on SCr changes over time.

Duration of Acute Kidney Injury

Rapidly reversible episodes of AKI within 48 hours of onset are epidemiologically distinct from those that last more than 48 hours for the association with short-term and long-term mortality. This has been demonstrated in observational studies including postoperative and critically ill patients with AKI.[42–45] Therefore, the terms "transient AKI" and "persistent AKI" are used for describing episodes of AKI of duration of less than and more than 48 hours, respectively.[19] Further, a minimum sustained AKI reversal for a period of 48 hours has been suggested by consensus for evaluation of recurrent or de novo AKI episodes. One should exert caution when interpreting these recommendations, as urine output data may be inaccurate in patients without urinary catheters and SCr is susceptible to specific clinical conditions such as sepsis, sarcopenia, and fluid overload/change in volume of distribution,[46–49] which can acutely affect SCr interpretation as a surrogate of kidney function.

The early recognition of "persistent AKI" may facilitate further evaluation of AKI etiology and interventions that can halt progression of kidney injury and its associated complications, including dependence on renal replacement therapy (RRT) and short-term and long-term mortality.[50,51] Importantly, many multimodal tools have been evaluated to identify patients at risk of "persistent AKI" over the past years, but standardized or fully validated risk-stratification tools are not yet available for clinical application.[19] The ability to combine pragmatic and readily available functional testing (eg, furosemide stress test),[52] kidney biomarkers of injury,[53,54] dysfunction[55] and repair,[56,57] functional imaging testing,[58] and novel methods of interrogation of "big data" (eg, machine learning)[59,60] shows promise, although challenges with reproducibility and access to external validation hinder applicability into clinical practice.

Assessment of Kidney Function

Iterative monitoring of kidney function is needed in hospitalized patients with AKI, particularly those patients in whom AKI persists for more than 48 hours. When assessing kidney function, it is important to consider that measurement of glomerular filtration rate (GFR) with inulin or iohexol, which yield high accuracy, is not practical for use in acute settings. Furthermore, estimation of GFR with equations routinely used in "steady-state" outpatient settings such as Modification of Diet in Renal Disease and Chronic Kidney Disease–Epidemiology Collaboration are not validated for use in acute settings of dynamic change in kidney function, particularly in the ICU.[61] Therefore, short-timed urine collection for measurement of creatinine clearance is a valid surrogate of kidney function, although overestimation of kidney function due to tubular secretion of creatinine limits its accuracy.[62] Alternative calculations of GFR based on volume of distribution and creatinine kinetics have shown promise in not "steady state" situations but further validation in larger studies is needed.[63–65] Measurement of GFR can be also obtained with optical fluorescence approaches using novel minimally invasive or noninvasive techniques that can quantify kidney function, independent of serum or urinary measurements.[66,67] Although these approaches hold promise to more comprehensively determine kidney function by measures of baseline and total GFR (whereas total GFR minus baseline GFR estimates renal reserve), reproducibility and validation in human studies are necessary.

Definition of Acute Kidney Disease

In an effort to provide more conceptual background to the AKI-to-CKD interaction, the 2012 KDIGO-AKI workgroup proposed the term "acute kidney disease" to define any acute condition that acutely decreases kidney function. The proposed term encompassed AKI, an absolute estimated GFR (eGFR) less than 60 mL/min per 1.73 m^2 or a decrease in eGFR by more than 35%, an increase in SCr of more than 50%, or any kidney damage lasting less than 3 months.[18] The ADQI 16 Workgroup further refined this definition by adding a staging criteria and proposing AKD to be defined as the post-AKI status of acute or subacute kidney damage/dysfunction manifested by persistence of AKI stage 1 or greater (KDIGO criteria) beyond 7 to 90 days after the initial AKI diagnosis. If criteria of AKI persist beyond 90 days, it is considered incident or progressive CKD according to baseline kidney function (see **Fig. 1**). It is important to note that the ADQI 16 Workgroup determined the period of AKD beyond 7 to 90 days after a known AKI initiating event. Patients with community-acquired AKI, those transferred from other facilities, or those with unmeasured baseline kidney function may have an ambiguous timeline of the initial AKI event and therefore the precise AKI, AKD, or CKD status of these patients may be difficult to ascertain. Hence, clinical rationale is highly recommended when diagnosing AKD in the inpatient setting.[19] Among survivors of the inciting AKI events, the period of AKD includes multiple outcomes that should be clearly differentiated and defined to guide tailored management and mitigate the burden of post-AKI complications. These outcomes include (1) recovery, (2) recurrence of AKI, and (3) persistence or progression of AKD.

Recovery

Recovery of AKD is defined as a reduction in peak AKI stage (KDIGO criteria) within 7 and 90 days after the initial AKI diagnosis. Understanding the caveats of isolated use of KDIGO criteria, additional information from trajectories of SCr,[68,69] real-time measurement of GFR, kidney biomarkers of injury/repair, and functional assessment of kidney function/reserve could assist in phenotyping the presence and degree of recovery of AKD.[32] The concept of defining recovery involves the quantification of the loss of baseline kidney function and the status of current residual kidney function and reserve, which conveys important prognostic information to risk-stratify patients.

Recurrent acute kidney injury

In cases in which AKI has resolved, meaning kidney function has returned back to baseline level for at least 48 hours, the incidence of a new episode of AKI (KDIGO criteria) within the period of AKD will be considered recurrent AKI.[19]

Persistence or progression of acute kidney disease

In cases in which AKI has not resolved, meaning kidney function has not returned back to baseline level, AKD may persist or worsen based on KDIGO criteria of AKI.

Subclinical Acute Kidney Injury and Acute Kidney Disease

An important consideration when examining AKD is the presence of subclinical AKI, which is not detected by traditional KDIGO criteria of AKI but with histologic, imaging, or biomarker evidence of kidney damage or dysfunction not included in current KDIGO definition of AKI.[70] Furthermore, subclinical AKD after AKI is also possible and detected when SCr remains above baseline but without reaching the threshold established by KDIGO to define persistence of AKI criteria. Observational studies have shown that patients who achieved a recovery SCr that remains 15% to 49% above baseline levels still carry an increased mortality risk than those with complete recovery to baseline levels.[71] The standardization of measurements of ongoing injury, status of kidney repair and/or regeneration or indicators of loss of glomerular or tubular reserve is needed to further characterize subclinical AKD.

Acute Kidney Disease Staging Criteria

Table 1 outlines proposed AKD staging criteria according to consensus by the ADQI 16 Workgroup.[19] The proposed definition can facilitate better phenotyping of AKI and AKD beyond initial AKI KDIGO diagnosis and staging, which can outline the natural course of kidney disease and assist the implementation of tailored surveillance and interventions (eg, follow-up care) that can mitigate progression of AKI to AKD and its detrimental complications. However, the proposed AKD definition and staging needs additional validation in large epidemiologic studies.

PATHOPHYSIOLOGY OF KIDNEY REPAIR AND REGENERATION

The transition from AKD to CKD is complex, as there are important a priori considerations. First, CKD is a strong risk factor for AKI, therefore an AKI event in a patient with preexisting CKD may serve to accelerate the underlying CKD in a different manner than incident de novo AKI in a patient who was previously healthy. Second, the type

Table 1
Proposed staging criteria of AKD

AKD Stage	Definition	Diagnosis
Stage 0	0A: Absence of criteria for B or C but susceptible to post-AKI complications 0B: Ongoing injury, repair/regeneration, or loss of glomerular/tubular reserve 0C: SCr <1.5 times baseline but not back to baseline levels 0B + C	In addition to examination of SCr, biomarkers/imaging studies (still under investigation) or clinical characteristics such as new-onset proteinuria, worsened proteinuria from baseline, new-onset hypertension, or worsening hypertension can be used for assessment of ongoing injury or loss of renal reserve
Stage 1	SCr 1.5–1.9 times baseline	SCr levels
Stage 2	SCr 2.0–2.9 times baseline	SCr levels
Stage 3	SCr 3.0 times baseline or increase in SCr to $\geq$353.6 μmol/L ($\geq$4.0 mg/dL)[a] or ongoing need for renal replacement therapy	SCr levels and need for renal replacement therapy

Abbreviations: AKD, acute kidney disease; AKI, acute kidney injury; SCR, serum creatinine.
[a] If baseline SCr is <353.6 μmol/L (<4.0 mg/dL) and an episode of AKI has occurred.

of injury (eg, ischemic vs nephrotoxic) may have important impacts on the AKI-to-AKD-to-CKD transition. Third, host factors related to preexisting chronic conditions, risk factors for CKD development, and genetic factors may all play important roles. Nonetheless, the main pathophysiologic pathways that have been identified in preclinical and supporting clinical investigations suggest broad "themes" of injury (eg, AKI) that then lead to dysregulated or maladaptive repair and impaired recovery that propagate the transition to incident or progressive CKD.[72]

In general, AKI most commonly targets tubular cells, and although the kidney tissue and proximal tubular cells in particular have prodigious capacity for repair and regeneration, most studies identified maladaptive repair processes and impaired recovery as a key driver of the transition to a fibrotic phenotype and ensuing CKD.[73] Proximal tubular cells depend on mitochondrial β-oxidation for source of ATP due to limited glycolytic activity and have the ability to differentiate and proliferate following injury.[73] Surviving and adjacent intact tubular epithelial cells are key contributors to the repair capacity of the kidney after AKI.[74,75] Resident fibroblasts crosstalk with tubular epithelial cells, migrate, and may promote tubular regeneration in early stages of injury.[76] However, maladaptive multimodal repair processes ensue in response to distinct microenvironment conditions leading to inflammation and fibrosis.[72] The key pathways of maladaptive repair leading to fibrosis and inflammation that have been identified are as follows (**Fig. 2**): (1) tubular cell cycle arrest (G2/M phase of cell cycle)[77]; (2) aberrant reactivation of developmental pathways[78,79]; (3) endothelial injury followed by peritubular capillary regression and rarefaction[80]; (4) mitochondrial dysfunction leading to excess of reactive oxygen species[81]; (5) phagocyte (fibroblast, macrophage) dysfunctional differentiation and migration[73]; and (6) dysfunctional immune

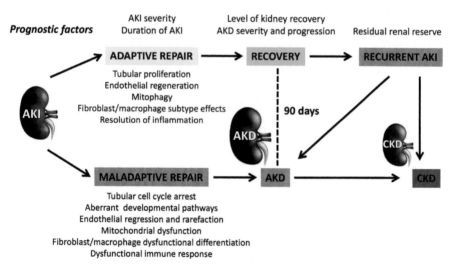

Fig. 2. Pathobiology of maladaptive repair following AKI that leads to CKD. The key pathways of maladaptive repair leading to fibrosis and inflammation that have been identified are (1) tubular cell cycle arrest (G2/M phase of cell cycle); (2) aberrant reactivation of developmental pathways; (3) endothelial injury followed by pericyte detachment from peritubular capillary vessels leading to capillary regression and rarefaction; (4) mitochondrial dysfunction leading to excess of reactive oxygen species; (5) phagocyte (fibroblast, macrophage) dysfunctional differentiation and migration; and (6) dysfunctional immune response with imbalance of more proinflammatory injury and less anti-inflammatory repair.

response with imbalance of more proinflammatory injury and less anti-inflammatory repair.[82–84]

EPIDEMIOLOGY OF ACUTE KIDNEY DISEASE

Since the ADQI 16 Workgroup consensus to redefine AKD, several observational studies examining epidemiology of AKD in different study populations have been published. A summary of these studies is presented in **Table 2**.[85–92] Multiple important aspects should be noted when reviewing these observational data, such as (1) the patient populations represented in these studies are mostly single-center and very heterogeneous, limiting generalizability; (2) the timeframe of observation of AKD incidence is sometimes a continuous period within 7 to 90 days following AKI or a cross-sectional observation within this time period, typically at 30 or 90 days following AKI, and therefore time-to-event is highly variable and the incidence of AKD ranges from ~5% to ~50%; (3) the diagnosis of AKD is dependent on SCr measures performed under routine clinical care, which is currently not standardized for AKI survivors; (4) some studies evaluated AKD following an AKI event detected by the KDIGO-AKI definition but others evaluated AKD in patients without a clinical diagnosis of AKI under the premise that subclinical AKI is common and not detected by the KDIGO-AKI definition, particularly in critical care settings; (5) most studies evaluated outcomes of mortality and kidney recovery associated with AKD but non–kidney-related outcomes of cardiovascular health, processes of post-AKI care, or patient-centered quality-of-life outcomes have not been yet comprehensively evaluated in AKI survivors to further define AKD epidemiology; and (6) the identification of clinical parameters associated with AKD is limited by selection bias and lack of external validation in the represented studies, therefore robust and potentially useful risk-stratification models of AKD are not yet available.

Most recent studies have adopted the proposed AKD definition by the ADQI 16 Workgroup,[85–88] whereas others have used variants of these consensus criteria to adapt to the specific study populations or limitations of data availability or both.[89–92] One important observation is the seldom use of urine output criterion to define AKI or evaluate kidney function within the 7-day to 90-day period post-AKI, which has shown relevance for diagnosis and prognosis of AKI, particularly in ICU settings.[38] Only the study by Peerapornratana and colleagues[85] used both SCr and urine output criteria for defining AKI and transition to AKD post-AKI in a specific group of critically ill septic patients. As a result of distinct study populations and definitions, the incidence of AKD has been variably reported in observational studies: critically ill septic patients (26.9%),[85] cardiac surgery patients (~5% to 47.6%),[86,87,90,92] patients on extracorporeal membrane oxygenation (ECMO) support (44.6%),[88] hematopoietic stem cell transplantation (HSCT) patients (15.7%),[91] and 32.5% in-hospital survivors of AKI followed in specialized clinics.[89] Albeit this is expected fluctuation in the observed incidence of AKD, it should be recognized as a frequent outcome following AKI in different clinical settings.

Another frequent observation in these studies is the association of AKD with scarce kidney recovery at hospital discharge in critically ill septic patients,[85] and the consistent association of AKD with short-term and long-term mortality outcome, particularly in patients who underwent cardiac surgery or received ECMO.[86–88,92] These studies generally exhibited a graded association between level of AKD and future risk of mortality. In addition, cardiac surgery patients transitioning from AKI to AKD exhibited lower chances of kidney recovery at 90 days and higher risk of further deterioration of kidney function up to 2 years following cardiac surgery, reflecting the association

Table 2
Observational studies of AKD published after consensus definition by the ADQI 16 Workgroup

Study	Population	Definition of AKD	Incidence of AKD	Outcomes	Comments
Peerapornratana et al,[85] 2020	1341 pts with septic shock *19.9% died first 7 d	AKI KDIGO (SCr/UOP) ≥1 × more than 7–90d from AKI onset	26.9%	9.3% of AKD pts recovered kidney function at discharge	• Male sex, black race, and CKD were more frequent in AKD pts • TIMP-2*IGFBP7, NGAL, KIM-1, L-FABP not useful to predict AKD
Chen et al,[86] 2020	269 pts in the coronary care unit *4.8% hospital mortality	AKI KDIGO (SCr) ≥1 × more than 7–90 d from AKI onset	47.6%	Mortality risk at 5 y correlated with AKD stages, particularly AKD 1–3	• Age, hemoglobin, ejection fraction, serum IL-18 associated with AKD
Matsuura et al,[87] 2020	3605 pts post cardiac surgery	AKI KDIGO (SCr) ≥1 × more than 7–90 d from AKI onset	11.2%	AKD → 90-d mortality (aOR: 63.0, 95% CI: 27.9–180.6) AKD → 50% eGFR decline at 2-y f/u in survivors (aOR: 3.56, 95% CI: 2.24–5.57)	• Renal recovery at 90-d was 54.8% in AKD patients
Hsu et al,[88] 2020	168 ECMO pts that survived >7 d	AKI KDIGO (SCr) ≥1 × more than 7–90 d from AKI onset	44.6%	AKD → up to 10-y mortality f/u (45.8% died within 90 d) Stage 1: aHR 2.58 (95% CI 1.27–5.23) Stage 2: aHR 2.35 (95% CI 1.10–5.51) Stage 3: aHR 5.25 (95% CI 2.71–10.16)	• Age, initial SOFA score, urine output on day 1 of ECMO associated with mortality

(continued on next page)

Table 2
(continued)

Study	Population	Definition of AKD	Incidence of AKD	Outcomes	Comments
Hines et al,[89] 2020	345 AKI survivors discharged from the hospital	AKI KDIGO (SCr) ≥1 at first clinic visit after a hospitalization complicated by AKI (median: 33 d from discharge)	32.5%	There was no difference in the rate of AKD in patients discharged vs not discharged on an ACEI/ARB (12.5 vs 15.0%, P = .530)	• Acute exposure to an ACEI/ARB during hospitalization was not associated with AKD at the time of first clinic visit
Sun Cho et al,[90] 2019	1190 cardiac surgery pts with preserved baseline kidney function (eGFR ≥60)	eGFR <60 or ESKD at 90 d after surgery	7.2%	AKD → CKD at 12 mo (aOR: 16.8; 95% CI: 8.2–34.2)	• Age and preoperative albumin level associated with AKD • Postoperative AKI increased the risk of AKD at 90 d, even if it resolved within 3 d
Mima et al,[91] 2019	108 pts undergoing HSCT	AKI KIDGO (SCr) ≥1 or GFR <60 or decrease in GFR by ≥35% or increase in SCr by >50% × <3 mo	15.7%	AKD → 100-d mortality AKD vs no AKD mortality (29.4% vs 20.2, respectively, P = .409)	• ABO-incompatible HSCT and acute GVHD after HSCT were more frequent in AKD pts
Mizuguchi et al,[92] 2018	2095 cardiac surgery pts *43% with CKD (preoperative eGFR <60)	Doubling of SCr 2–4 wk after surgery	4.4% in patients with preserved kidney function and 4.8% in patients with CKD	Pts with AKD had higher hospital and 30-d mortality than those without AKD, both in patients with and without CKD at baseline	• Stages of AKI predicted AKD in a graded manner

Abbreviations: ACEI, angiotensin-converting enzyme inhibitor; aHR, adjusted hazard ratio; AKI, acute kidney injury; aOR, adjusted odds ratio; ARB, angiotensin-II receptor blocker; CKD, chronic kidney disease; CI, confidence interval; ECMO, extracorporeal membrane oxygenation; eGFR, estimated glomerular filtration rate; ESKD, end-stage kidney disease; f/u, follow-up; GVHD, graft vs host disease; HSCT, hematopoietic stem cell transplantation; IL-18, interleukin 18; KDIGO, Kidney Disease: Improving Global Outcomes; KIM-1, kidney injury molecule-1; L-FABP, liver fatty acid-binding protein; NGAL, neutrophil gelatinase-associated lipocalin; pts, patients; SCr, serum creatinine; SOFA, Sequential Organ Failure Assessment; TIMP-1*IGFBP7, product of tissue metalloproteinase inhibitor 2 and the insulin growth factor–binding protein 7; UOP, urine output.

between AKD and the risk of CKD.[87,90] Despite observational data support that AKI begets AKD even when accompanied by an apparent complete return of SCr to baseline level,[7,8,93] kidney injury biomarkers measured in the first 24 hours of ICU admission, such as the product of tissue metalloproteinase inhibitor 2 and the insulin growth factor–binding protein 7 (TIMP-1*IGFBP7), kidney injury molecule-1 (KIM-1), neutrophil gelatinase-associated lipocalin (NGAL), and liver fatty acid-binding protein (L-FABP) were not useful to predict AKD in patients with septic shock.[85] Only 1 study reported that levels of serum interleukin-18 (IL-18) measured close to coronary care unit admission were associated with subsequent AKD. Limited data using kidney biomarkers are currently available. Furthermore, time-varying biomarker data may be more informative that single time-point measurements for recalibrating risk of AKD, which may be influenced by a myriad of events occurring in the first 7 days of hospital or ICU admission. In addition, utilization of biomarkers more reflective of kidney repair and regeneration processes are needed to be able to accurately stratify the individual risk of AKD in susceptible populations. Among these biomarkers, urinary C–C motif chemokine ligand 14 (CCL14)[56] and urinary klotho[57] have shown promise as potential biomarkers of kidney recovery risk-stratification but further study for validation and clinical application is needed. Moreover, the combination of tailored panels of kidney biomarkers of tubular injury or repair with functional tubular testing (eg, furosemide stress test) hold promise for further evaluation in the context of AKD.[52,53]

Among summarized studies in **Table 2**, the most consistent clinical parameter associated with AKD was age, whereas other notable parameters inconsistently associated with AKD in different studies included male gender, black race, prevalent CKD, hemoglobin levels, left ventricular ejection fraction, Sequential Organ Failure Assessment (SOFA) score, and urine output on day 1 of admission. The use of "big data" with proper external validation may help reconcile these parameters and underpin others that can inform risk-stratification tools that can be useful and widely used.[32] The importance of early recognition and risk-stratification of AKD is beyond diagnostic purposes, as it may assist timely interventions that can mitigate detrimental post-AKI complications. However, there is a dire need to further define AKD epidemiology and its clinical course as well as standardize its definition, risk-stratification, and clinical application. Furthermore, the evaluation of processes of health care and patient-centered outcomes across the trajectory of AKI-to-AKD-to-CKD is fundamental to ameliorate the burden of kidney and non–kidney-related complications and the overall health-related quality of life of AKI survivors.[94] This is a critical aspect for improving the care of patients with AKI that has ongoing collaborative research initiatives in the scientific nephrology and critical care community.

MANAGEMENT OF ACUTE KIDNEY DISEASE

The management of AKI has been traditionally supportive based on KDIGO-bundle recommendations focusing on hemodynamic support and monitoring, optimization of fluid management and organ perfusion pressure, avoidance of nephrotoxic agents and hyperglycemia, tailored diagnostic workup that warrants specific intervention, and timely RRT initiation when appropriate.[18] Although there are no specific widely effective therapies that prevent or drastically ameliorate AKI in clinical practice, timely implementation of the KDIGO-bundle in high-risk patients, identified with assistance of biomarkers of kidney injury, significantly attenuated the incidence of postoperative AKI following cardiac surgery.[95,96] Therefore, timely kidney-protective approaches centered in 3 key aspects, such as fluid management, exposure to nephrotoxic agents, and follow-up care may have a big impact in AKD management and outcomes.

Fluid Management

The main goal of fluid management is the timely recognition of fluid responsiveness and type of fluid to be administered during resuscitation and optimization phases of fluid therapy, while preventing iatrogenic fluid overload during stabilization and deescalation phases of fluid therapy.[97–99] Fluid overload is a state of impaired homeostasis characterized by fluid retention, often detrimentally in the interstitial compartment, caused by either impaired kidney function and/or iatrogenic excessive fluid administration. Several observational studies have found fluid overload to be associated with increased mortality and increased ventilator dependence in critically ill patients.[39,100–105] Interventions to prevent or limit fluid overload include conservative fluid management after resuscitation, optimal diuretic use, and timely RRT when appropriate and extracorporeal fluid removal is desired.[97,102,105,106] Fluid overload also has been associated with increased mortality and reduced kidney recovery, including RRT dependence, in patients with AKI.[39–41,102,107,108] Being that fluid therapy is a dynamic target in hospitalized patients with AKI and AKD, particularly in those critically ill in the ICU, iterative assessment and adjustment in goals of fluid therapy are required. In this context, a physiologic-based approach to administration of diuretics,[109,110] as well as patient selection for RRT and timely initiation of RRT are crucial.[111] Evolving evidence from randomized clinical trials suggests that accelerated initiation of RRT may increase the risk of RRT dependence and RRT-related adverse events supporting a more conservative strategy of vigilant waiting in critically ill patients with regard to RRT initiation.[112–114] However, individualized risk-stratification to timely address modifiable risk factors such as fluid overload is recommended while protocol-based approaches of de-resuscitation are more widely tested. Furthermore, multiple RRT-specific factors may have an impact on AKI-to-AKD-to-CKD transition and require further study (eg, hypotension during RRT or the acute impact on nutritional status and early mobilization/rehabilitation).[19]

Limiting Exposure to Nephrotoxic Agents

The incidence of AKI related to exposure to nephrotoxic agents accounts for approximately 1 of 5 cases of community-acquired AKI in developed countries and approximately 1 of 4 cases of AKI occurring in the ICU.[115–117] Importantly, drug-associated AKI has similar rates of mortality and RRT dependence than AKI resulting from other etiologies.[116] Careful examination of ambulatory and inpatient medication exposure is necessary when evaluating a patient with AKI and AKD to limit continued exposure if a plausible and causal temporal relationship is determined.[18] The incremental association between number of nephrotoxic agents and risk of AKI has been well established in observational studies,[118,119] whereas some combinations affecting renal plasma flow (eg, diuretics, nonsteroidal anti-inflammatory drugs [NSAIDs] and angiotensin-converting enzyme inhibitors [ACEI] or angiotensin-II receptor blockers [ARB]) may be particularly detrimental to the kidneys, particularly when tissue perfusion is already compromised by hypovolemia, intra-abdominal hypertension, or peripheral vasodilation.[120] The exposure to NSAIDs was shown as high as 20% after AKI in one observational study.[121]

Time-varying drug dosing according to kidney functional recovery and changes in volume of distribution and metabolic status are needed during the AKD period.[19] It is important to recognize that medication dosing during AKD has been seldom studied and is challenging given the difficulties in evaluating kidney functional status in a standardized and validated fashion. Furthermore, drug-to-drug interactions such as specific type of macrolide antibiotics (clarithromycin or erythromycin) together with a 3-

hydroxy 3-methylglutaryl-coenzyme A (HMG-CoA) reductase inhibitor (statin) for the risk of rhabdomyolysis-related AKI should be considered, among multiple others.[122]

The use of ACEI/ARB in the context of AKD is controversial. The traditional approach is to routinely hold these medications during an AKI episode, but the evidence for this is lacking, particularly in mild to moderate cases without severe hypotension or hyperkalemia.[18] Furthermore, questions related to risk-stratification of patients that can benefit from these drugs and the best timing for reinitiating these drugs during the period of AKD is unclear.[123] Overall, evidence suggests that exposure to an ACEI/ARB may be associated with absent or small risk of AKI that may be confounded by indication, and mostly functional AKI rather than structural damage to the kidneys.[124,125] Furthermore, a recent study found that acute exposure to an ACEI/ARB ($\geq$48 hours) before or during an AKI episode was not associated with AKD at the time of first postdischarge clinic visit (median follow-up of 33 days from hospital discharge).[89] Another recent population-based study found that survivors of AKI with exposure to an ACEI/ARB (new or continued use) within 6 months of discharge had greater 2-year survival. The use of ACEI/ARB within 6 months of discharge was associated with an increased risk of hospitalization for kidney-related events (AKI or hyperkalemia), but no increased risk of ESKD or doubling of SCr during the 2-year follow-up.[126] In a different study including critically ill survivors of AKI, an association between ACEI/ARB prescription and a lower 1-year mortality rate was described.[127] It has also been demonstrated that holding these medications during a hospitalization may lead to an inadvertent nonresumption after hospitalization, therefore depriving patients of important therapy for their chronic conditions, including the known kidney- and heart-protective effects of these drugs.[89] The use/exposure to ACEI/ARB during AKD constitutes an area of post-AKI intervention that needs further study to develop evidence-guided approaches.

An example of feasibility of improvement in processes of care for patients with AKD is the recently published quality improvement initiative (The Nephrotoxic Injury Negated by Just-in time Action [NINJA]) developed to prevent nephrotoxic drug exposure in hospitalized children.[128] This clinical decision support tool continuously screened high-risk children exposed to multiple nephrotoxic drugs and recommended providers to obtain daily SCr measurements throughout the identified exposure period and to consider alternative less nephrotoxic options when possible. Importantly, this tool dramatically decreased drug-induced AKI in hospitalized children by 23.8% at a multicenter level.[128] The successful implementation of the NINJA program holds promise for similar interventions in the adult population throughout the spectrum of heterogeneity of the AKI-to-AKD-to-CKD conundrum.

Follow-up Care

Adequate and accessible postdischarge AKD care is essential for reducing the AKI-to-CKD transition and CKD progression. It is well recognized that AKI is associated with incident and progressive CKD, including risk of ESKD,[7,8] and is a novel risk factor for cardiovascular disease.[11,13] The exacerbation of traditional risk factors such as hypertension and proteinuria, which frequently occurs after AKI,[14,36,37] may partially explain the observed association, although precise mechanisms and therapeutic targets are not fully elucidated. Furthermore, incomplete kidney recovery and/or impairment of kidney functional reserve may render the kidney more susceptible to subsequent insults and recurrent AKI, as demonstrated in observational studies showing exceedingly high rates of rehospitalizations within the first year after discharge.[34,35]

Furthermore, processes of care are far beyond optimal to address challenges of timely recognition and management of risk factors for incident or progression of

AKD, limitation of nephrotoxic drug exposure, appropriate initiation or reinitiation of kidney-protective and heart-protective medications, and evaluation and management of patient-centered outcomes, such as impairments in cognitive and functional status and debilitating symptoms hindering health-related quality of life in survivors of AKI.[129] Despite that KDIGO guidelines recommend that all survivors of AKI should have their kidney function evaluated at 3 months after discharge to determine kidney recovery and progression of kidney disease,[18] up to one-third of AKI survivors were shown not to have a single SCr measurement postdischarge. Similarly, proteinuria was seldom examined despite being a potentially modifiable risk factor of progressive kidney disease after AKI.[37,130] Furthermore, only 8% of veterans who experience AKI were referred to see a nephrologist after hospitalization in the VA Healthcare System, despite studies demonstrating that referral may improve outcomes.[131]

Importantly, poor patient knowledge and awareness of AKI have been demonstrated in different studies of AKI survivors.[132,133] However, patients' self-perceived knowledge about AKI significantly increased following a single postdischarge clinic encounter, which included education about AKI.[133] The latter finding highlights potential interventions tailoring processes of postdischarge care as a way to mitigate the burden of AKD and its complications, as the quality of care provided to patients with or at risk for AKD is highly variable and may contribute to poor outcomes. One option is to develop and implement postdischarge AKI care bundles that can be applied to high-risk patients by incorporating simple, straightforward processes of care that can be reproduced and sustained across multiple centers with a wide range of available logistics and resources, and improve clinical and patient-centered outcomes beyond that which would be expected when applied individually.[134,135] Limited observational data and, most importantly, absence of interventional studies hinder evidence-based practices for postdischarge AKI/AKD care but represent a key area of active research to ameliorate the global burden of kidney disease.

SUMMARY

Both AKI and CKD represent a public health problem due to their high occurrence, economic impact, and burden of morbidity and mortality. These 2 clinical syndromes are interconnected. AKI and CKD predispose to each other in a vicious circle and may exert negative impacts independently or synergistically. In an effort to provide more conceptual background to the AKI-to-CKD interaction, the term AKD has emerged and is defined as the post-AKI status of acute or subacute kidney damage/dysfunction manifested by persistence of AKI stage 1 or greater (KDIGO criteria) beyond 7 to 90 days after the initial AKI diagnosis. If criteria of AKI persist beyond 90 days, it is considered incident or progressive CKD according to baseline kidney function.

The transition from AKD to CKD is complex, as there are important a priori considerations. First, CKD is a strong risk factor for AKI, therefore an AKI event in a patient with preexisting CKD may serve to accelerate the underlying CKD in a different manner than incident de novo AKI in a patient who was previously healthy. Second, the type of injury (eg, ischemic vs nephrotoxic) may have important impacts on the AKD-to-CKD transition. Third, host factors related to preexisting chronic conditions, risk factors for CKD development, and genetic factors may all play important roles. Pathways of maladaptive repair predisposing to inflammation and fibrosis leading to CKD have been identified and include cell cycle arrest, endothelial injury followed by capillary regression and rarefaction, mitochondrial dysfunction, fibroblast/macrophage-aberrant differentiation and function, and the immune response with imbalance of more proinflammatory injury and less anti-inflammatory repair.

Limited clinical data exist with regard to AKD epidemiology. Studies published after AKD was formally defined have limited generalizability, as they represent heterogeneous populations with distinct timeframes of observation to determine AKD. Using current aggregate observational data, at least 1 of 4 AKI survivors developed AKD by 90 days of follow-up. Useful risk-stratification tools to predict risk of AKD and its prognosis are needed for bedside management and to test interventions on modifiable risk factors. Timely kidney-protective approaches centered in aspects, such as fluid management, exposure to nephrotoxic agents, and follow-up care, may have a big impact in AKD management and outcomes.

CLINICS CARE POINTS

- AKI and CKD are common interconnected syndromes that represent a public health problem.
- AKD is the persistence of AKI KDIGO stage 1 or greater beyond 7 to 90 days after the initial AKI diagnosis.
- Multifaceted repair pathways after AKI has been identified but therapeutic interventions to promote AKI recovery are still limited.
- Risk-classification tools to predict risk of AKD and its prognosis are needed.
- Fluid management, avoidance of nephrotoxins, and follow-up care are important aspects to mitigate AKI-to-CKD progression.

ACKNOWLEDGMENTS

Dr Neyra is currently supported by grants from NIDDK (R56 DK126930 and P30 DK079337) and NHLBI (R01 HL148448-01 and R21 HL145424-01A1).

DISCLOSURE

The authors have nothing to disclose.

REFERENCES

1. Coresh J, Selvin E, Stevens LA, et al. Prevalence of chronic kidney disease in the United States. JAMA 2007;298(17):2038–47.
2. National Center for Health Statistics (US). Health, United States, 2015: With Special Feature on Racial and Ethnic Health Disparities. Hyattsville (MD): National Center for Health Statistics (US); 2016.
3. Hu M, Zhu Y, Taylor JM, et al. Using Poisson mixed-effects model to quantify transcript-level gene expression in RNA-Seq. Bioinformatics 2012;28(1):63–8.
4. Chawla LS, Kimmel PL. Acute kidney injury and chronic kidney disease: an integrated clinical syndrome. Kidney Int 2012;82(5):516–24.
5. Lewington AJ, Cerda J, Mehta RL. Raising awareness of acute kidney injury: a global perspective of a silent killer. Kidney Int 2013;84(3):457–67.
6. Hoste EA, Bagshaw SM, Bellomo R, et al. Epidemiology of acute kidney injury in critically ill patients: the multinational AKI-EPI study. Intensive Care Med 2015; 41(8):1411–23.
7. Heung M, Steffick DE, Zivin K, et al. Acute kidney injury recovery pattern and subsequent risk of CKD: an analysis of veterans health administration data. Am J kidney Dis 2016;67(5):742–52.

8. Coca SG, Singanamala S, Parikh CR. Chronic kidney disease after acute kidney injury: a systematic review and meta-analysis. Kidney Int 2012;81(5):442–8.

9. Wu VC, Wu CH, Huang TM, et al. Long-term risk of coronary events after AKI. J Am Soc Nephrol 2014;25(3):595–605.

10. Wu VC, Wu PC, Wu CH, et al. The impact of acute kidney injury on the long-term risk of stroke. J Am Heart Assoc 2014;3(4).

11. Odutayo A, Wong CX, Farkouh M, et al. AKI and long-term risk for cardiovascular events and mortality. J Am Soc Nephrol 2017;28(1):377–87.

12. Gammelager H, Christiansen CF, Johansen MB, et al. Three-year risk of cardiovascular disease among intensive care patients with acute kidney injury: a population-based cohort study. Crit Care 2014;18(5):492.

13. Bansal N, Matheny ME, Greevy RA Jr, et al. Acute kidney injury and risk of incident heart failure among US veterans. Am J kidney Dis 2018;71(2):236–45.

14. Hsu CY, Hsu RK, Yang J, et al. Elevated BP after AKI. J Am Soc Nephrol 2016; 27(3):914–23.

15. Hsu CY, Ordonez JD, Chertow GM, et al. The risk of acute renal failure in patients with chronic kidney disease. Kidney Int 2008;74(1):101–7.

16. Lafrance JP, Djurdjev O, Levin A. Incidence and outcomes of acute kidney injury in a referred chronic kidney disease cohort. Nephrol Dial Transplant 2010;25(7): 2203–9.

17. Chawla LS, Eggers PW, Star RA, et al. Acute kidney injury and chronic kidney disease as interconnected syndromes. N Engl J Med 2014;371(1):58–66.

18. Kidney Disease: Improving Global Outcomes (KDIGO) Acute Kidney Injury Work Group. Kidney disease: improving global outcomes (KDIGO) clinical practice guideline for acute kidney injury. Kidney Int Suppl 2012;2:1–138.

19. Chawla LS, Bellomo R, Bihorac A, et al. Acute kidney disease and renal recovery: consensus report of the acute disease quality initiative (ADQI) 16 workgroup. Nat Rev Nephrol 2017;13(4):241–57.

20. Waikar SS, Liu KD, Chertow GM. Diagnosis, epidemiology and outcomes of acute kidney injury. Clin J Am Soc Nephrol 2008;3(3):844–61.

21. Wald R, Quinn RR, Adhikari NK, et al. Risk of chronic dialysis and death following acute kidney injury. Am J Med 2012;125(6):585–93.

22. Lafrance JP, Miller DR. Acute kidney injury associates with increased long-term mortality. J Am Soc Nephrol 2010;21(2):345–52.

23. Chawla LS, Amdur RL, Amodeo S, et al. The severity of acute kidney injury predicts progression to chronic kidney disease. Kidney Int 2011;79(12):1361–9.

24. Thakar CV, Christianson A, Himmelfarb J, et al. Acute kidney injury episodes and chronic kidney disease risk in diabetes mellitus. Clin J Am Soc Nephrol 2011;6(11):2567–72.

25. Chertow GM, Burdick E, Honour M, et al. Acute kidney injury, mortality, length of stay, and costs in hospitalized patients. J Am Soc Nephrol 2005;16(11): 3365–70.

26. Hsu RK, McCulloch CE, Dudley RA, et al. Temporal changes in incidence of dialysis-requiring AKI. J Am Soc Nephrol 2013;24(1):37–42.

27. Siew ED, Davenport A. The growth of acute kidney injury: a rising tide or just closer attention to detail? Kidney Int 2014;87(1):46–61.

28. Rewa O, Bagshaw SM. Acute kidney injury—epidemiology, outcomes and economics. Nat Rev Nephrol 2014;10(4):193–207.

29. Bouchard J, Acharya A, Cerda J, et al. A prospective international multicenter study of AKI in the intensive care unit. Clin J Am Soc Nephrol 2015;10(8): 1324–31.

30. Silver SA, Long J, Zheng Y, et al. Cost of acute kidney injury in hospitalized patients. J Hosp Med 2017;12(2):70–6.
31. Shah S, Leonard AC, Harrison K, et al. Mortality and recovery associated with kidney failure due to acute kidney injury. Clin J Am Soc Nephrol 2020;15(7): 995–1006.
32. Neyra JA, Leaf DE. Risk prediction models for acute kidney injury in critically ill patients: opus in progressu. Nephron 2018;140(2):99–104.
33. Grams ME, Matsushita K, Sang Y, et al. Explaining the racial difference in AKI incidence. J Am Soc Nephrol 2014;25(8):1834–41.
34. Siew ED, Parr SK, Abdel-Kader K, et al. Predictors of recurrent AKI. J Am Soc Nephrol 2016;27(4):1190–200.
35. Goldstein SL, Jaber BL, Faubel S, et al. Acute kidney injury advisory group of American Society of Nephrology. AKI transition of care: a potential opportunity to detect and prevent CKD. Clin J Am Soc Nephrol 2013;8(3):476–83.
36. Matheny ME, Peterson JF, Eden SK, et al. Laboratory test surveillance following acute kidney injury. PloS one 2014;9(8):e103746.
37. Parr SK, Matheny ME, Abdel-Kader K, et al. Acute kidney injury is a risk factor for subsequent proteinuria. Kidney Int 2018;93(2):460–9.
38. Kellum JA, Sileanu FE, Murugan R, et al. Classifying AKI by urine output versus serum creatinine level. J Am Soc Nephrol 2015;26(9):2231–8.
39. Bouchard J, Soroko SB, Chertow GM, et al. Fluid accumulation, survival and recovery of kidney function in critically ill patients with acute kidney injury. Kidney Int 2009;76(4):422–7.
40. Neyra JA, Li X, Canepa-Escaro F, et al. Cumulative fluid balance and mortality in septic patients with or without acute kidney injury and chronic kidney disease. Crit Care Med 2016;44(10):1891–900.
41. Woodward CW, Lambert J, Ortiz-Soriano V, et al. Fluid overload associates with major adverse kidney events in critically ill patients with acute kidney injury requiring continuous renal replacement therapy. Crit Care Med 2019;47(9): e753–60.
42. Brown JR, Kramer RS, Coca SG, et al. Duration of acute kidney injury impacts long-term survival after cardiac surgery. Ann Thorac Surg 2010;90(4):1142–8.
43. Perinel S, Vincent F, Lautrette A, et al. Transient and persistent acute kidney injury and the risk of hospital mortality in critically ill patients: results of a multi-center cohort study. Crit Care Med 2015;43(8):e269–75.
44. Coca SG, King JT Jr, Rosenthal RA, et al. The duration of postoperative acute kidney injury is an additional parameter predicting long-term survival in diabetic veterans. Kidney Int 2010;78(9):926–33.
45. Sood MM, Shafer LA, Ho J, et al. Early reversible acute kidney injury is associated with improved survival in septic shock. J Crit Care 2014;29(5):711–7.
46. Doi K, Yuen PS, Eisner C, et al. Reduced production of creatinine limits its use as marker of kidney injury in sepsis. J Am Soc Nephrol 2009;20(6):1217–21.
47. Thongprayoon C, Cheungpasitporn W, Kashani K. Serum creatinine level, a surrogate of muscle mass, predicts mortality in critically ill patients. J Thorac Dis 2016;8(5):E305–11.
48. McLean S, Nurmatov U, Liu JL, et al. Telehealthcare for chronic obstructive pulmonary disease. Cochrane database Syst Rev 2011;(7):Cd007718.
49. Macedo E, Bouchard J, Soroko SH, et al. Fluid accumulation, recognition and staging of acute kidney injury in critically-ill patients. Crit Care 2010;14(3):R82.

50. Korenkevych D, Ozrazgat-Baslanti T, Thottakkara P, et al. The pattern of longitudinal change in serum creatinine and 90-day mortality after major surgery. Ann Surg 2016;263(6):1219–27.

51. Kellum JA, Sileanu FE, Bihorac A, et al. Recovery after acute kidney injury. Am J Respir Crit Care Med 2017;195(6):784–91.

52. Koyner JL, Davison DL, Brasha-Mitchell E, et al. Furosemide stress test and biomarkers for the prediction of AKI severity. J Am Soc Nephrol 2015;26(8): 2023–31.

53. Matsuura R, Komaru Y, Miyamoto Y, et al. Response to different furosemide doses predicts AKI progression in ICU patients with elevated plasma NGAL levels. Ann Intensive Care 2018;8(1):8.

54. Kashani K, Al-Khafaji A, Ardiles T, et al. Discovery and validation of cell cycle arrest biomarkers in human acute kidney injury. Crit Care 2013;17(1):R25.

55. Gharaibeh KA, Hamadah AM, El-Zoghby ZM, et al. Cystatin C predicts renal recovery earlier than creatinine among patients with acute kidney injury. Kidney Int Rep 2018;3(2):337–42.

56. Hoste E, Bihorac A, Al-Khafaji A, et al. Identification and validation of biomarkers of persistent acute kidney injury: the RUBY study. Intensive Care Med 2020; 46(5):943–53.

57. Neyra JA, Li X, Mescia F, et al. Urine klotho is lower in critically ill patients with versus without acute kidney injury and associates with major adverse kidney events. Crit Care Explor 2019;1(6).

58. Zhou HY, Chen TW, Zhang XM. Functional magnetic resonance imaging in acute kidney injury: present status. Biomed Res Int 2016;2016:2027370.

59. Siew ED, Ikizler TA. Continuous prediction of future acute kidney injury: a step forward. Kidney Int 2020;97(6):1094–6.

60. Rashidi P, Bihorac A. Artificial intelligence approaches to improve kidney care. Nat Rev Nephrol 2020;16(2):71–2.

61. Carlier M, Dumoulin A, Janssen A, et al. Comparison of different equations to assess glomerular filtration in critically ill patients. Intensive Care Med 2015; 41(3):427–35.

62. Hoste EA, Damen J, Vanholder RC, et al. Assessment of renal function in recently admitted critically ill patients with normal serum creatinine. Nephrol Dial Transplant 2005;20(4):747–53.

63. Jelliffe R. Estimation of creatinine clearance in patients with unstable renal function, without a urine specimen. Am J Nephrol 2002;22(4):320–4.

64. Bouchard J, Macedo E, Soroko S, et al. Comparison of methods for estimating glomerular filtration rate in critically ill patients with acute kidney injury. Nephrol Dial Transplant 2010;25(1):102–7.

65. Pianta TJ, Endre ZH, Pickering JW, et al. Kinetic estimation of GFR improves prediction of dialysis and recovery after kidney transplantation. PloS one 2015;10(5):e0125669.

66. Molitoris BA, Reilly ES. Quantifying glomerular filtration rates in acute kidney injury: a requirement for translational success. Semin Nephrol 2016;36(1): 31–41.

67. Wang E, Meier DJ, Sandoval RM, et al. A portable fiberoptic ratiometric fluorescence analyzer provides rapid point-of-care determination of glomerular filtration rate in large animals. Kidney Int 2012;81(1):112–7.

68. Bhatraju PK, Mukherjee P, Robinson-Cohen C, et al. Acute kidney injury subphenotypes based on creatinine trajectory identifies patients at increased risk of death. Crit Care 2016;20(1):372.

69. Bhatraju PK, Zelnick LR, Chinchilli VM, et al. Association between early recovery of kidney function after acute kidney injury and long-term clinical outcomes. JAMA Netw Open 2020;3(4):e202682.

70. Ronco C, Kellum JA, Haase M. Subclinical AKI is still AKI. Crit Care 2012; 16(3):313.

71. Pannu N, James M, Hemmelgarn B, et al. Association between AKI, recovery of renal function, and long-term outcomes after hospital discharge. Clin J Am Soc Nephrol 2013;8(2):194–202.

72. Ferenbach DA, Bonventre JV. Mechanisms of maladaptive repair after AKI leading to accelerated kidney ageing and CKD. Nat Rev Nephrol 2015;11(5): 264–76.

73. Sato Y, Takahashi M, Yanagita M. Pathophysiology of AKI to CKD progression. Semin Nephrol 2020;40(2):206–15.

74. Kusaba T, Lalli M, Kramann R, et al. Differentiated kidney epithelial cells repair injured proximal tubule. Proc Natl Acad Sci U S A 2014;111(4):1527–32.

75. Schiessl IM, Grill A, Fremter K, et al. Renal interstitial platelet-derived growth factor receptor-beta cells support proximal tubular regeneration. J Am Soc Nephrol 2018;29(5):1383–96.

76. Nakamura J, Sato Y, Kitai Y, et al. Myofibroblasts acquire retinoic acid-producing ability during fibroblast-to-myofibroblast transition following kidney injury. Kidney Int 2019;95(3):526–39.

77. Yang L, Besschetnova TY, Brooks CR, et al. Epithelial cell cycle arrest in G2/M mediates kidney fibrosis after injury. Nat Med 2010;16(5):535–43, 531p following 143.

78. Ding H, Zhou D, Hao S, et al. Sonic hedgehog signaling mediates epithelial-mesenchymal communication and promotes renal fibrosis. J Am Soc Nephrol 2012;23(5):801–13.

79. Zhou D, Li Y, Lin L, et al. Tubule-specific ablation of endogenous beta-catenin aggravates acute kidney injury in mice. Kidney Int 2012;82(5):537–47.

80. Ohashi R, Shimizu A, Masuda Y, et al. Peritubular capillary regression during the progression of experimental obstructive nephropathy. J Am Soc Nephrol 2002; 13(7):1795–805.

81. Bhargava P, Schnellmann RG. Mitochondrial energetics in the kidney. Nat Rev Nephrol 2017;13(10):629–46.

82. Sato Y, Yanagita M. Immune cells and inflammation in AKI to CKD progression. Am J Physiol Renal Physiol 2018;315(6):F1501–12.

83. D'Alessio FR, Kurzhagen JT, Rabb H. Reparative T lymphocytes in organ injury. J Clin Invest 2019;129(7):2608–18.

84. Rabb H, Griffin MD, McKay DB, et al. Inflammation in AKI: current understanding, key questions, and knowledge gaps. J Am Soc Nephrol 2016;27(2):371–9.

85. Peerapornratana S, Priyanka P, Wang S, et al. Sepsis-associated acute kidney disease. Kidney Int Rep 2020;5(6):839–50.

86. Chen YT, Jenq CC, Hsu CK, et al. Acute kidney disease and acute kidney injury biomarkers in coronary care unit patients. BMC Nephrol 2020;21(1):207.

87. Matsuura R, Iwagami M, Moriya H, et al. The clinical course of acute kidney disease after cardiac surgery: a retrospective observational study. Sci Rep 2020; 10(1):6490.

88. Hsu CK, Wu IW, Chen YT, et al. Acute kidney disease stage predicts outcome of patients on extracorporeal membrane oxygenation support. PloS one 2020; 15(4):e0231505.

89. Hines A, Li X, Ortiz-Soriano V, et al. Use of angiotensin-converting enzyme inhibitors/angiotensin receptor blockers and acute kidney disease after an episode of AKI: a multicenter prospective cohort study. Am J Nephrol 2020;51(4): 266–75.

90. Cho JS, Shim JK, Lee S, et al. Chronic progression of cardiac surgery associated acute kidney injury: intermediary role of acute kidney disease. J Thorac Cardiovasc Surg 2019. https://doi.org/10.1016/j.jtcvs.2019.10.101.

91. Mima A, Tansho K, Nagahara D, et al. Incidence of acute kidney disease after receiving hematopoietic stem cell transplantation: a single-center retrospective study. PeerJ 2019;7:e6467.

92. Mizuguchi KA, Huang CC, Shempp I, et al. Predicting kidney disease progression in patients with acute kidney injury after cardiac surgery. J Thorac Cardiovasc Surg 2018;155(6):2455–2463 e2455.

93. Bucaloiu ID, Kirchner HL, Norfolk ER, et al. Increased risk of death and de novo chronic kidney disease following reversible acute kidney injury. Kidney Int 2012; 81(5):477–85.

94. Macedo E, Bihorac A, Siew ED, et al. Quality of care after AKI development in the hospital: consensus from the 22nd acute disease quality initiative (ADQI) conference. Eur J Intern Med 2020;80:45–53.

95. Meersch M, Schmidt C, Hoffmeier A, et al. Prevention of cardiac surgery-associated AKI by implementing the KDIGO guidelines in high risk patients identified by biomarkers: the PrevAKI randomized controlled trial. Intensive Care Med 2017;43(11):1551–61.

96. Gocze I, Jauch D, Gotz M, et al. Biomarker-guided intervention to prevent acute kidney injury after major surgery: the prospective randomized BigpAK study. Ann Surg 2018;267(6):1013–20.

97. Hoste EA, Maitland K, Brudney CS, et al. Four phases of intravenous fluid therapy: a conceptual model. Br J Anaesth 2014;113(5):740–7.

98. Self WH, Semler MW, Wanderer JP, et al. Balanced crystalloids versus saline in noncritically III adults. N Engl J Med 2018;378(9):819–28.

99. Semler MW, Self WH, Wanderer JP, et al. Balanced crystalloids versus saline in critically III adults. N Engl J Med 2018;378(9):829–39.

100. Goldstein SL, Currier H, Graf C, et al. Outcome in children receiving continuous venovenous hemofiltration. Pediatrics 2001;107(6):1309–12.

101. Goldstein SL, Somers MJ, Baum MA, et al. Pediatric patients with multi-organ dysfunction syndrome receiving continuous renal replacement therapy. Kidney Int 2005;67(2):653–8.

102. Sutherland SM, Zappitelli M, Alexander SR, et al. Fluid overload and mortality in children receiving continuous renal replacement therapy: the prospective pediatric continuous renal replacement therapy registry. Am J Kidney Dis 2010; 55(2):316–25.

103. Liu KD, Thompson BT, Ancukiewicz M, et al. Acute kidney injury in patients with acute lung injury: impact of fluid accumulation on classification of acute kidney injury and associated outcomes. Crit Care Med 2011;39(12):2665–71.

104. Payen D, de Pont AC, Sakr Y, et al. A positive fluid balance is associated with a worse outcome in patients with acute renal failure. Crit Care 2008;12(3):R74.

105. National Heart L, Blood Institute Acute Respiratory Distress Syndrome Clinical Trials N, Wiedemann HP, et al. Comparison of two fluid-management strategies in acute lung injury. N Engl J Med 2006;354(24):2564–75.

106. Selewski DT, Goldstein SL. The role of fluid overload in the prediction of outcome in acute kidney injury. Pediatr Nephrol 2016;33(1):13–24.

107. Heung M, Wolfgram DF, Kommareddi M, et al. Fluid overload at initiation of renal replacement therapy is associated with lack of renal recovery in patients with acute kidney injury. Nephrol Dial Transplant 2012;27(3):956–61.
108. Prowle JR, Bellomo R. Fluid administration and the kidney. Curr Opin Crit Care 2013;19(4):308–14.
109. Bissell BD, Donaldson JC, Morris PE, et al. A narrative review of pharmacologic de-resuscitation in the critically ill. J Crit Care 2020;59:156–62.
110. Bissell BD, Laine ME, Thompson Bastin ML, et al. Impact of protocolized diuresis for de-resuscitation in the intensive care unit. Crit Care 2020;24(1):70.
111. Neyra JA, Goldstein SL. Optimizing renal replacement therapy deliverables through multidisciplinary work in the intensive care unit. Clin Nephrol 2018; 90(1):1–5.
112. Investigators. Canadian Critical Care Trials Group; Australian and New Zealand Intensive Care Society Clinical Trials Group; United Kingdom Critical Care Research Group; Canadian Nephrology Trials Network, et al. Timing of initiation of renal-replacement therapy in acute kidney injury. N Engl J Med 2020;383(3): 240–51.
113. Gaudry S, Hajage D, Schortgen F, et al. Initiation strategies for renal-replacement therapy in the intensive care unit. N Engl J Med 2016;375(2): 122–33.
114. Barbar SD, Clere-Jehl R, Bourredjem A, et al. Timing of renal-replacement therapy in patients with acute kidney injury and sepsis. N Engl J Med 2018;379(15): 1431–42.
115. Wu TY, Jen MH, Bottle A, et al. Ten-year trends in hospital admissions for adverse drug reactions in England 1999-2009. J R Soc Med 2010;103(6): 239–50.
116. Mehta RL, Pascual MT, Soroko S, et al. Spectrum of acute renal failure in the intensive care unit: the PICARD experience. Kidney Int 2004;66(4):1613–21.
117. Uchino S, Kellum JA, Bellomo R, et al. Acute renal failure in critically ill patients: a multinational, multicenter study. JAMA 2005;294(7):813–8.
118. Cartin-Ceba R, Kashiouris M, Plataki M, et al. Risk factors for development of acute kidney injury in critically ill patients: a systematic review and meta-analysis of observational studies. Crit Care Res Pract 2012;2012:691013.
119. Rivosecchi RM, Kellum JA, Dasta JF, et al. Drug class combination-associated acute kidney injury. Ann Pharmacother 2016;50(11):953–72.
120. Lapi F, Azoulay L, Yin H, et al. Concurrent use of diuretics, angiotensin converting enzyme inhibitors, and angiotensin receptor blockers with non-steroidal anti-inflammatory drugs and risk of acute kidney injury: nested case-control study. BMJ 2013;346:e8525.
121. Lipworth L, Abdel-Kader K, Morse J, et al. High prevalence of non-steroidal anti-inflammatory drug use among acute kidney injury survivors in the southern community cohort study. BMC Nephrol 2016;17(1):189.
122. Patel AM, Shariff S, Bailey DG, et al. Statin toxicity from macrolide antibiotic co-prescription: a population-based cohort study. Ann Intern Med 2013;158(12): 869–76.
123. Tomson C, Tomlinson LA. Stopping RAS inhibitors to minimize acute kidney injury: more harm than good? Clin J Am Soc Nephrol 2019;14(4):617–9.
124. Mansfield KE, Nitsch D, Smeeth L, et al. Prescription of renin-angiotensin system blockers and risk of acute kidney injury: a population-based cohort study. BMJ Open 2016;6(12):e012690.

125. Palevsky PM, Zhang JH, Seliger SL, et al. Incidence, severity, and outcomes of AKI Associated with dual renin-angiotensin system blockade. Clin J Am Soc Nephrol 2016;11(11):1944–53.

126. Brar S, Ye F, James MT, et al. Association of Angiotensin-converting enzyme inhibitor or angiotensin receptor blocker use with outcomes after acute kidney injury. JAMA Intern Med 2018;178(12):1681–90.

127. Gayat E, Hollinger A, Cariou A, et al. Impact of angiotensin-converting enzyme inhibitors or receptor blockers on post-ICU discharge outcome in patients with acute kidney injury. Intensive Care Med 2018;44(5):598–605.

128. Goldstein SL, Dahale D, Kirkendall ES, et al. A prospective multi-center quality improvement initiative (NINJA) indicates a reduction in nephrotoxic acute kidney injury in hospitalized children. Kidney Int 2020;97(3):580–8.

129. Johansen KL, Smith MW, Unruh ML, et al. Predictors of health utility among 60-day survivors of acute kidney injury in the Veterans Affairs/National institutes of health acute renal failure trial network study. Clin J Am Soc Nephrol 2010;5(8):1366–72.

130. Hsu CY, Chinchilli VM, Coca S, et al. Post-acute kidney injury proteinuria and subsequent kidney disease progression: the assessment, serial evaluation, and subsequent sequelae in acute kidney injury (ASSESS-AKI) study. JAMA Intern Med 2020;180(3):402–10.

131. Harel Z, Wald R, Bargman JM, et al. Nephrologist follow-up improves all-cause mortality of severe acute kidney injury survivors. Kidney Int 2013;83(5):901–8.

132. Siew ED, Parr SK, Wild MG, et al. Kidney disease awareness and knowledge among survivors ofacute kidney injury. Am J Nephrol 2019;49(6):449–59.

133. Ortiz-Soriano V, Alcorn JL 3rd, Li X, et al. A survey study of self-rated patients' knowledge about aki in a post-discharge AKI clinic. Can J kidney Health Dis 2019;6. 2054358119830700.

134. Hoste EA, De Corte W. Implementing the kidney disease: improving global outcomes/acute kidney injury guidelines in ICU patients. Curr Opin Crit Care 2013;19(6):544–53.

135. Bagshaw SM. Acute kidney injury care bundles. Nephron 2015;131(4):247–51.

Printed and bound by CPI Group (UK) Ltd, Croydon, CR0 4YY

03/10/2024

01040481-0006